# Practical Radiotherapy

# PRACTICAL RADIOTHERAPY

## PHYSICS AND EQUIPMENT

**Second Edition**

Edited by

**Pam Cherry MSc TDCR**
*Senior Lecturer*
*Department of Radiography*
*City University*
*London*

**Angela M. Duxbury MSc FCR TDCR**
*Professor of Therapy Radiography and Principal Lecturer*
*Faculty of Health and Wellbeing*
*Sheffield Hallam University*
*Sheffield*

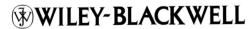
**WILEY-BLACKWELL**
A John Wiley & Sons, Ltd., Publication

This edition first published 2009
© 2009 Blackwell Publishing Ltd

Blackwell Publishing was acquired by John Wiley & Sons in February 2007. Blackwell's publishing programme has been merged with Wiley's global Scientific, Technical, and Medical business to form Wiley-Blackwell.

*Registered office*
John Wiley & Sons Ltd, The Atrium, Southern Gate, Chichester, West Sussex, PO19 8SQ, United Kingdom

*Editorial offices*
9600 Garsington Road, Oxford, OX4 2DQ, United Kingdom
2121 State Avenue, Ames, Iowa 50014-8300, USA

For details of our global editorial offices, for customer services and for information about how to apply for permission to reuse the copyright material in this book please see our website at www.wiley.com/wiley-blackwell.

*Library of Congress Cataloging-in-Publication Data*

Practical radiotherapy : physics and equipment / edited by Pam Cherry, Angela M. Duxbury. – 2nd ed.
       p. ; cm.
   Includes bibliographical references and index.
   ISBN 978-1-4051-8426-7 (pbk. : alk. paper)
   1. Medical physics.   2. Radiotherapy–Equipment and supplies.   I. Cherry, Pam.   II. Duxbury, Angela.
   [DNLM:   1. Radiotherapy–instrumentation.   2. Health Physics. WN 250 P896 2009]

   R920.P73 2009
   615.8'42–dc22
                                                                                        2008052868

A catalogue record for this book is available from the British Library.

Set in 10/12.5 pt Sabon by SNP Best-set Typesetter Ltd., Hong Kong
Printed and bound in Singapore by Fabulous Printers Pte Ltd

1  2009

# CONTENTS

# LIST OF CONTRIBUTORS

**Dr Christopher M Bragg**
Physicists, Weston Park Hospital, Sheffield

**Mr Pete Bridge**
Senior Lecturer, Faculty of Health and
Wellbeing, Sheffield Hallam University, Sheffield

**Dr Fiona Chamberlain**
Senior Lecturer, Department of Radiography,
Faculty of Health and Social Care, University
of the West of England, Glenside Campus,
Bristol

**Mrs Janette Chianese**
Senior Lecturer, Department of Radiography,
Faculty of Health and Social Care, University
of the West of England, Glenside Campus,
Bristol

**Ms Katheryn Churcher**
Section Head, Radiation Therapy Austin
Health Radiation Oncology Centre, Heidelberg,
Victoria, Australia

**Dr John Conway**
Principal Physicist, Weston Park Hospital,
Sheffield

**Ms Kathryn Cooke**
Planning Superintendent, Cromwell Hospital,
London

**Mr David Duncan**
Lecturer, Department of Radiography,
City University, London

**Mr David Flinton**
Senior Lecturer, Department of Radiography,
City University, London

**Mr Tony Flynn**
Previous Head of Brachytherapy Physics,
Cookridge Hospital, Leeds

**Ms Cath Holborn**
Senior Lecturer, Faculty of Health and
Wellbeing, Sheffield Hallam University,
Sheffield

**Mrs Anne Jessop**
Senior Lecturer, Department of Clinical
Oncology, Princess Royal Hospital, Hull

**Mrs Elizabeth Miles**
Lecturer, Department of Radiography,
City University, London

**Mr Jonathan McConnell**
Senior Lecturer (Medical Imaging), Department
of Medical Imaging and Radiation Sciences,
Monash University, Clayton, Victoria,
Australia

**Mr Alan Needham**
Advanced Practitioner (Simulator Technology),
Department of Radiotherapy, St James's
Institute of Oncology, Leeds

**Dr Elaine Ryan**
Lecturer, Department of Medical Radiation
Sciences, Faculty of Health Sciences, University
of Sydney, Australia

**Dr Bruce Thomadsen**
Medical Physics, University of Wisconsin,
Madison, Wisconsin, USA

**Mrs Helen White**
Senior Lecturer in Radiotherapy, Division of
Radiography, Birmingham City University,
Birmingham

**Mr Nick White**
Senior Lecturer in Radiotherapy, Division of
Radiography, Birmingham City University,
Birmingham

**Ms Caroline Wright**
Senior Lecturer (Radiation Therapy),
Department of Medical Imaging and Radiation
Sciences, Monash University, Victoria,
Melbourne, Australia

# PREFACE

This book was written primarily for the undergraduate therapeutic radiographer, but it is hoped that medical physicists, nurses and clinical oncologists will also find it useful.

Our main aims for the book were to fulfil a current need for such a text and to produce a 'reader-friendly' book on radiotherapy physics and equipment.

This second edition has been influenced by feedback on the first edition mainly from student therapy radiographers, from those who have a passion for physics and those who find this subject a challenge, so we hope that we have met the needs of all students.

The contributors to the book are from different backgrounds; some work in academic settings, others as practitioners in their specialist fields. Subsequently, each chapter has its own style, reflecting that of the author.

The book is intended to complement others currently on the market in order to provide the undergraduate with a broad and comprehensive database. Each chapter offers a 'further reading' section and so aims to provide a coherent whole on any particular subject.

*Pam Cherry and Angela Duxbury.*
*London and Sheffield, 2009*

# ACKNOWLEDGEMENTS

The editors would like to thank all the contributors who have written chapters for this book. Also we would like to thank the following authors whose work has been incorporated from the first edition: Sue Huggett, David Biggs, Euan Thomson, Michelle Cook, Julie O'Boyle, Andy Moloney, Jill Stief, Glenys Payne and Tony Flynn who, sadly, is now deceased.

We would like to thank the equipment manufacturers and application specialists for supplying up-to-date information for the text.

Angela would like to thank her husband, David and her children Sophie and Hayden and Pam would like to thank her husband, Gordon and her children Laura and Simon, for their support and patience whilst working on the editing of this book.

# Chapter 1

# BASIC SKILLS FOR RADIOTHERAPY PHYSICS

Elaine Ryan

## Aims and objectives

The aim of this chapter is to provide a review of the mathematics and basic physics that will help with the understanding of radiotherapy physics. This section aims to serve as a quick reference guide to help when confronted with problems further in the book.

After completing this chapter the reader should:
- have a clear understanding of the basic mathematical skills required to understand the physics of radiotherapy
- be able to complete simple mathematical problems applied to radiotherapy physics
- understand the theories and concepts of basic physics
- be able to perform simple calculations using basic physics formulae.

## Mathematical skills relevant to radiotherapy

### Fractions

A fraction is one number divided by another. The top number, $a$, is the numerator and the bottom number, $b$, is the denominator:

$$x = \frac{a}{b}$$

### Addition

To add two fractions together:

$$\frac{a}{b} + \frac{c}{d} = \frac{a \times d}{b \times d} + \frac{c \times d}{b \times d} = \frac{(a \times d) + (c \times d)}{b \times d}$$

---

### Example

Question: add together two-thirds and four-fifths:

Answer:

$$\text{two-thirds} + \text{four-fifths} = \frac{2}{3} + \frac{4}{5}$$
$$= \frac{2 \times 5}{3 \times 5} + \frac{4 \times 3}{3 \times 5}$$
$$= \frac{(2 \times 5) + (4 \times 3)}{3 \times 5}$$
$$= \frac{22}{15} = 1\frac{7}{15}$$

---

### Subtraction

To take one fraction away from another:

$$\frac{a}{b} - \frac{c}{d} = \frac{a \times d}{b \times d} - \frac{c \times b}{b \times d} = \frac{(a \times d) - (c \times b)}{b \times d}$$

1

**Example**

Question: take three-tenths away from four-ninths:

Answer:

$$\text{four-ninths} - \text{three-tenths} = \frac{4}{9} - \frac{3}{10}$$

$$= \frac{4 \times 10}{9 \times 10} - \frac{3 \times 9}{9 \times 10}$$

$$= \frac{(4 \times 10) - (3 \times 9)}{9 \times 10}$$

$$= \frac{13}{90}$$

## Multiplication

To multiply two fractions together:

$$\frac{a}{b} \times \frac{c}{d} = \frac{a \times c}{b \times d}$$

**Example**

Question: multiply together two-thirds and three-fifths

Answer:

$$\frac{2}{3} \times \frac{3}{5} = \frac{2 \times 3}{3 \times 5} = \frac{6}{15} = \frac{2}{5}$$

## Division

To divide one fraction by another, you have to invert one fraction and then multiply them together:

$$\frac{a}{b} \div \frac{c}{d} = \frac{a}{b} \times \frac{d}{c} = \frac{a \times d}{b \times c}$$

**Example**

Question: divide two-fifths by three-eighths
Answer:

$$\frac{2}{5} \div \frac{3}{8} = \frac{2}{5} \times \frac{8}{3} = \frac{2 \times 8}{5 \times 3} = \frac{16}{15} = 1\frac{1}{15}$$

## Ratios

A ratio is another way of expressing a fraction, but is more useful when trying to compare two quantities. A ratio is expressed as $m:n$ (the ratio of $m$ to $n$)

To divide a quantity $A$ into a ratio $m:n$ to find $p:q$:

$$p = \frac{A}{(m+n)} \times m$$

$$q = \frac{A}{(m+n)} \times n$$

**Example**

Question: a treatment regimen with a total dose of 20 Gy must be given in two phases. The ratio of the dose in each phase is 3:1. What dose must be given for each phase?
Answer:

$$\text{Phase 1 dose} = \frac{20}{6+2} \times 6 = 15\,\text{Gy}$$

$$\text{Phase 2 dose} = \frac{20}{6+2} \times 2 = 5\,\text{Gy}$$

The ratio of the phase 1 to phase 2 dose is 15:5.

To find a ratio in the form $p:1$ or $1:q$:

$$q = \frac{n}{m}$$

$$p = \frac{m}{n}$$

### Example

Question: if an anterior field of length 4 cm appears as 3 cm on a simulator film find the film magnification.
Answer: the measurements are in the ratio 4 : 3, so the magnification is:

$$1 : \frac{4}{3} = 1 : 0.75$$

## Proportionality

If two quantities are linearly proportional, then they have a constant scaling or multiplication factor, $k$. When $a \, \alpha \, b$ then $a = kb$ where $k$ is a constant of proportionality.

### Example

Question: a treatment machine delivers a dose of 0.75 Gy in 15 seconds. How long will it take to deliver a dose of 2 Gy?
Answer:

$$k = 15/0.75 = 20 \, (\text{s/Gy})$$

$$t = k \times 2 = 40 \, \text{s}$$

### Example

Question: a CT plan shows a 95% coverage of the prostate on 21 slices out of 30. What percentage of the prostate volume is covered by the 95% isodose?

Answer: $x = \left( \dfrac{21}{30} \times \dfrac{100}{1} \right) \% = 70\%$

To work out $x\%$ of $y$:

$$x\% = \frac{x}{100} \times \frac{y}{1}$$

### Example

Question: the spinal cord is covered by the 90% isodose in a plan. If the patient is given 1.75 Gy for the first fraction, what dose did the spinal cord receive?

Answer: $z = \left( \dfrac{90}{100} \times \dfrac{1.75}{1} \right) = 1.575 \, \text{Gy}$

To find $z$, an increase of $y$ by $x\%$:

$$z = \left( \frac{x}{100} \times y \right) + y$$

### Example

Question: a field size of 30 cm needs to be increased by 12% in order to allow for organ motion. What is the correct enlarged field size?

Answer: $z = \left( \dfrac{12}{100} \times 30 \right) + 30 = 33.6 \, \text{cm}$

## Percentages

Percentages are often used to indicate the amount by which a value has changed or by how much a value should be changed. Per cent means 'per 100' or 1/100. Therefore 50% = 50/100 or one half.

To change a fraction $(a/b)$ to a percentage $(x)$:

$$x = \left( \frac{a}{b} \times \frac{100}{1} \right) \%$$

## Standard form

A very large or very small number needs to be expressed in standard form, or scientific notation. A number in standard form has a number between 1 and 10 multiplied by 10 raised to a power. The power is easy to work out by counting the number of times that you shift the significant figure.

## Examples

Question: find 0.0895 in standard form.
Answer: move the decimal place twice to the right so the power = $-2$: $8.95 \times 10^{-2}$
Question: find 800 000 in standard form.
Answer: move the decimal place five places to the left so the power = 5: $8.0 \times 10^5$
Question: find 47 000 000 000 in standard form.
Answer: move the decimal point a total of 10 places to the left so the power = 10: $4.7 \times 10^{10}$

Multiplying numbers in standard form:

$$(a \times 10^x) \times (b \times 10^y) = (a \times b) \times 10^{(x+y)}$$

## Example

Question: find $6.4 \times 10^8$ multiplied by $7.2 \times 10^4$.
Answer: $(6.4 \times 10^8) \times (7.2 \times 10^4) = (6.4 \times 7.2) \times 10^{(8+4)} = 46.08 \times 10^{12} = 4.608 \times 10^{13}$

Dividing numbers in standard form:

$$(a \times 10^x) \div (b \times 10^y) = \left(\frac{a}{b}\right) \times 10^{(x-y)}$$

## Example

Question: Find $6.4 \times 10^8$ divided by $8.0 \times 10^{-4}$.
Answer: $(6.4 \times 10^8) \div (8.0 \times 10^{-4}) = (6.4/8) \times 10^{(8--4)} = 0.8 \times 10^{12} = 8.0 \times 10^{11}$

## Logarithms

A log is just a way of expressing a number as the 'power' of another number (the 'base').

For the general equation:

$$y = b^x \quad \log_b y = x$$

If $b$ is given the value 10, then $y = 10^x$. Now, if $x$ is given the values 1, 2, 3, etc.:

| y | $10^x$ | x |
|---|---|---|
| 10 | $10^1$ | 1 |
| 100 | $10^2$ | 2 |
| 1000 | $10^3$ | 3 |
| 10 000 | $10^4$ | 4 |
| 100 000 | $10^5$ | 5 |

This is a 'log' table to the 'base' 10. Therefore:

- $\log_{10} 10 = 1$
- $\log_{10} 100 = 2$
- $\log_{10} 1000 = 3$.

The value for $y$ gets very large, but when it is expressed as a logarithm it stays small.

## Exponentials

A special logarithmic case is 'e', where a constant change in $x$ results in the same fractional change in $y$. The example, $y = e^x$ can also be expressed as $\log_e y = x$ or as $\ln y = x$. A log to base e is a 'natural logarithm' (ln) and 'e' has the value 2.718:

| $e^x$ | x | y |
|---|---|---|
| $e^1$ | 1 | 2.718 |
| $e^2$ | 2 | 7.389 |
| $e^3$ | 3 | 20.086 |
| $e^4$ | 4 | 54.598 |
| $e^5$ | 5 | 148.413 |

If $e^x$ is plotted against $x$, an exponential curve is obtained. This type of curve describes many naturally occurring events such as radioactive decay. Any number would produce a similarly shaped curve, but, with 'e', the gradient at any point is proportional to the value of $x$, i.e. if the value of $x$ is halved the rate of decrease of $y$ is also halved.

## Similar triangles

If one triangle is an enlargement of another they are similar triangles. The triangles must have the same corresponding angles. Figure 1.1 shows two similar triangles.

In radiotherapy, similar triangles are used in three ways: field size; inverse square law; and magnification.

### Field size

To find the field size (FS) variation with the source to skin distance (SSD).

In Figure 1.2 the ratio $SSD_1 : SSD_2$ is equal to the ratio $FS_1 : FS_2$, therefore:

$$\left(\frac{SSD_2}{SSD_1}\right) = \left(\frac{FS_2}{FS_1}\right)$$

Provided that any three of these variables are known, it is possible to calculate the fourth, unknown value.

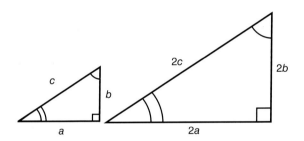

**Figure 1.1** Two similar triangles.

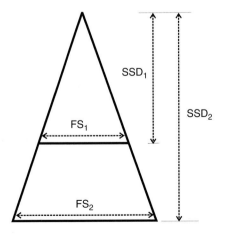

**Figure 1.2** Similar triangles to illustrate how field size changes with source to skin distance (SSD).

---

**Example**

Question: at an SSD of 100 cm, the field length is 12 cm. What is the field length if the SSD is increased to 150 cm?
Answer:

$$\left(\frac{SSD_2}{SSD_1}\right) = \left(\frac{FS_2}{FS_1}\right)$$

$$FS_2 = FS_1\left(\frac{SSD_2}{SSD_1}\right) = 12 \times \left(\frac{150}{100}\right) = 18 \, cm$$

---

### The inverse square law

This relationship considers similar triangles in three dimensions. In Figure 1.3 the top of the object is a point source of X-rays. All photons travel in straight lines. Photons in the shaded area 'A' have come from the point source, are at a distance '$d$' from it and are travelling directly away from it. Photons in the shaded area 'B' are further away from the point source at a distance '$2d$', but the number of photons in area B is the same as in area A. Therefore, the number of photons per unit area, or the intensity, is less in B than in A. The decrease in intensity can be derived using similar triangles.

In Figure 1.3, if the distance from the source is doubled, then all sides of the triangles will double. Therefore:

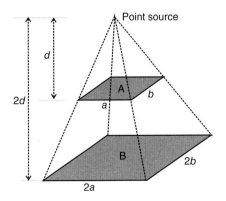

**Figure 1.3** A diagram of the inverse square law.

$$Area\ 1 = a \times b = ab$$

$$Area\ 2 = 2a \times 2b = 4ab.$$

Therefore, the area is four times greater but the number of photons is the same and:

$$I = \frac{I_0}{4}$$

where $I$ is the intensity and $I_0$ is the initial intensity of the beam.

$$I = I_0 \times \left( \frac{a \times b}{4 \times a \times b} \right)$$

If the distance is increased from $d$ to $10d$:

$$Area\ 1 = a \times b = ab$$

$$Area\ 2 = 10a \times 10b = 100ab$$

$$I = I_0 \times \left( \frac{a \times b}{100 \times a \times b} \right)$$

When the distance from the source increases, $I$ always decreases by:

$$I = I_0 \times \left( \frac{d_1}{d_2} \right)^2$$

or it can be said that $I$ is inversely proportional to $d^2$.

$$I \propto \left( \frac{1}{d} \right)^2$$

For the inverse square law to work, all photons must be travelling from the same point and in a straight line. Therefore, there must be a point source and no scatter (change of direction).

## Magnification

Figure 1.4 shows an object being imaged onto a film using a point source. The magnification ($M$) is defined as

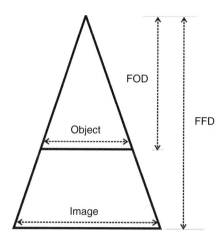

**Figure 1.4** An object being imaged using a point source.

$$M = \frac{\text{size of image } (I)}{\text{size of object } (O)}$$

Where FFD is the focus to film distance and FOD is the focus to object distance, similar triangles can be used to work out dimensions, if three quantities are known.

$$M = \frac{I}{O} = \frac{FFD}{FOD}$$

## Pythagoras's theorem

For a right-angled triangle the longest side is called the hypotenuse. The square of the hypotenuse is equal to the sum of the squares of the other two sides. For the triangle shown in Figure 1.5:

$$a^2 + b^2 = c^2$$

**Example**

For a triangle with sides $a = 3.5\,cm$ and $b = 4.2\,cm$, what is the length of the hypotenuse?

$$c = \sqrt{(3.5)^2 + (4.2)^2} = 5.5\,cm$$

## Trigonometry

A right-angled triangle has a hypotenuse, an adjacent side and an opposite side.

   If one of the angles apart from the right angle is chosen as the marked angle (θ), then the sides are as follows: the hypotenuse is opposite the right angle. It is always the longest side. The adjacent side joins θ to the right angle. The opposite side is opposite θ.

   The trigonometric ratios for calculating unknown sides or angles are as follows:

$$\mathrm{Sin}\,\theta = \frac{\text{opposite}}{\text{hypotenuse}}$$

$$\mathrm{Cos}\,\theta = \frac{\text{adjacent}}{\text{hypotenuse}}$$

$$\mathrm{Tan}\,\theta = \frac{\text{opposite}}{\text{adjacent}}$$

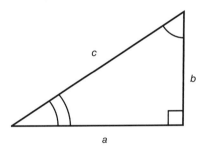

**Figure 1.5** Pythagoras's theorem.

---

### Example 1

Question: in Figure 1.6a–c find the length of the side marked $x$

Answer:

(a)  $\mathrm{Sin}\,\theta = \dfrac{\text{opp}}{\text{hyp}}$

therefore opp = Sin θ × hyp = Sin 37 94.2 = 56.7

(b)  $\mathrm{Cos}\,\theta = \dfrac{\text{adj}}{\text{hyp}}$

therefore $\mathrm{hyp} = \dfrac{\text{adj}}{\mathrm{Cos}\theta} = \dfrac{58.2}{\mathrm{Cos}24} = 63.7$

(c)  $\mathrm{Tan}\,\theta = \dfrac{\text{opp}}{\text{adj}}$

therefore opp = adj × Tanθ = 30.7 × Tan52 = 39.3

### Example 2

Question: in Figure 1.6d,e find the unknown angle θ.

Answer:

(d)  $\mathrm{Sin}\,\theta = \dfrac{\text{opp}}{\text{hyp}}$

therefore $\theta = \mathrm{Sin}^{-1}\left(\dfrac{\text{opp}}{\text{hyp}}\right) = \mathrm{Sin}^{-1}\left(\dfrac{54.2}{67.8}\right) = 53°$

(e)  $\mathrm{Tan}\,\theta = \dfrac{\text{opp}}{\text{adj}}$

therefore $\theta = \mathrm{Tan}^{-1}\left(\dfrac{\text{opp}}{\text{adj}}\right) = \mathrm{Tan}^{-1}\left(\dfrac{38.4}{42.9}\right) = 42°$

---

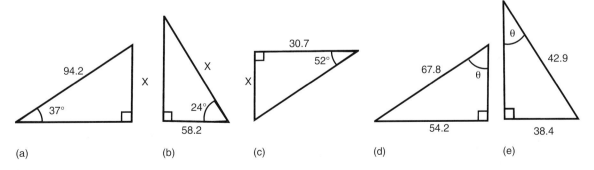

**Figure 1.6** Examples of trigonometry.

# Basic physics relevant to radiotherapy

## Units of measurement

It is often necessary to present the results of measurements or calculations in a numerical fashion. The number used to do this requires two parts: a pure number and the unit in which the quantity has been measured or calculated, e.g. 100 Gy where the unit is the 'gray' and the pure number is 100. There are, however, some basic units on which all measurements are based and a number of derived units that are based on combinations of the basic units.

### Basic units
All measurements used in science are based on three basic units of measurement (Table 1.1). These are the basic units of measurement because they are independent of each other and cannot be converted from one to another.

### Derived units
Any physical quantities other than mass, length or time are measured in derived units, some of which are listed in Table 2.2, Chapter 2.

**Table 1.1** Basic units of measurement

| Unit | Symbol | SI unit |
|------|--------|---------|
| Mass | $m$ | kilogram (kg) |
| Length | $l$ | metre (m) |
| Time | $t$ | second (s) |

**Table 1.2** Common prefixes

| | | | | | |
|---|---|---|---|---|---|
| pico | p | $10^{-12}$ | kilo | k | $10^{3}$ |
| nano | n | $10^{-9}$ | mega | M | $10^{6}$ |
| micro | μ | $10^{-6}$ | giga | G | $10^{9}$ |
| milli | m | $10^{-3}$ | tera | T | $10^{12}$ |

### Prefixes
As discussed earlier, it is easier to present very large or small numbers in standard form. A way of simplifying this further is by the use of universal prefixes. Table 1.2 shows common prefixes.

For example, $0.000007 \, m = 7 \times 10^{-6} = 7 \, \mu m$ and $3000 \, m = 3 \times 10^{3} = 3 \, km$.

### Suffixes
Suffixes are used to identify a specific value of a given quantity. For example, the activity of a radionuclide may be denoted using the symbol $A$. The activity of the radionuclide will decay over a period of time and it may be necessary to specify the activity at a given time. Time may be denoted using the symbol $t$ and activity at time $t$ is identified as $At$.

A special case is the suffix '0' which is normally used to indicate the initial value of a quantity. The initial activity of the radionuclide would therefore be $A_0$.

## Classical mechanics (Table 1.3)

Classical, or newtonian, mechanics is the study of the connection of matter, forces and motion.

**Table 1.3** A summary of units used in classical mechanics

| Unit | Symbol | Equation | SI Unit |
|------|--------|----------|---------|
| Velocity | $v$ | $v = l/t$ | m/s |
| Acceleration | $a$ | $a = v/t$ | m/s$^2$ |
| Weight | $w$ | $w = mg$ | newton (N) |
| Force | $F$ | $F = ma$ | newton (N) |
| Work and energy | $E$ | $E = Fl$ | joule (J) |
| Power | $P$ | $P = E/t$ | watt (W) |

### Velocity
The average velocity ($v$) of a body in motion is the total distance ($l$) travelled by the body divided by the time ($t$) taken for this travel in a given direction. It is given as:

$$v\left(\frac{m}{s}\right) = \frac{l(m)}{t(s)}$$

Although the SI units for distance and time are metres and seconds, respectively, velocity can be expressed in units such as miles per hour or kilometres per hour.

## Acceleration

Linear acceleration ($a$) is the rate of change in velocity ($v$) or the ratio of a change in velocity to a corresponding change in time ($t$). This is when a body in motion is speeding up or slowing down. It is given as:

$$a\left(\frac{m}{s^2}\right) = \frac{v\left(\frac{m}{s}\right)}{t(s)}$$

Acceleration is expressed in units of metres per second squared (m/s²).

## Force

Force ($F$) is the mass ($m$) of a body multiplied by the acceleration ($a$) acting on it, which is expressed as:

$$F(\mathrm{N}) = m(\mathrm{kg}) \times a(\mathrm{m/s^2}).$$

This is Newton's second law of motion.

Weight is the name given to the force exerted on a body by the gravitational acceleration of the earth, $g$. Therefore, weight is given as:

$$W(\mathrm{N}) = m(\mathrm{kg}) \times g(\mathrm{m/s^2})$$

and is just a special case of Newton's second law of motion. This gravitational acceleration is measured as about 10 m/s². Force is expressed in newtons (N), where $1\,\mathrm{N} = 1\,\mathrm{kg\,m/s^2}$.

It is important to distinguish between mass and weight. If something is weighed as 0.5 kg, this is actually its mass. The weight of this body is 0.5 kg × 10 m/s² = 5 N.

## Work, energy and power

Work is defined as force ($F$) multiplied by the distance ($d$) moved, i.e. if a force is applied to a body then work is performed:

$$W(\mathrm{J}) = F(\mathrm{N}) \times d(\mathrm{m}).$$

The unit of work is the joule (J) and 1 J of work is performed when a force of 1 N moves through a distance of 1 m: 1 newton metre or joule = $1\,\mathrm{kg\,m^2/s^2}$.

Energy is defined as the ability to do work. Two special forms of energy must be considered: potential and kinetic.

*Potential energy* (PE) is the energy a body possesses by virtue of its condition or state. Potential energy is therefore 'stored' energy such as that in a battery or coiled spring. A body's potential energy is equal to the amount of work that has been performed to put it in its particular position, i.e. the force applied multiplied by the distance moved. For a body of mass $m$ above the ground by a distance $h$ and under the effect of gravity, $g$, its potential energy = mgh.

*Kinetic energy* (KE) is the energy that a body possesses by virtue of its motion. A body's kinetic energy is that energy that would have to be applied to the body to bring it completely to rest. A body of mass $m$ moving at a velocity $v$ will have kinetic energy

$$= \frac{1}{2}mv^2$$

*Power* is defined as the rate of doing work or the rate at which energy is used. The unit of power is the watt (W) and 1 watt (W) = $1\,\mathrm{J\,s^{-1}}$.

## Waves

Electromagnetic waves all travel in a vacuum with a velocity equal to the speed of light ($c$) where $c = 3 \times 10^8$ m/s. All waves have a wavelength, $\lambda$, the distance travelled in one cycle, and a frequency, $v$, the number of cycles per second, measured in hertz (Hz). Figure 1.7 shows the

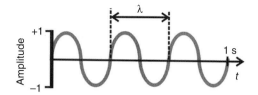

**Figure 1.7** The wavelength, frequency and amplitude of a wave.

wavelength, frequency and amplitude of a wave. The wave in this example has a frequency of 3 Hz.

For all waves the speed *(c)* is equal to the frequency, $v$, times the wavelength, $\lambda$:

$$c(\text{m/s}) = \lambda(m) \times v(1/\text{s}).$$

## Electricity, magnetism and electromagnetic radiation

Electricity and magnetism are very important to the understanding of radiation. The movement of charges in an electric field and the combination of electric and magnetic fields in the form of electromagnetic waves underpin X-ray production and interactions.

### Electric fields

Separate but similar charges repel each other and unlike charges attract each other. As two electrons are both negatively charged they repel each other. The force with which they do this is the same as the force between any two charges ($q_1$ and $q_2$), and is given as:

$$F_\varepsilon(N) = k\frac{q_1 q_2}{r^2}$$

with units of newtons (N).

The electric field strength at a point in space is given by:

$$\varepsilon\left(\frac{N}{C}\right) = \frac{F_\varepsilon(N)}{q(C)}$$

An electric field can be created across two electrodes – a cathode, which is positive, and an anode, which is negative – with the application of a potential.

### Current

Current is the motion of electrons from one electrode to another through a conductor. Current is defined as the net charge ($Q$) flowing through an area $A$ per unit time ($t$), which is expressed as

$$I(A) = \frac{Q(C)}{t(s)}$$

The unit of current is the ampere ($A$), which is equal to Coulombs per second ($C/s$). This is shortened to 'amp'. Currents in X-ray tubes are of the magnitude of milliamps (mA).

### Voltage

The force that drives current around a circuit is the potential difference. This is measured in volts. An electron moving through a potential difference experiences a net change in energy, measured in electron-volts. This effect is analogous to a mass falling through a given height difference in a gravitational field. One electron volt is the energy required by an electron to move through a potential difference of 1 V.

### Resistance

The voltage of a circuit divided by its current is known as the resistance of the circuit. This is given as:

$$R(\Omega) = \frac{V(V)}{I(A)}$$

This is Ohm's law. The unit of resistance is the ohm ($\Omega$), which is equal to 1 volt per ampere ($V/A$).

## Magnetism

A magnetic field produced by a magnet has a north and a south pole. As with electric charges, opposite poles attract and like poles repel; however, unlike electric charges the opposite charges in a magnet cannot be isolated, but always come in pairs. The magnetic field lines produced by a magnet run from north to south.

## Electromagnetic induction

When a magnet is moved through a coil of wire, a current is induced in the coil. The opposite is also true: a current passing through a coil generates a magnetic field through the centre of the coil. This is known as electromagnetic induction.

## Electromagnetic waves

The phenomenon of electromagnetic induction tells us that electric and magnetic fields that vary with time are not independent – one affects the other. When a magnetic field moves with time it induces an electric field perpendicular to it, and the same is true of the inverse situation when a time-varying electric field induces a magnetic field. Electromagnetic waves are so called because they are waves of energy transmitted by oscillating interdependent electric and magnetic fields. As an electromagnetic wave is energy radiating away from an oscillating source it is also called electromagnetic radiation.

Radio waves, microwaves, ultraviolet light, infrared light, visible light, X-rays and gamma rays are all types of electromagnetic radiation. Electromagnetic radiation can be considered to behave as both a wave and a particle because it demonstrates both wave- and particle-like properties.

### Wave-like properties

Electromagnetic radiation is usually thought of as being a wave. How is it known that it behaves like a wave? If visible light is considered, it can be demonstrated that visible light can undergo reflection, refraction, diffraction, interference, etc., all of which are properties of waves. Experimental work with mass spectrometers has also demonstrated the diffraction of X-rays.

### Particle-like properties

Some phenomena associated with electromagnetic radiation, such as the photoelectric effect and Compton scattering, cannot be explained by the wave theory. To explain these phenomena, electromagnetic radiation must be considered to behave as particles or packets of energy rather than as waves.

### Wave particle duality

The wave- and particle-like properties of electromagnetic radiation can be related. From the wave-like properties, it is known that the wave can be described by the following relationship:

$$E = v\lambda$$

If particle-like properties are considered, it can be shown that the energy carried by the particles or photons is given by:

$$E = hv$$

where $E$ is the energy of the photon, expressed in joules, $h$ is known as Planck's constant and is equal to $6.62 \times 10^{-34}$ Js, and $v$ is the frequency expressed in cycles per second.

These two equations can be combined because it is known that $v = c/\lambda$ and we can therefore substitute for $v$ in the equation $E = hv$ which results in the relationship:

$$E = \frac{hc}{\lambda}$$

It is also known that $h = 6.62 \times 10^{-34}$ Js and $c = 3 \times 10^{8}$ m s$^{-1}$ and, if energy is converted to electron volts, where $1\,eV = 1.602 \times 10^{-19}$ J, then the relationship simplifies to:

$$E = 1.24 \times 10^{-6}/\lambda$$

where $E$ is expressed in electron volts (eV) and $\lambda$ is expressed in metres (m). From this relationship it can be seen that, as the energy increases, the wavelength will decrease.

## The electromagnetic spectrum

The electromagnetic spectrum includes radiation from the longest radio waves to the shortest X-rays. All forms of electromagnetic radiation have an associated frequency and energy. It should be noted that there is often a degree of overlap between the radiation types and that there are therefore no distinct boundaries between them. Figure 1.8 shows the electromagnetic spectrum.

All radiation types share some common properties:

- They are composed of transverse electric and magnetic waves.
- They travel at the speed of light in a vacuum.
- In free space they travel in straight lines.
- In free space they obey the inverse square law.

## Atomic structure

The atom is the basic component of an element and elements are the individual entities from which all matter is composed. An atom consists of a central nucleus, which is positively charged. It also has electrons orbiting this nucleus, which are negatively charged.

## Nucleus

The nucleus can be broken down further and is composed of two kinds of elementary particles or nucleons: protons and neutrons. Protons (p) are positively charged with a charge of $1.602 \times 10^{-19}$ C whereas neutrons (n) have no charge, thus giving the nucleus its overall positive charge. The electrons (e) orbiting the nucleus are negatively charged and their charge is equal in magnitude to that of the proton, i.e. $-1.602 \times 10^{-19}$ C. The number of electrons orbiting the atom is equal to the number of protons in the nucleus and the overall charge of the atom is therefore balanced.

The mass of a proton is the same as that of a neutron and is $1.67261 \times 10^{-27}$ kg, while the mass of an electron is much less, $9.109 \times 10^{-31}$ kg, which is approximately 1/1840 of the mass of the proton or neutron.

## Mass numbers and atomic numbers

For an element X, with mass number $A$ and atomic number $Z$, its chemical symbol is written as:

$$^{A}_{Z}X$$

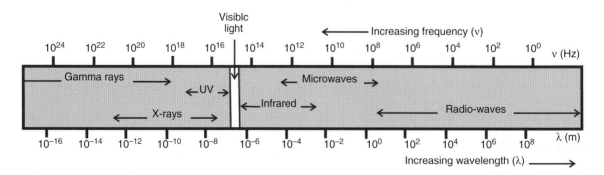

**Figure 1.8** The effect on the tube spectrum when filtration has been added to the exit beam.

$A$ is equal to the number of nucleons, i.e. the total number of protons and neutrons in the nucleus, whereas $Z$ denotes the total number of protons in the nucleus. As the number of protons and electrons is equal, the atomic number also indicates the number of electrons outside the nucleus. For example, an atom of carbon would be written as:

$$^{12}_{6}C$$

where the mass number 12 indicates that the total number of protons and neutrons in the nucleus is 12 and the atomic number 6 indicates that there are 6 protons (and 6 electrons). As the mass number indicates that there are a total of 12 nucleons, and from the atomic number it is known that there are 6 protons, it can be calculated that there are also 6 neutrons.

### Isotopes

Atoms of the same element can exist with different mass numbers but the same atomic number, i.e. the number of neutrons present in the nucleus is different but the number of protons remains the same. Such elements are known as isotopes. For example, cobalt has 11 isotopes, of which two are $^{59}_{27}Co$ and $^{60}_{27}Co$. Of the 11 isotopes, only $^{59}_{27}Co$ is stable. $^{60}_{27}Co$ is used in cobalt treatment machines and some brachytherapy afterloading machines. The other isotopes are also radioactive.

The important point to remember about isotopes is that, as the number of protons and therefore the number of electrons is unchanged, the chemical properties of the element are unchanged. When the imbalance in the number of protons and neutrons becomes too great, the atom and therefore the isotope may become radioactive and the isotope is called a radioisotope.

### Electron orbits

Within the atom, the electrons orbiting the nucleus are arranged in shells, each being identi-

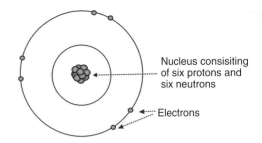

**Figure 1.9** Representation of the particles in a carbon atom.

fied by a letter K, L, M, etc. starting from the shell closest to the nucleus. Each shell has a limit to the number of electrons that it can contain and the inner shells are always occupied first. The K-shell can accept up to 2 electrons, the L-shell up to 8, the M-shell up to 18, etc. For example, carbon with its atomic number of 6 has 2 electrons in the K-shell and the remaining 4 electrons in the L-shell. A diagram of a carbon atom is illustrated in Figure 1.9.

The electron configuration of the atom determines its chemical properties. Neon ($Z = 10$), for example, is chemically inert because both the K- and L-shells are full. Fluorine ($Z = 9$), however, has one electron missing from its outer shell and is chemically reactive. Another example, argon ($Z = 18$), suggests the presence of subshells. It is chemically inert but has only eight electrons in its M-shell, suggesting that atoms are also stable when subshells are full.

### Atomic energy levels

Electron orbits also have an energy associated with them. This is known as the binding energy and is dependent on the force of attraction between the nucleus and the orbiting electrons. The binding energy associated with the K-shell is greater than for shells further away from the nucleus because the force of attraction on the K-shell electrons will be greater.

It is the binding energy that must be overcome if an electron is to be removed from its shell. The potential energy associated with shells further from the nucleus will be greater than for those shells close to the nucleus, which is analogous to the greater potential energy associated with an object the further it is away from the earth.

## Heat and temperature

### Heat

The atoms and molecules of any material are in constant motion. The type of motion varies depending on the form of the material. Within a solid, particles vibrate about a fixed position, whereas in liquids and gases motion is much more random as the particles have much greater freedom of movement. All materials therefore possess kinetic energy due to this motion. Heat is the form of kinetic energy possessed by a material resulting from the motion of its particles and, as heat is a form of energy, the SI unit for it is the joule.

### Temperature

Temperature is a measure of the level of kinetic energy of the atoms and molecules of a material. As the speed of vibrations increases within a body, so the kinetic energy due to these vibrations will increase and the material will increase in temperature. The temperature determines the direction of heat flow when one object is brought into thermal contact within another. Heat will flow from a region of higher to a region of lower temperature.

Temperature can be expressed in several units of measurement:

• Celsius (C): a temperature scale based on certain properties of water. By definition, water freezes at 0 °C and boils at 100 °C.
• Kelvin (K): water freezes at 273K and boils at 373K. This is known as the absolute or Kelvin temperature scale and is important because at

0K all particles within a material should be a rest. Therefore, at 0K, or absolute zero, a body will have no heat energy.

Conversion between the Kelvin and Celsius scales can be made using the following relationship:

Temperature (K) = temperature (°C) + 273.
• Fahrenheit (F): water freezes at 32 °F and boils at 212 °F.

Conversion between the Fahrenheit and Celsius scales can be made using the following relationship:

Temperature (°F) = (temperature (°C) + 32) × (8/5).

### Heat transfer

Heat energy can be transferred from one body to another by the processes of conduction, convection and radiation.

#### Conduction

This process applies principally to solids or objects that are in direct contact with each other. Transfer of heat is by collision of particles in one body with those in the other body. If the temperature of one end of a body is increased, this heat will flow along the body due to the collisions of neighbouring particles. The flow of heat in a body will be affected by a number of physical factors: cross-sectional area and length of the body and the difference in temperature between the two ends of the body.

Heat flow ∝ cross-sectional area ($A$)

Heat flow ∝ 1/length ($l$)

Heat flow ∝ temperature difference ($T_1 - T_2$)

Heat flow is also dependent on the material itself, in particular its thermal conductivity ($k$). The rate of heat flow in a body is given by:

$$\frac{kA(T_2 - T_1)}{l}$$

## Convection

Convection is the main process by which heat is transferred in a fluid (liquids and gases). Heat energy is moved around by circulation of the heated fluid. As a fluid is heated it becomes less dense and will therefore rise. As it rises, it is replaced by cooler fluid, which is then heated and rises, so the process continues creating convection currents in the fluid by virtue of this movement.

## Radiation

This is the only form of heat transfer that can take place in a vacuum. As no particles are present in a vacuum, transfer due to neither collision of particles nor convection currents can take place. As particles in a body vibrate they emit energy in the form of electromagnetic waves. Heat radiation occurs in the electromagnetic spectrum just beyond the red part of the visible spectrum. One of the properties of electromagnetic radiation is that it can travel in a vacuum. Therefore it is possible to transfer heat across a vacuum. It is by this process that heat from the sun is felt, because it has to pass through a vacuum before it reaches the earth.

Examples of these processes of heat transfer can be seen in the cooling of the anode/target of a fixed anode X-ray tube. By one route heat builds up in the tungsten target and is transferred by conduction to the copper anode. From the copper anode, the heat is transferred to the surrounding oil and from there by convection to the surrounding housing. Heat is conducted through the housing and then transferred by convection to the air. Heat will also be radiated from the tungsten target across the inside of the evacuated glass envelope to the wall of the glass envelope, from where it is transferred by conduction to the oil surrounding the glass envelope.

### Self-test questions

1. The spinal cord is covered by the 90% isodose in a plan. If the patient is given 2.00 Gy for their first fraction, what dose did the spinal cord receive?
2. The electromagnetic spectrum includes radiation from the longest radio waves to the shortest X-rays. List three common properties.
3. Define the term electromagnetic induction.
4. What is wave particle duality?
5. What is meant by electron-binding energy?

## Further reading

Bomford CK, Kunkler IH, Sherriff S. *Walter and Miller's Textbook of Radiotherapy*, 6th edn. Edinburgh: Churchill Livingstone, 2003.

Graham DT, Cloke P. *Principles of Radiological Physics*, 4th edn. Edinburgh: Churchill Livingstone, 2003.

Meredith WJ, Massey JB. *Fundamental Physics of Radiology*, 3rd edn. Chichester: John Wright & Sons, 1977.

Williams JR, Thwaites DI. *Radiotherapy Physics in Practice*, 2nd edn. Oxford: Oxford University Press, 2000.

## Chapter 2

# X-RAY PRODUCTION

Elaine Ryan

## Aims and objectives

The aim of this chapter is to provide an overview of how X-rays are produced within an X-ray tube, the mechanisms of X-ray production within the tube target and how these relate to the output spectrum of the tube.

After studying this chapter the reader should be able to:

- describe the components of an X-ray tube
- understand the physics behind the design of each component
- understand how electrons are interacting with the X-ray tube target to produce X-rays
- relate electron interaction processes to the appearance of an X-ray emission spectrum, with reference to characteristic X-rays and Bremsstrahlung
- outline the factors affecting the output intensity of an X-ray tube
- outline the factors affecting the quality of an X-ray spectrum.

## The X-ray tube

Within an X-ray tube, X-rays are produced when electrons with kinetic energy impact upon a high-density target. Each component part of the X-ray tube has been designed with the desire to produce electrons, supply them with energy and enable an efficient as possible interaction with a target. The aim is to provide a small area on the target, where X-rays are emitted (the focal spot), with a high-intensity beam. This has to be traded off with the large amount of heat produced in the anode as a byproduct. This section looks at the function of each component of an X-ray tube.

Figure 2.1 shows a diagram of the components of an X-ray tube. This tube consists of a cathode and an anode enclosed within an evacuated glass or metal envelope. This is all contained within lead-shielded housing, which also contains oil to remove heat from the X-ray tube. A high voltage is applied across the tube by a generator.

## Cathode

The cathode is the negatively charged electrode, where electrons are released into the X-ray tube. This is the start of the X-ray production process and consists of two parts: a filament and a focusing cup. The filament is a coil of tungsten wire, which is about 2 mm in diameter. It is tightly coiled, similar to the heating element in a bar heater or a toaster, in order to increase the surface area of the metal. A very high current is passed through this coil, which heats the metal to such an extent that the outer electrons of the tungsten atoms are boiled off, and ejected from the surface of the coil. This phenomenon is known as thermionic emission. Tungsten is a good material for

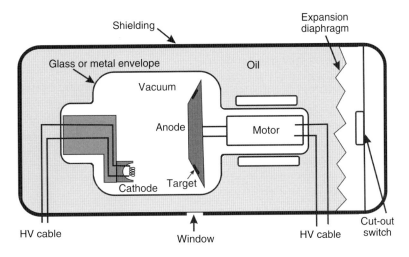

**Figure 2.1** A diagram of an X-ray tube.

this purpose because it has a high melting point and high thermal conductivity. This means that it can heat and cool quickly, allowing it to be heated rapidly for thermionic emission, and it can withstand high temperatures without becoming damaged. The rate at which the electrons are emitted by the cathode is directly related to the tube current.

When electrons are produced by the cathode coil they spread out, because their negative charges electrostatically repel each other. This would result in some electrons not reaching the target, which would reduce the efficiency of the tube. To stop this from happening a focusing cup is used, which is a negatively charged block of nickel that shapes the electrons coming from the filament into a focused beam, and hence a small area on the target.

### High voltage

The tube current flows from the cathode to the positively charged anode. A high voltage is supplied across the tube in order to accelerate the electrons and increase their kinetic energy. This voltage is the kilovolt (kV) setting of the tube and is supplied by a generator, which is separate from the X-ray tube.

### Anode

The anode is the positively charged electrode, directly opposing the cathode. It consists of a high-density metal target, embedded in a copper disc. The electrons from the cathode hit the target area of the anode and interact. Tungsten is usually chosen as a target material. This is due to the useful properties of this material. First, it has a high density, which increases the number of interactions per projectile electron. It also has a high melting point, allowing the target to become very hot without becoming damaged, and last it has a high thermal conductivity. This means the heat generated in the target is quickly dissipated to the surrounding copper, which acts as a heat sink for the anode.

Most tubes have a rotating anode. This is to increase the efficiency of removing heat from the target area during the production of X-rays, which makes it possible to produce a higher-intensity beam without damaging the area of the anode struck by the projectile electrons. Some industrial, dental and small mobile units have stationary anodes. A stationary anode tube is cheaper to manufacture and easier to maintain; however, it cannot be used when a high power output is needed.

## Focal spot size

The area where the electron current hits the target is known as the focal spot. The smaller the focal spot, the greater the resolution of the image produced with the tube. However, with a small focal spot the amount of heat transferred to the target by the electrons becomes concentrated in a small area. If the heat from the target cannot be dissipated fast enough the target may become damaged and crack, causing the tube to fail. Apart from using a rotating anode a good way to reduce the focal spot size is to utilise the angle of the anode.

The actual focal spot size is the area of the target that interacts with the electron beam. The angle of the anode means that the X-ray beam exiting the tube is much smaller than this area. This is called the line focus principle and is illustrated in Figure 2.2. The angle marked θ is known as the target angle.

## Envelope

The cathode and anode are housed inside a glass or metal envelope. The envelope is sealed, and maintained at vacuum pressure. This is necessary so that the electrons can travel from the cathode to the anode without losing any energy during unwanted interactions with air molecules. The envelope was traditionally made of glass, because this is an easy material to mould and it is resistant to high temperatures. More modern tubes have housing made from metal. This does not degrade over time in the same way that glass does and so increases the lifetime of the tube.

## Housing

The envelope is in turn contained inside sturdy housing, which has several purposes. It provides protection and support for the components of the X-ray tube. There is a low attenuation window where the radiation beam exits towards the patient. The housing is filled with oil, which is used to dissipate heat from the anode. The oil expands as it heats up, and if this expansion becomes too great a cut-off switch is activated to prevent the tube from overheating. The housing is also coated in lead to provide shielding, and prevent radiation from being given off in any direction except the window. Finally filters and collimators can be attached to this housing.

## Motor

The motor rotates the anode using electromagnetic induction. This type of motor allows the anode to be powered, while the envelope containing the anode can still be sealed.

## X-ray production

The X-ray tube is designed to accelerate a large number of electrons in a focused manner from the cathode to the anode, such that when they arrive they have acquired kinetic energy. When these electrons hit the anode they interact, transferring their kinetic energy to the target atoms. These interactions take place in a very small depth of penetration into the target

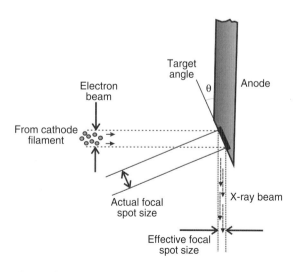

**Figure 2.2**  The effective focal spot size of an X-ray tube.

(0.25–0.5 mm). They result in either the conversion of kinetic energy into thermal energy, in the form of heat, or electromagnetic energy in the form of X-rays.

## Electron interactions within the target

As discussed in Chapter 1, an atom consists of a nucleus and surrounding electron orbits. The nucleus contains protons and neutrons and hence is positively charged. The surrounding electrons occupy set energy levels called shells and there are a maximum number of electrons that can exist in each shell. The inner shell is known as the K-shell and can have a maximum of 2 electrons, the next L-shell can have 8, the M-shell 18 and the N-shell 32.

An incoming electron can interact with any of these orbiting electrons causing excitation, where the incoming electron transfers enough energy to raise the orbiting electron to a higher orbit, or ionisation, in which the incoming electron completely removes the electron from the atom.

## Characteristic radiation

Ionisation results in an electron being ejected from the atom and leaving a hole in its place. If this hole is in an inner shell, this is a very unnatural state for the target atom to be in and the hole is very quickly filled by one of the outer electrons. The electron that moves from an outer to an inner shell has excess energy, which is emitted as an X-ray photon. This X-ray has an energy equal to the difference between the binding energies (BEs) of the electrons involved. Figure 2.3a shows an atom being ionised by an incoming projectile electron with high energy. The target electron has been ejected and has left a space in the K-shell. In Figure 2.3b an electron from the M-shell has moved into the vacancy, emitting a characteristic X-ray photon with an energy of 66.7 keV.

For this interaction to occur in a tungsten atom, the energy of the emitted X-ray is calcu-

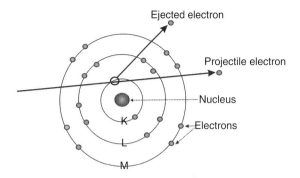

(a)

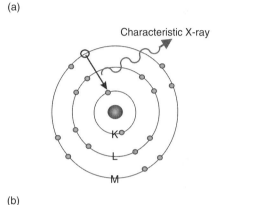

(b)

**Figure 2.3** (a) An atom being ionised when a K-shell electron is ejected by an energetic projectile electron. (b) The vacancy in the K-shell, resulting from ionisation of the atom, is filled by an M-shell electron. A characteristic X-ray is given off.

lated as 69.5 keV (BE of K-shell) – 2.8 keV (BE of M-shell) = 66.7 keV.

Similarly, the resultant X-ray energies can be calculated if an M, N, O or P electron fills this space, but all are called K X-rays because they result from an ionisation of the K-shell. In the above example, the M-shell electron would also be replaced by an electron from an outer orbit and so on, producing a cascade of replacements with each one emitting a photon of energy equal to the difference in the binding energies. This emission spectrum of the material is known as Characteristic radiation because it is characteristic of the target element. It is a line spectrum of these discrete energy X-rays.

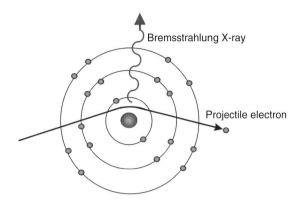

**Figure 2.4** An incoming electron changing direction, due to the atomic nucleus, and giving off a Bremsstrahlung X-ray.

## Bremsstrahlung

The closer a projectile electron gets to the nucleus of a target atom the more it is influenced by the electrostatic field of the nucleus. As it passes close to the nucleus it is slowed down and it changes course, leaving in a different direction with reduced kinetic energy. This loss of kinetic energy appears as an X-ray, as shown in Figure 2.4.

These X-ray photons are known as Bremsstrahlung, which comes from the German for 'braking' (*brems*) and 'radiation' (*strahlung*). The electron may loose all or any intermediate amount of its kinetic energy, resulting in X-rays being emitted with a spread of energies, ranging from 0 to the maximum energy of the electron beam, which is the kilovolt setting on the console.

A low-energy Bremsstrahlung X-ray is produced when the incoming electron is only slightly influenced by the nucleus, producing a low-energy X-ray photon and then continuing with reduced energy. A high-energy Bremsstrahlung X-ray is produced when the electron loses all its energy and stops. The intensity ($I$) with which Bremsstrahlung radiation is produced increases with the atomic number ($Z$) of the target and the energy of the electrons ($E$):

$$I \propto ZE^2 \qquad (2.1)$$

Equation 1 also illustrates why heavy metal targets, such as tungsten, are used, because the efficiency of bremsstrahlung production is directly proportional to the atomic number of the target material.

## Heat

Most of the kinetic energy of the electron beam hitting the target is converted into heat. The projectile electrons interact with outer shell electrons of the target atoms but do not transfer enough energy to remove (ionise) them and only raise them to a higher energy level. These outer electrons immediately drop back down to their normal energy state with the emission of heat. This happens frequently, making the X-ray tube very inefficient, because this energy has effectively been wasted. The probability of X-rays being emitted from the target is only around 1–5%. The remaining 95–99% of emissions result in the kinetic energy of the electron beam being converted into heat.

In the next section we look at the emission spectra of an X-ray tube and how they relate to each interaction within the target.

## The X-ray spectrum

As described above, either characteristic X-rays, which have discrete photon energies, or Bremsstrahlung X-rays, which can have any photon energy up to the maximum kinetic energy of the electron hitting the target, can be produced. This X-ray spectrum can be represented graphically as a plot of the frequency with which X-rays are emitted as a function of their energy. Figure 2.5 shows the characteristic X-ray line spectrum superimposed on top of the continuous spectrum for the Bremsstrahlung X-rays.

The characteristic line spectrum is so called because the lines represent high intensities of single energy X-rays. Only the K X-rays are shown because these are the only characteristic

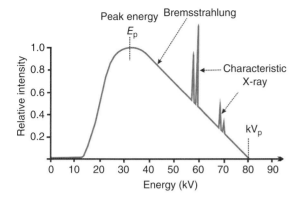

**Figure 2.5** An X-ray emission spectrum for a tungsten target tube, with an operating voltage of 80 kV and a current of 400 mA.

emission from tungsten with sufficient energy to be of value in diagnostic radiology.

The general shape of the X-ray spectrum is the same for all X-ray machines. The maximum energy of the X-ray photons is equal to the voltage across the tube, which is set by the operator. This setting is actually the peak kilovoltage ($kV_p$). The low-energy radiation is decreased in intensity as a result of the self-absorption of the anode itself. The average energy of the X-ray beam is about one-third of the maximum X-ray energy and its total intensity is given by the area under the curve. The maximum energy of the X-ray photons is inversely proportional to the wavelength ($\lambda$):

$$\lambda(m) = \frac{1.24 \times 10^{-10}(keV \cdot m)}{kV_p(keV)} \quad (2.2)$$

For example, the minimum wavelength associated with the X-rays emitted from a unit operated at $100\,kV_p$ is 0.0124 nm.

## X-ray output intensity

The X-rays produced at the target are given off in all directions. Most are absorbed by the target itself or the surrounding shielding. The small amount of X-rays that leave the tube through the window is called the exit beam, and these are the useful X-rays. A measure of the amount of these X-rays is the output intensity, which is the number of photons in the useful beam.

The intensity of the beam is determined by the number of X-rays given off at the target. This is influenced by the number of electrons arriving at the target, i.e. the tube current, the kinetic energy that they have when they hit the target, i.e. the voltage across the tube, and whether anything is in the beam that may absorb any X-rays when they exit the window. Therefore, when these factors are altered, the output intensity of the useful beam changes. Intensity is defined as the X-ray energy passing through unit area per unit time and is measured in roentgens or expressed as air kerma in grays.

The intensity of the X-ray tube is equal to the tube efficiency multiplied by the tube power.

$$\text{Tube power} \propto (W)$$
$$= \text{voltage}\,(KV_p) \times \text{current}\,(mA) \quad (2.3)$$

$$\text{Efficiency} \propto \text{voltage}\,(kV_p) \quad (2.4)$$

therefore

$$\text{Intensity}\,(I) \propto (kV_p)^2 \times mA \quad (2.5)$$

## Beam quality

It is difficult to quote an energy for the spectrum that comes from an X-ray tube, due to the fact that it is polyenergetic. This means it has a spread of energies between zero and the maximum kilovoltage of the tube, with the shape of a bremsstrahlung spectrum. As a polyenergetic beam travels through material, lower-energy photons are attenuated more than higher-energy ones. This means that the spread of energies present in the beam will determine how far it will travel in a material, or how penetrating it is. This is the beam quality.

## Half-value layer

This is a way to measure beam quality. The output of a well-collimated output beam is measured and thin aluminium foils, usually of 1-mm thickness, placed into the beam until the intensity is half its original value. The thickness of aluminium producing this 50% reduction is called the half-value layer of the beam (HVL). The HVL is found by plotting the series of readings on a graph and is quoted as millimetres of Al. The HVL is measured at 80 kVp for a standard X-ray tube. It gives a measure of the penetrability of the beam, and can be monitored over time to ensure that an X-ray tube is not deteriorating.

## Factors affecting the output intensity and quality of the beam

### Tube current

Changing the current of the X-ray tube (the milliamps or mA) changes the number of electrons hitting the target. If you increase the mA by a factor of 2 then the number of X-rays emitted at each energy will also increase by a factor of 2. The shape of the output spectrum does not change, only the amplitude. This is illustrated in Figure 2.6, which shows what happens when the mA are doubled and all other factors are kept constant. This shows that $I \propto mA$, where

$I$ is the total intensity, shown by the area under the curve. Changing the current of the X-ray tube does not affect the quality of the beam, as the energy spread and hence effective energy stays the same.

### Peak tube voltage

Changing the voltage across the tube increases the kinetic energy of the electrons that reach the target. This means that the amount of bremsstrahlung produced increases, as well as the average energy and the maximum energy of the X-rays produced. This is shown in Figure 2.7, which shows two spectra, one with a peak tube voltage ($kV_p$) of 70 kV and one with 80 kV. All other factors have been kept the same. The output intensity increases by a factor proportional to the $kVp^2$, as shown by equation 2.5. The quality of the beam has also increased, because the effective energy of the beam has increased.

### Filtration

Applying a filter over the exit window will alter the number of X-rays in the useful beam and also their energy. A filter such as aluminium will filter out more of the lower-energy X-rays because these are attenuated more easily by the metal, whereas the higher-energy X-rays will pass through. The beam coming out of the tube will

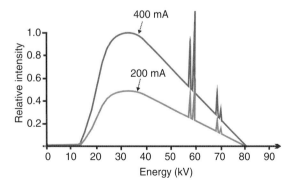

**Figure 2.6** The effect on the tube spectrum when the mA has been halved.

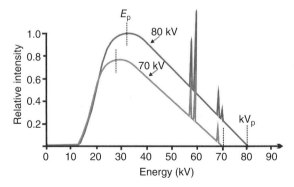

**Figure 2.7** The effect on the tube spectrum when the kV has been reduced from 80 kV to 70 kV.

always have some effect of filtering, because the exit window and any inherent filtration will attenuate some low-energy photons. Figure 2.8 shows the effect of adding filtration into the exit beam. The highest energy of the spectrum (the kVp) stays the same, as the maximum energy of the X-rays coming out of the tube has not changed and some of these will always pass through all filtering unattenuated. The effective energy shifts to a higher kilovoltage as the number of lower energy X-rays has decreased.

Filtration is used in X-ray tubes to reduce the patient dose, because lower energy X-rays will always be absorbed by the patient without giving any useful information to the medical image produced.

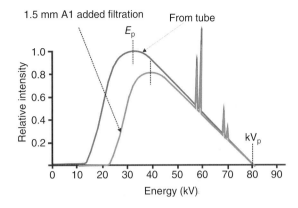

**Figure 2.8** The effect on the tube spectrum when filtration has been added to the exit beam.

## Self-test questions

1. Describe the main function of the following parts of an X-ray tube:
   (a) cathode
   (b) anode
   (c) housing.

2. What makes tungsten a good choice for both the filament and the target material?

3. What is the difference between the actual focal spot size and the effective focal spot size?

4. Describe the process of thermionic emission.

5. Why is it necessary to maintain the glass/metal envelope at vacuum pressure?

6. How are Characteristic X-rays produced?

7. How are Bremsstrahlung X-rays produced?

8. Why are X-ray tubes thought of as inefficient?

9. What is the X-ray output intensity of an X-ray tube dependent on?

10. What is the quality of an X-ray spectrum?

11. How do you measure the quality of an X-ray tube?

12. What does the kV setting on a console control?

13. What happens within the X-ray tube if the kV setting on the console is increased?

14. What does the mA setting on a console relate to?

15. What happens within the X-ray tube if the mA setting on the console is increased?

16. Calculate the change in intensity of an X-ray tube if the original intensity was 75 μGy after:
    (a) the $kV_p$ has been increased from 80 kV to 100 kV
    (b) the mA has been decreased from 500 mA to 300 mA.

17. (a) Draw the spectrum from an X-ray tube operated at 80 kV and 300 mA with no added filtration.
    (b) On the same graph draw the output from the same tube if the setting were changed to 70 kV and 200 mA (with no added filtration).

18. How has the intensity from the tube changed in the above example, if the original intensity of the tube was 100 μGy?

19. (a) Draw the spectrum from an X-ray tube without any filtration.
    (b) On the same graph draw the output from the same tube if 1.5 mm of Al has been added over the exit window.

20. What would happen if an X-ray tube were clinically operated with no added filtration in the beam?

## Further reading

Bomford CK, Kunkler IH. *Walter and Miller's Text-book of Radiotherapy*, 6th edn. Edinburgh: Churchill Livingstone, 2003.

Meredith WJ, Massey JB. *Fundamental Physics of Radiology*, 3rd edn. Chichester: John Wright & Sons, 1977.

Dowsett DJ, Kenny PA, Johnston RE. *The Physics of Diagnostic Imaging*, 2nd edn. London: Hodder Arnold, 2006.

# Chapter 3
# RADIATION DOSIMETRY

Janette Chianese and Fiona Chamberlain

**Aims and objectives**

The aim of this chapter is to provide an introduction to the theory of dose measurement and
give an overview of the design and operation of
practical dosimeters encountered in the modern
radiotherapy department.

After studying this chapter the reader should be
able to:

• describe the unit of absorbed dose and
exposure
• understand the physical principles and design
of devices used to detect and measure radiation
dose.

## The unit of absorbed dose

There is no definition of a fundamental unit of
radiation that causes known responses in different biological models because of the disparate
interaction properties of different particles and
qualities of radiation. It is possible, however, to
relate the damage mechanisms of radiation to the
amount of ionising energy deposited in tissues.
Although the precise microscopic distribution of
this energy deposition has a profound effect on
the overall biological response, for particles and
qualities producing similar interactions (such as
electrons and photons in the range 0.05–10 MeV)
the constant of proportionality remains the same.
It is impractical to measure microscopic distribu-

tion and so a macroscopic assessment of absorbed
energy is made quantified by the SI unit of
absorbed dose – the gray.

The gray is defined as: 'The absorbed dose ($D$)
is the quotient of d$e$ by d$m$, where d$e$ is the mean
energy imparted by ionising radiation to matter
of mass d$m$.'

$$D = \frac{de}{dm}$$

1 gray = 1 joule per kilogram (1 Gy = 1 J kg$^{-1}$).

## Measuring the gray

The National Physical Laboratory (NPL) houses
specialist equipment that measures absorbed
dose under controlled conditions, enabling an
absolute standard to be produced (the primary
standard). Dosimeters across the country are sent
to this centre for comparison and subsequent
calibration against this standard and are therefore known as secondary standards. Dosimeters
calibrated against secondary dosimeters are
termed tertiary standards. Calibration of the
local standard against the primary standard is
recommended every 2 years.[1]

## Calorimetry

Calorimetry is one method of measuring absorbed
dose whereby the precise quantification of minute

temperature changes in irradiated samples are used to produce direct evidence of the energy absorbed during the process, because the heat energy absorbed by a sample is proportional to the absorbed dose. Calibration of local ionisation detectors against a national calorimetric standard also exists for a range of megavoltage photon qualities; however, calorimetry is not always practicable because it suits the measurement of large absorbed quantities of radiation under very controlled conditions. Therefore there are other preferred methods for less energetic X-rays and electrons.

The first step is to specify a unit of ionisation that is compatible with absorbed dose.

## Exposure

Exposure is defined as: 'The exposure $(X)$, is the quotient of $dQ$ by $dm$ where the value of $dQ$ is the absolute value of the total charge of the ions of one sign produced in air when all the electrons (negatrons and positrons) liberated by photons in air of mass dm are completely stopped in air.'[2] The SI unit of exposure is coulombs per kilogram $(C\,kg^{-1})$.

This definition explicitly defines exposure for photons interacting with a defined mass of air and no other radiation particles or irradiated medium. To determine the exposure at some point within any other medium, it is necessary to replace a small part of that material with a volume of air small enough to prevent disruption of the photon field. The process covered by this definition thus comprises two stages. First, photons interact with the air to produce electrons (by photoelectric absorption or Compton scatter) or electrons and positrons (by pair production). Second, these electrons and positrons diffuse though the air causing more ionisation. Exposure is thus the collection of all the ions of one sign when the energy of all subsequent particles has been completely dissipated. It should be noted that some of the secondary particles will lose a small amount of energy by the bremsst-

rahlung process, which in turn may cause further ionisation, and this must be excluded from the total charge contributing to the definition of exposure.

As absorbed dose in $(D_{air}) = X\dfrac{W}{E}$, where $E$ = the charge on an electron and $W$ = the mean energy expended in the formation of one ion-pair, and exposure $(X)$

$$= \frac{dQ}{dm}$$

and $D_{air} = \dfrac{W_{air}}{e} \times \dfrac{dQ}{dm} = \dfrac{W_{air}}{e} \times X$

Absorbed dose in material $(D_{mat})$
$$= \frac{A_{mat}}{A_{air}} \times \frac{W_{air}}{e} \times X \qquad (3.1)$$

where $W_{air}$ = average energy absorbed in the production of a single ion-pair in air (33.85 eV); $e$ = charge on each ion; $W_{air}/e$ = 33.85 J C$^{-1}$; $A_{mat}$ = mass energy absorption coefficient for material; and $A_{air}$ = mass energy absorption coefficient for air.

Although the concept of exposure satisfies the mathematical requirements of the derivation of dose, there are obvious practical problems when attempting to irradiate a defined mass of air while leaving a surrounding volume sufficient to attenuate the secondary particles, unirradiated. The practical solution is the free air chamber that utilises charged particle equilibrium to circumvent this dilemma.

## Free air ionisation chamber

The theory and operation of this exposure device may be explained by considering the schematic diagram in Figure 3.1. A collimated photon beam enters the chamber through the diaphragms on the left-hand side exiting through the opposite wall. Within the body of the chamber, a parallel

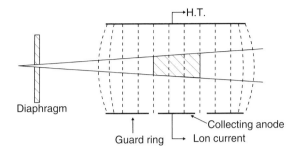

**Figure 3.1** The 'free-air' ionisation chamber.

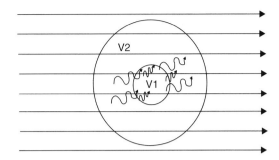

**Figure 3.2** Principle of the 'air-wall'.

plate electrode assembly is mounted with guard wires and a concentric guard ring arranged to define a volume of air from which secondary charged particles are collected. The separation of the plates is chosen to ensure that any remaining kinetic energy of the secondary particles is dissipated before their arrival at the collecting electrode, while being sufficiently close for the applied polarising voltage to collect all the ions produced within the defined volume. In order to satisfy the conditions imposed by the definition of exposure, the ions generated within the collection boundary (shaded area) that are lost to the periphery must be balanced with externally generated ions entering this critical volume. This is the state of electronic equilibrium. Corrections are required for lack of saturation in the ionisation current, the presence of any water vapour, and ionisation resulting from bremsstrahlung and scattered radiation or leakage through the primary collimators.

## Cavity chamber (cylindrical or thimble chamber)

The free air chamber is capable of accurately determining exposure for energies up to 300 kV. Above this energy the separation of the electrodes demands prohibitive polarising voltages to collect the charges produced. Although the free-air chamber enables a definitive measurement of exposure, by utilising the concept of

electronic equilibrium, it is not a practical piece of equipment for everyday clinical use due to its large size. More portable dosimeters have been designed that are more practical for use in the high-energy ranges used in radiotherapy. These portable devices have small detectors capable of measuring exposure 'in phantom' without agitating the radiation fluence. To achieve this goal the 'air–wall' concept is used (Figure 3.2).

Consider the small volume of air, $V_1$, completely surrounded by a larger and concentric volume of air, $V_2$, uniformly irradiated by a photon radiation field. If $V_2$ is sufficiently large such that the energies of the secondary particles produced within $V_1$ are dissipated before leaving $V_2$, then the geometric requirements for achieving electronic equilibrium are satisfied. If $V_2$ is then compressed to 1/1000 of its original volume, the diameter can be reduced without compromising the electronic equilibrium and, if central and peripheral electrodes are incorporated, an ionisation detector with similar performance characteristics to the free air chamber can be achieved. In practice, $V_2$ is not actually compressed but is replaced by a material of similar atomic number but greater density, e.g. graphite; this has the added benefit of being a conductor and can therefore act as one of the electrodes. The complete assembly is known as the thimble chamber (Figure 3.3).

Using this device it is possible to extend the estimation of exposure across a greater range of energies (typically the Farmer-type chambers can

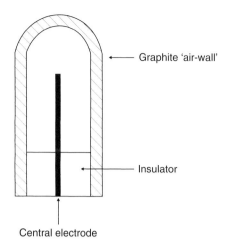

**Figure 3.3** The thimble chamber.

measure up to 50 MeV) with equipment that is essentially portable and suited to the rigors of practical radiotherapy output measurements.

## Parallel plate (pancake) chambers

Parallel plate chambers, as the name suggests, are constructed of two parallel plates of material (plastic) that forms the walls of the chamber. These walls are coated with a conducting layer that forms the positive and negative electrodes. A layer of gas between the walls acts as the collecting volume. The electrodes lie close together so that the air cavity can be constructed very thinly, leading to very little noticeable perturbation. Guard electrodes (rings) create uniform field lines by minimising settling time of the chamber. Parallel plate chambers must be used when the mean electron energy is greater than 5 MeV at any depth.[1] These chambers can measure a range of energies up to 50 MeV electrons. Desirable properties of these chambers are that they should be waterproof and their construction as homogeneous and water equivalent as possible. It is important to check the polarity of the chamber routinely because this may change during the lifetime of the chamber.

## Air kerma

The term 'kerma' originates from the acronym 'kinetic energy released per unit mass'. This term is not complete without specifying the material concerned.

It is formally defined as: 'the quotient $dE_{tr}$ by $dm$, where $dE_{tr}$ is the sum of the initial kinetic energies of all the charged ionising particles liberated by uncharged ionising particles in a material of mass $dm$'.[2]

Therefore:

$$K = dE_{tr}/dm.$$

Kerma is therefore an energy equivalent to exposure and is measured in joules/kilogram and therefore has the same dimensions as absorbed dose, the gray, being related by the expression:

$$\text{Absorbed dose} = \frac{A_{mat}}{T_{air}} \times \text{air kerma (Gy)}$$

where $A_{mat}$ = mass energy absorption coefficient for material; $T_{air}$ = mass energy transfer coefficient for air; and $A_{mat}/T_{air} \approx 1.1$.

The difference between the quantity of energy transferred and the eventual energy absorbed is only 0.4% and is due to bremsstrahlung production,

## Dosimetry of megavoltage photons

Unlike the traditional approach to exposure measurement, where the electronic equilibrium conditions are satisfied entirely within the detector body and the unit acts as a 'photon probe', consideration must be given to the charge balance at a single point in a large medium exposed to uniform photon irradiation in which a gas cavity has been introduced. In this case, if the cavity is sufficiently small to prevent the disturbance of the particle fluence within the medium, the same number and energy of electrons traverse this volume, whether gas or medium, and the ratio of the electron energies lost per unit mass of gas to medium is the same as the ratio of the two mass stopping powers (S), to the energy lost (dE) by the charged particles in traversing a small distance (dl) divided by its density (μ), i.e.

$$S = \frac{dE/dl}{\mu}$$

If this absorbed energy in the gas produces a charge J, then the energy required to produce this ionisation is given by JWg/e, where Wg is the mean energy required to produce one ionisation in air and e is the charge on the electron, the equivalent absorbed dose ($D_m$) within the medium is given by:

$$D_m = S_{mg} \times J \times Wg/e \qquad (3.2)$$

where $S_{mg}$ is the stopping power ratio of medium to gas. This equation summarises the hypotheses proposed initially by Bragg (1912)[3] and then refined by Gray (1929, 1936),[4,5] and relies for its validity on four basic assumptions:

1. Charged particle equilibrium exists in the absence of the cavity.
2. The particle fluence is not disturbed by the cavity presence.
3. The mass stopping power ratio is constant over the energy spectrum.
4. The secondary particles lose their energy by a large number of small interactions.

Equation 3.2 is analogous to the low energy photon version expressed in equation 3.1, but with the ratio of the mass energy absorption coefficients replaced by the stopping power ratio $S_{mg}$.

As discussed previously the ionisation chamber:

- is generally calibrated in terms of air kerma rather than charge itself
- has a minimal effect on particle fluence

- disturbs the continuity of the material by its very presence.

Therefore, in terms of the reading, R, of an instrument calibrated in air kerma, the formula[7] for deriving absorbed dose to water ($D_w$) is:

$$D_w = R \times N \times C\lambda$$

where R is the dosimeter reading corrected for temperature and pressure; N is the calibration factor converting the reading R to grays in air kerma; and Cλ is the factor converting air kerma to absorbed dose for the photon energy of use.

Cλ brings together the conversion from exposure to air kerma at 2 MV, the calibration energy and the variation sensitivity with energy of the secondary standard ionisation chamber for which Cλ is calculated. So, in summary, Cλ is the factor that allows a secondary standard to be used instead of the primary one.

## Electrons

The Bragg–Gray cavity theory is also used in electron dosimetry, but there is a fundamental difference in the way that dose is derived from ionisation measurements compared with that used for photons. The energy spectrum of a photon beam does not change significantly with increasing depth of penetration in water; the factors relating absorbed dose to ionisation remain effectively constant, because electrons are absorbed within a medium. However, the average energy of their spectrum decreases approximately linearly with increasing depth, reducing to zero at their maximum penetration, $R_p$.

If the mean incident energy of the electrons is denoted $E_0$ then the approximate mean spectral energy can be calculated at any depth (d) by the equation:

$$E_d = E_0(1 - d/R_p).$$

Derivation of the dose at any depth therefore involves two stages: first, determination of the mean incident energy from a half-value thickness in water measurement; and second, application of the corresponding correction factors for the particular energy at depth to the ionisation values measured under appropriate clinical conditions.

## Calorimetry

Although dose derivation using the Bragg–Gray approach, under conditions of charged particle equilibrium, is accepted, there are several assumptions enshrined within the theory that are difficult to measure directly and will always introduce unacceptable margins of uncertainty. To remove these errors of uncertainty, a more direct measurement of energy deposition is required, which to date has been achieved for megavoltage photons using a graphite calorimeter (Figure 3.4).

Although graphite has a specific thermal capacity some six times greater than that of water, the temperature increase resulting from a typical radiotherapy fraction is still only a few thousandths of a degree Celsius, and certainly negligible compared with the changes in the surrounding ambient temperature. To determine these fluctuations accurately and to improve on the alternative methods of dosimetry, the measuring system must be capable of discriminating temperature changes of one-millionth of a degree. To measure these minuscule temperature changes resulting from absorbed radiation dose the

sample, or, in this case, graphite 'core', must be thermally isolated from the local environment. This is partially achieved by mounting the core inside an evacuated 'jacket' of equal mass and material, which is in itself thermally isolated from the surrounding 'mantle' by a vacuum gap. To compensate for any thermal transfer from core to jacket the system is calibrated by heating the core using a known amount of electrical energy and observing the temperature changes in the jacket. As each component of the calorimeter has both heaters and thermocouples embedded within it, the whole assembly can be heated and maintained at a stable temperature to minimise any thermal transfer to and from the surrounding environment. More recently the NPL has developed a portable calorimeter that can be used on site in clinical departments.[6]

## Radiation detection and measurement

Table 3.1 lists the effects of radiation that form the basis of various detectors and dosimeters.

Some of the devices are best suited to direct measurement of doses received by patients and clinical staff and others to measurement of doses from treatment machines (at commissioning, acceptance and routine quality assurance testing).

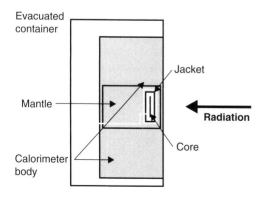

**Figure 3.4** The absorbed dose calorimeter.

**Table 3.1** Properties of radiation which form the basis of measuring devices

| Effects of radiation | Example of dosimeter/detector |
| --- | --- |
| Heat | Calorimeter |
| Photographic effect | Film badge |
| Ionisation | Thimble chamber, semiconductor detectors Geiger Muller tube |
| Chemical effect | Fricke dosimeter |
| Scintillation | Scintillation counter |
| Thermoluminescence | Thermoluminescent dosimeter |

It is recommended that all patients receiving radiotherapy have their first treatment dose checked with a dosimeter[1] and the most commonly used device for this purpose is a semiconductor device. Other devices used in the radiotherapy department to measure absorbed dose are ionisation chambers, film and thermoluminescent dosimeters (TLDs). Ionisation chambers have already been discussed. Photographic film, although used in quality assurance programmes, e.g. field size and beam flatness determination, is not generally used to quantify radiation dose at therapeutic levels. The exception to this, however, is environmental and personal monitoring where the sensitive response of film to a wide range of radiation qualities is a desirable feature.

To be useful in a radiotherapy department a detector must satisfy certain basic requirements. It should:

- be accurate
- be sensitive
- exhibit a linear response to dose
- be mechanically robust
- have a suitable physical size.

## Semiconductor detectors

These have three uses in radiotherapy:

1. Relative dosimetry of photon and electron beams
2. In vivo dosimetry of photon and electron beams
3. Quality assurance measurements.

### Principles of operation

A semiconductor has electrical conducting properties somewhere between those of a conductor and those of an insulator. The most commonly used semiconductor material is silicon, which is a group IV element in the periodic table. Silicon has four electrons in its outer valence band. In pure silicon, these valence electrons are covalently bonded with valence electrons in adjacent silicon atoms to form a crystal lattice. If the crystal absorbs energy, the covalent bonds can be broken, resulting in a free electron and a positive hole where the electron once was. The electron can then move through the crystal. If the positive hole takes up an electron from a neighbouring atom, the hole also moves. If impurities are added to silicon, a process known as doping, semiconductors with excess electrons or excess positive holes can be created (n- and p-type semiconductors, respectively).

A p-type semiconductor consists of silicon to which has been added a substance from group III of the periodic table, such as boron or aluminium. Group III elements have three electrons in their valence band that are able to form covalent bonds with the silicon atoms; however, one bond is not completed and thus a positive hole is created. In an n-type semiconductor an element is added from group V of the periodic table, such as phosphorus or arsenic. Group V elements have five electrons in their valence band. Four of these are able to take part in covalent bonds with silicon atoms, the fifth being free to move though the crystal (Figure 3.5).

If the device is irradiated, electrons and positive holes are created. The electrons are attracted towards the positively charged impurity in the n-type silicon and the positive holes diffuse towards the negatively charged impurity in the p-type silicon. This constitutes an ionisation current that is proportional to the incident dose rate and can be measured using an electrometer.

In practice, semiconductor dosimeters comprise a large portion of one type (p or n) and a smaller part of the other type. The dosimeter is then classified as either a p- or n-type detector according to the larger constituent part; n-type detectors show a sensitivity decrease and become non-linear with respect to dose rate as a result of radiation damage; p-type semiconductors do not suffer this drawback and also demonstrate a slower sensitivity decrease after irradiation, and for this reason are preferred for most clinical applications.

N-type                                    P-type

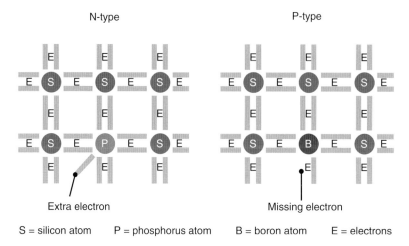

Extra electron                    Missing electron

S = silicon atom    P = phosphorus atom    B = boron atom    E = electrons

**Figure 3.5** Principles of thermoluminescence.

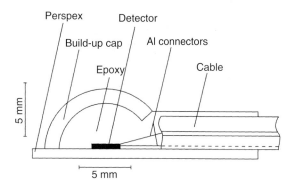

**Figure 3.6** Scanditronix p-Si patient dosimetry detector. (Reproduced by permission Scanditronix Medical AB.)

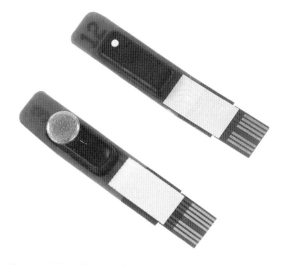

**Figure 3.7** Wireless detectors.

### Detector design

The detector consists of a small silicon detector crystal (external dimensions 2.5 mm × 2.5 mm × 0.4 mm) mounted on a Perspex plate (Figure 3.6). It is connected via aluminium foils to a coaxial cable (wireless detectors are also now available – Figure 3.7), and it is encapsulated in a protective sheath. A build-up cap is also incorporated and the type of material from which it is made and its thickness depend on the radiation quality being measured.

### Advantages

The semiconductor detector has the following advantages:

- High electrical signal: this means that the device is very sensitive – approximately 18 000 times more sensitive than an ionisation chamber.

- Small physical size: this is possible because of the high sensitivity, which means that the measuring volume can be small. This has the added advantage that the effective measuring point can be located close to the surface of the detector, providing a high degree of spatial resolution.

- Mechanically stable.
- Independent of atmospheric pressure – therefore no pressure correction factor is required.
- The small stopping power variation with energy in electron beams makes the detector suitable for measuring electron beams.
- Immediate read-out available.

### Limitations

The semiconductor detector has the following limitations:

- The sensitivity of the detector varies with temperature (in clinical practice, this variation is of the order of 1–3%), this is a consideration when in vivo measurements are made. The temperature of the detectors will rise when in contact with the patient's skin. To account for this the detectors may be placed on the patient 3–4 minutes before treatment starts to allow time for the detector to reach a steady state. A correction factor is then applied to take into account the change in sensitivity due to temperature (usually an increase). Alternatively, the detector may be calibrated at body temperature using a phantom at a raised temperature.
- The sensitivity also varies with accumulated radiation dose. Above a certain accumulated dose, the sensitivity stabilises and for this reason detectors are often supplied pre-irradiated.
- Radiation damage is a particular problem in n-type detectors that progressively exhibit a non-linear response with dose rate; p-type detectors are less susceptible to this effect. The amount of damage inflicted on the detector is related not only to the total radiation dose but also to the quality of radiation.

## Thermoluminescent dosimeters

These have four uses in radiotherapy:

- Relative dosimetry of electron and photon beams
- In vivo dosimetry of electron and photon beams
- Personal monitoring
- Environmental monitoring.

### Principles of operation

The electrons in orbit around an atom occupy a series of discrete energy levels. In a crystal, interactions between neighbouring atoms result in these energy levels being broadened into a series of continuous energy bands. The highest filled band is called the valence band and it is separated from the conduction band by an energy gap of a few electron-volts. Electrons in the conduction band are free to move within that band. The energy gap separating the conduction and valence bands is sometimes referred to as the forbidden zone.

If impurities are introduced into the crystal, intermediate energy levels are formed within the forbidden zone and these are referred to as electron traps. If the crystal is irradiated, electrons in the valence band may receive sufficient energy for them to be raised to the conduction band. Electrons may then fall back to the valence band or get caught in an electron trap (Figure 3.8). Electrons caught in the traps are unable to escape until the crystal is heated. When sufficient heat is applied the electrons gain thermal energy and

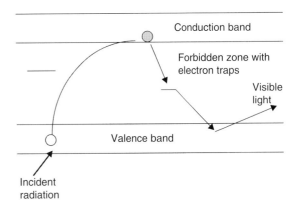

**Figure 3.8** Principles of thermoluminescence.

fall back from the electron trap to the valence band; in doing so the electrons emit energy in the form of light photons. The total light output is proportional to the number of trapped electrons, which in turn is proportional to the energy absorbed from the radiation beam.

## Detector design

There are a number of different crystalline materials that exhibit thermoluminescent properties. The most commonly used within radiotherapy are those based on lithium fluoride (LiF) because LiF is approximately tissue equivalent (effective atomic number of 8.2 compared with 7.4 for tissue) and almost energy independent in the range 100 keV–1.3 MeV gamma radiation. Other TLD materials include those based on lithium borate ($LiBO_4$), calcium fluoride ($CaF_3$) and calcium sulphate ($CaSO_4$). Each of these materials has specific advantages with regard to sensitivity, measuring range or tissue equivalence, but LiF has the best overall properties for most purposes within radiotherapy.[8]

TLD materials are supplied in powder form and as solid discs, rods and chips (Figure 3.9). Discs can be encapsulated in Teflon for use in personal dosimeters, which may incorporate built-in filters to enable energy discrimination of radiation dose received.

Read-out of dose is achieved using specialised instrumentation. The TLD material is heated either by direct contact with a heated tray or by hot gas. Light emitted by the TLD material is measured using a photomultiplier, which converts the light into a current signal, which is then amplified and displayed. It should be noted that the read-out count is dependent on the temperature and duration of the annealing cycle and the section of the glow curve sampled during read-out. It is essential, therefore, that both of these are predetermined and fixed for any particular batch of TLDs used. There are advantages to using TLDs but also some limitations that should be considered (Table 3.2).

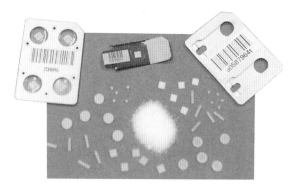

**Figure 3.9** The variety of physical forms of thermoluminescent dosimeter (TLD) materials available. (Reproduced courtesy of Harshaw/Bicon NE Technology Ltd.)

**Table 3.2** Advantages and limitations of thermoluminescent dosimeters (TLDs)

| Advantages | Limitations and disadvantages |
|---|---|
| Re-usable | Precision can be affected by poor handling and storage |
| Automated read out | Immediate read out is not possible |
| Energy independent over a wide range of the energies | 'Fading'– unintentional release of trapped electrons, may be caused by exposure to heat or light (particularly ultraviolet) |
| Similar atomic number to soft tissue (except those containing calcium) | Some types may liquefy if left in humid conditions |
| Capable of measuring over a wide range of doses | Scratches on the surface of the TLD or reduction in mass will affect the light emission characteristics |
| Small physical size | May become contaminated by grease or adhesives |

## Self-test questions

1. What unit is absorbed dose measured in?
2. What property does the calorimetry process use to measure the absorbed dose?
3. What do you need to know to convert from absorbed dose to kerma?
4. What is a secondary standard dosimeter?
5. Explain the acronym kerma.
6. What is the process known as doping with respect to the construction of semi-conductor materials?
7. Name types of dosimeter used for in vivo measurements.
8. What dosimeter/detectors directly measure the ionisation properties of radiation?
9. What are the three processes of photon interaction in air?
10. By what process do secondary particles lose a small amount of energy during an exposure?
11. Why is a free air ionisation chamber not routinely used in clinical practice?
12. What is a better method to use in respect of 11 above?
13. Name the theory utilised in electron and mega-voltage dosimetry.
14. What is the typical energy measurement range for a parallel plate chamber?
15. Why is it important that the chamber be tissue equivalent?
16. List three essential requirements of any radiation detector used in a radiotherapy department.
17. Explain the term thermoluminescence.
18. Which TLD material is typically used for dose measurements in radiotherapy?
19. What properties make this material ideal for this purpose?
20. List advantages and disadvantages of using TLDs for in vivo dosimetry?

## References

1. Institute of Physics and Engineering in Medicine (IPEM). Code of Practice for Electron Dosimetry for Radiotherapy Beams of Initial Energy from 4-25 MeV based on an absorbed dose to water calibration. *Physics in Medicine and Biology* 2003; **48**: 2929–70.
2. International Commission on Radiation Units and Measurements. *Radiation Quantities and Units.* ICRU Report 33. Washington DC: ICRU, 1980.
3. Bragg WH. *Studies in Radioactivity.* London: Macmillan, 1912.
4. Gray LH. The Absorption of Penetrating Radiation. *Proceedings of the Royal Society* 1929; **A122**: 647.
5. Gray LH. The Absorption of Penetrating Radiation. *Proceedings of the Royal Society* 1936; **A156**: 578.
6. McEwen MR, Duane SA. Portable graphite calorimeter for measuring absorbed dose in the radiotherapy clinic. *Physics in Medicine and Biology* 2000; **45**: 3675–691.
7. Greene D, Williams PC. *Linear Accelerators for Radiation Therapy*, 2nd edn. London: IOP Publishing Ltd, 1997.
8. Derreumaux S, Chavaudra J, Bridier A, Rossetti V, Dutreix A. A European quality assurance network for radiotherapy: dose measurement procedure. *Physics in Medicine and Biology* 1995; **40**: 1191–208.

## Further reading

Greening JR. *Fundamentals of Radiation Dosimetry.* London: IOP Publishing, 1992.
Khan FM. *The Physics of Radiation Therapy*, 3rd edn. Baltimore, MA: Lippincott Williams & Wilkins, 2003.
Institute of Physical Sciences in Medicine (IPSM). Code of Practice for High Energy Photon Therapy based on the NPL absorbed dose calibration service. *Physics in Medicine and Biology* 1990; **35**: 1355–60.
McKinlay AF. *Thermoluminescence Dosimetry.* Bristol: Adam Hilger, 1981.
Williams JR, Thwaites DI. *Radiotherapy Physics in Practice*, 2nd edn. Oxford: Oxford University Press, 2000.
Williams AJ, Rosser, Thomson NJ, DuSautoy AR. Recent advances in water calorimetry at NPL. In: *Proceedings of the 22nd Annual EMBS International Conference*, 23–28 July 2000, Chicago IL.

# Chapter 4
# X-RAY INTERACTIONS WITH MATTER

Kathryn Cooke

### Aims and objectives

- To explain the following terms: attenuation, attenuation coefficient and half-value layer.
- To describe the three interaction processes that occur when ionising radiation interacts with a medium within the energy ranges relevant to radiotherapy.
- To outline the practical relevance of the interaction processes to radiotherapy

## Introduction

There are several interaction processes that occur when ionising radiation interacts with matter. These depend on the nature and energy of the primary radiation beam and the structure of the medium through which the radiation beam passes. It is beyond the scope of this chapter to describe all possible interaction processes, so only the three that occur within the X-ray energy ranges utilised in radiotherapy are presented later: photoelectric process, Compton scatter and pair production.

## Attenuation

It is important to understand how the intensity of the X-ray beam is affected when ionising radiation interacts with a medium.

When a beam of X-rays traverses matter, there is a reduction in the intensity of that beam. *Intensity* is defined as the rate of flow of photon energy through a unit area lying at right angles to the path of the beam. This reduction in intensity is referred to as *attenuation* and involves a process of absorption, scattering or a combination of both.

*Absorption* is the transference of energy from the primary X-ray beam to the atoms of the medium through which the X-ray beam is passing. It is defined as the energy deposited in the material per unit mass. The transferred energy is converted into kinetic energy of the electrons within the medium, enabling them to move through the medium. The electrons may interact with other atoms in the medium causing *ionisation* and *excitation* (see Chapter 2). This results in the chemical and biological changes important to radiotherapy.

*Scattering* occurs following a collision interaction between the primary X-ray beam and the atoms of the medium through which the X-ray beam is passing. The incident photon is deflected out of the path of the primary beam and travels onward in a new direction. This collision may or may not involve transference of energy from the incident photon to the medium.

The size of the nucleus of an atom is extremely small compared with the overall size of the atom and so most of the atom is considered as space.

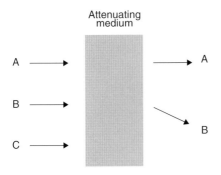

**Figure 4.1** Process of attenuation. A. transmission; B. scattering; C. absorption.

Therefore, there is a high probability that some X-rays will pass straight through a medium without undergoing absorption or scattering (Figure 4.1). The X-rays are said to be transmitted and it is these X-rays that play a part in the production of a radiographic image and contribute to the exit dose of a beam of X-rays used for radiation treatment.

## Exponential relationship

Although it is impossible to predict which photons will interact with the medium, it is possible to predict the fraction of total photons that will undergo interaction. Experimentally it can be shown that for a narrow, homogeneous beam of X-rays, i.e. a beam of photons of similar energy, the intensity of radiation transmitted is reduced in an 'exponential' manner (Figure 4.2). Equal thicknesses of uniform attenuating material placed in the path of the beam produce equal fractional reductions in the intensity of radiation transmitted, e.g. a thickness of attenuator (*t*) reduces the intensity of the beam initially by 50% (100% reduced to 50%), then again by 50% (50% reduced to 25%). This is referred to as an exponential relationship and is represented by the equation:

$$I_t = I_0 e^{\mu t}$$

where $I_t$ = intensity with medium of thickness (*t*) inserted in the path of the beam; $I_0$ = intensity

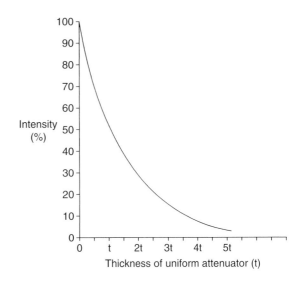

**Figure 4.2** Exponential relationship between intensity of transmitted radiation and thickness of attenuator for a homogeneous beam of X-rays.

with no medium in path of beam; *e* = exponential coefficient; μ = total linear attenuation coefficient; *t* = thickness of stated medium.

Due to this exponential relationship it is not possible to attenuate an X-ray beam completely, although the intensity may be reduced to an insignificant level.

## Half-value layer

An important descriptor known as the half-value layer (HVL) can be related to the exponential relationship between the attenuator and the intensity of the beam. The HVL is the thickness of a stated medium that will reduce the intensity of a narrow beam of X-rays to exactly half of its original value.

The first HVL is indicated in Figure 4.2 by the value of the thickness of attenuator that reduces the intensity of the beam from 100% to 50%; the second HVL is the thickness that reduces the intensity of the beam from 50% to 25%. For a homogeneous beam of radiation, these values will always be equal, e.g. referring to Figure 4.2, the HVL is 't'. However, an X-ray beam is heterogeneous and comprises photons of differing energies, so successive values of HVL cannot be the same due to filtration of the lower energy photons in the beam by the initial attenuation. The beam increases in homogeneity as filtration occurs and later values of HVL will become equivalent.

By definition, if the intensity of a beam of X-rays is reduced to 50% of the original intensity by a stated material of thickness HVL, it can be said that:

$$I_0 \div I_{HVL} = 2.$$

By inserting this value in the exponential equation, it is found that the HVL is related to the linear attenuation coefficient ($\mu$) by:

$$\mu = 0.693 \div HVL.$$

The HVL and related tenth value layer (TVL) are terms commonly used when discussing radiation protection materials. TVL is the thickness of a stated medium that will reduce the intensity of a narrow beam of X-rays to exactly one-tenth of its original value.

## Attenuation coefficients

An attenuation coefficient indicates the attenuating ability of a medium. The *linear attenuation coefficient* used previously is defined as the fractional reduction in intensity of a parallel beam of radiation per unit thickness of the attenuating medium traversed, and is awarded the SI unit of $m^{-1}$. It is essential that the beam of radiation is parallel (non-divergent), so that it is not affected by the inverse square law (refer to Chapter 1).

Attenuation of an X-ray beam involves an interaction between a photon and an atom of the attenuating medium. Therefore, the possibility of an interaction occurring increases as the number of atoms per unit volume of the medium increases; conversely it decreases as the number of atoms per unit volume of the medium decreases. The definition of the linear attenuation coefficient ($\mu$) suggests that it is dependent on the actual thickness of traversed medium but does not take into account the actual number of atoms within the traversed thickness. Therefore, any change of state in the same thickness of medium, e.g. solid to gaseous state, involving a decrease in the number of atoms per unit volume, i.e. change in density, is not accounted for by the linear attenuation coefficient.

To relate the dependence of attenuation to the number of atoms present in the medium, the *total mass attenuation coefficient* is used ($\mu/\rho$). This is defined as the fractional reduction in intensity in a parallel beam of radiation of cross-section area per unit mass of attenuating material and is awarded the SI unit $m^2 kg^{-1}$. This coefficient takes account of the possible different densities of an attenuating material and the value is therefore constant unless the elemental composition of the attenuating medium is altered. As presented below, there are several ways in which an X-ray beam may be attenuated, depending on the nature and energy of the primary radiation and the structure of the medium through which the X-ray beam passes. Each attenuation process has a related attenuation coefficient and the total linear or mass attenuation coefficient is the sum of these individual attenuation coefficients.

## X-ray interaction processes

There are approximately 12 different interaction processes that may occur when ionising radiation interacts with matter, but within the X-ray energy ranges utilised in radiotherapy only three are thought to be relevant: photoelectric process, Compton scatter and pair production.

*Elastic scattering* occurs at X-ray energies below those utilised in radiotherapy but is worthy of note as a comparison to Compton scatter. In addition, an attenuation process known as *photonuclear disintegration* occurs at very high-megavoltage photon energies, resulting in the

**Table 4.1** Relationship of interaction processes to atomic number, electron density and beam energy

|  | **Photoelectric process** | **Compton scatter** | **Pair production** |
|---|---|---|---|
| Atomic number | Proportional to $Z^3$ | Not dependent on $Z$ | Proportional to $Z$ |
| Electron density | Not dependent on electron density | Proportional to electron density | Not dependent on electron density |
| Beam energy | Proportional to 1 keV$^3$ | Proportional to 1 keV | Only occurs at energies >1.022 MeV |

ejection of a particle (usually a neutron) from the nucleus of the atom. These interactions occur over a small range of high photon energies and are outside the scope of this chapter.

A summary of the main X-ray interaction processes is presented in Table 4.1.

## Elastic scattering

This interaction process occurs at very low photon energies, below those useful for radiation treatment. It involves a collision interaction between the incident photon and an electron orbiting the nucleus of an atom in the attenuating medium. The energy of the incident photon is considered insignificant when compared with the binding energies of the electrons. This inhibits the transfer of energy from the incident photon to the electron. The consequence of the collision is that the incident photon continues to travel through the medium but in a different direction, i.e. it is scattered. The interaction is considered 'elastic' because there is no resultant loss of energy from the X-ray beam.

## Photoelectric absorption

Photoelectric absorption occurs at the X-ray energies utilised for diagnostic imaging, radiotherapy kilovolt imaging, and superficial and orthovoltage radiation therapy. Within these X-ray energy ranges, i.e. 50–500 kV, the energy of the incident photon is equal to or slightly greater than the binding energy of the inner orbital electrons of the atoms through which the X-ray beam passes. This is a requirement for

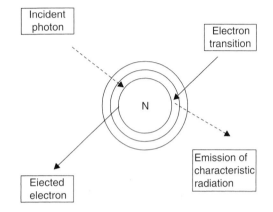

**Figure 4.3** Photoelectric absorption.

photoelectric absorption, summarised below, to occur:

- Incident photon interacts with an inner shell electron, transferring all of its energy to that electron (Figure 4.3).
- The incident photon no longer exists as a result of this interaction, i.e. it has been absorbed.
- The transferred energy from the incident photon overcomes the binding energy of the orbiting electron, causing it to be ejected from the atom.
- The ejected electrons, referred to as *photoelectrons*, are emitted at all angles. The higher the energy of the incident photon, the smaller the angle of photoelectron emission in order to conserve momentum and energy in the interaction.
- All remaining energy is converted to kinetic energy of the photoelectron, allowing it to travel through the attenuating material.

- The photoelectrons dissipate their kinetic energy in the atoms of the attenuating material until they are brought to rest.
- Ejection of the photoelectron from the atom leaves a vacancy in the inner electron shell, causing the atom to be unstable.
- The vacancy is filled by electron transition from an outer shell (see Chapter 2).
- The atom produces a photon of radiation, referred to as characteristic radiation, the energy of which is related to the binding energies of the two electron shells involved in the transition.
- The characteristic radiation is reabsorbed by the medium.

The characteristic radiation is so called because it is characteristic not only of the transitional shells but also of the particular element. It usually possesses less energy than the binding energies of the electrons of that medium, so is unlikely to interact further by photoelectric absorption. It is more probable that the characteristic radiation will be reabsorbed very close to the interaction in the same medium. This may not be the case with high atomic number materials because the characteristic radiation emitted will have a greater energy and may be transmitted if produced near to the surface of the medium. This is not of importance in soft tissue, however, and the photoelectric process is usually regarded as one of total absorption as the energy of the incident photon is completely absorbed by the medium.

Conservation of energy in this interaction is shown by the equation:

$$Ep = Eb + (mv^2/2)$$

where $Ep$ = energy of incident photon, $Eb$ = binding energy of electron, $m$ = mass of photoelectron and $v$ = velocity of photoelectron.

During the photoelectric interaction the atom recoils slightly in order to conserve momentum in the system. It is not possible for the incident photon to interact with 'free' electrons by the photoelectric process as energy and momentum could not be conserved in the interaction.

The probability of the interaction taking place increases with the atomic number ($Z$) of the attenuating medium and is approximately proportional to $Z^3$, i.e. if the atomic number of the element is doubled; the probability of photoelectric absorption occurring at a specific energy is increased eightfold.

Given that the binding energy associated with a particular electron orbit is dependent on the atomic number of the atom, the K-shell absorption limit is reached at lower energies in atoms of lower atomic number. Therefore, for materials of low atomic number, e.g. soft tissue (comprising mainly fat, water and muscle, creating an effective Z of approximately 7.5), the photoelectric process occurs over a lower energy range than for a material of high atomic number, e.g. lead (Z = 82).

At very low photon energies, e.g. >10 keV for tungsten where the binding energy for the L-shell is 12.1 keV, photoelectric absorption is able to occur only in the outer M and N orbits. As the energy of the incident photon increases and becomes equal to the binding energy of the L- and K-shells, photoelectric absorption preferentially occurs in the inner shells. As the photon energy increases above the limit for the K-shell, attenuation by photoelectric absorption becomes less likely and Compton scatter becomes the dominant process. Indeed, the probability of photoelectric absorption occurring decreases dramatically as the energy of the incident photon increases and in general is considered to be inversely proportional to the cube of the kiloelectron-volts ($keV^3$).

In reality, the above statement is a simplification of the dependence of the photoelectric process on the energy of the primary beam. As previously stated, the probability of M-shell transition decreases in an inverse relationship to the $keV^3$ as the incident photon energy increases. This continues until the incident photon energy becomes close to the binding energy associated with the L-shell. Preferential absorption now occurs in the L-shell and the probability of photoelectric absorption and L-shell transition occurring abruptly rises. This is contrary to the general relationship between the probability of photoelectric absorption and the energy of the primary beam. As the incident photon energy continues to increase above the binding energies of the L-shell, the probability of photoelectric absorption occurring decreases, again in an inverse relationship to the keV$^3$. This principle occurs within each separate electron shell. The point at which the attenuation suddenly increases is known as the *absorption edge* and is an important phenomenon with implications for the choice of quality filters used in orthovoltage treatment units (see Chapter 9).

### Practical relevance of photoelectric absorption to radiotherapy

The differential blackening and great contrast between areas of soft tissue and bone observed on a simulator localisation or verification radiograph occurs as a result of the photoelectric process being the predominant attenuation process at these lower energies, typically 50–120 kV. The partial mass attenuation coefficient of this process is dependent on the atomic number of the medium traversed and, as bone has a higher effective atomic number (approximately 13) than soft tissue (approximately 7.5), the absorption in bone will be many times higher than in soft tissue, resulting in less X-ray transmission reaching the film through bone than soft tissue.

The above principle is again applied at these lower energies when attempting to achieve contrast between particular anatomical structures, e.g. bladder or kidney, and surrounding areas of soft tissue of similar atomic number. An artificial agent possessing a high atomic number, e.g. iodine ($Z = 53$) or barium ($Z = 56$), may be introduced into the body to outline these particular structures. Due to the differential absorption between the 'positive contrast agent' and the surrounding soft tissue, a varied intensity pattern of transmitted X-rays is produced, allowing visualisation of the required anatomy.

Air within the respiratory tract may be considered a negative contrast agent. It possesses a lower density than soft tissue, allowing production of a varied intensity pattern of transmitted X-rays. Air may also be artificially introduced as a negative contrast agent, in addition to positive contrast agents in 'double-contrast' studies such as barium enemas.

When using X-rays in the superficial and orthovoltage energy ranges, it is imperative to remember the dependence of the photoelectric process on the atomic number of the substance. When treating tumours lying directly beneath the bone, the preferential absorption in bone produces a reduced dose at the tumour site itself. When treating tumours arising in cartilaginous areas, e.g. the pinna of the ear, the cartilage may receive a greater dose than planned due to its higher atomic number and consequent preferential absorption, ultimately leading to cartilage necrosis. Electron therapy, which is independent of the atomic number of the material traversed, may be more appropriate in the management of tumours arising in these areas.

A further practical relevance is highlighted in the choice of materials used in the radiation protection of diagnostic imaging and radiation treatment rooms, and this is discussed later with the practical relevance of the other attenuation processes.

### Compton scattering

The interaction process of Compton scattering is also referred to as inelastic or modified scattering and may be compared with the previous description of elastic scattering. The Compton process involves a collision interaction between the incident photon and a 'free electron', resulting in both absorption (transfer of energy from the X-ray beam to the atoms of the attenuating medium) and scattering (path of the incident photon is altered).

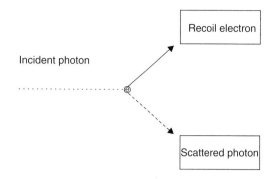

**Figure 4.4**   Compton scattering.

As the energy of the incident photon increases, the binding energy of the orbital electrons in the attenuating material becomes almost insignificant in comparison. The electron is no longer bound and is considered to be a 'free electron'. During a Compton scatter interaction the following steps occur:

- The incident photon collides with a free electron and transfers some of its energy to the free electron in the form of kinetic energy.
- The electron recoils from the collision, and is ejected at speed from the atom in either a forward or a side direction to travel through the attenuating material (Figure 4.4).
- The electron undergoes many electron–particle interactions, dissipating its kinetic energy before coming to rest.
- Radiation damage occurs as a result of electron–particle interactions.
- The incident photon continues but is deflected from its original path (Figure 4.4), and possesses less energy as it has transferred an amount to the electron.
- The scattered photon has a reduced frequency and increased wavelength compared with the incident photon.

Given that the total energy in a system must remain constant, it follows that the energy of the electron plus that of the scattered photon must be equal to the total energy of the incident photon. The electron and scattered photon therefore have an inverse relationship, i.e. if the electron recoils with a large kinetic energy then the scattered photon has an associated small amount of energy. This produces a spectrum of electron and scattered photon energies. Momentum is also conserved in this collision interaction by the electron removing some of the momentum of the incoming photon.

It follows therefore that the energy and the angles of travel of the recoil electron and the scattered photon are interconnected by this need for conservation of energy and momentum. In a situation of maximum energy transfer, i.e. a direct hit, the electron is ejected in the direction of travel of the incident photon whereas the scattered photon is deflected through 180°. Conversely, in a situation of minimum energy transfer, the electron recoils at an angle of 90° to the original direction of travel of the incident photon with minimal scattering of the photon. Most collisions lie somewhere between these two extremes.

It is known that incident photons of low energy lose only a small amount of energy on collision and therefore the electron travels through the medium with low kinetic energy whereas the amount of scattered radiation is high. This is in comparison to interactions involving incident photons of high energy where a larger energy transfer ensues, enabling the ejection of an electron possessing a higher kinetic energy. As an adjunct to this, it is important to note that less scattered radiation occurs in interactions involving higher energy X-rays.

In practice, low energy photons are scattered equally in all directions whereas high-energy photons are primarily scattered in a forward direction. In addition to the effects of differing electron ranges for orthovoltage and megavoltage X-ray beams (see below), this occurrence contributes to a difference in the position of the maximum dose for the respective X-ray beams. Comparison of the isodose curves shows that the orthovoltage beam dose is maximum at the surface of the attenuator, and at a point at a depth below the surface of the attenuator (dependent on the actual beam energy) for a megavoltage beam. This is known as the 'build-up region'. The 'back scatter' produced by Compton interaction at orthovoltage energies contributes significantly to the dose at the surface of the attenuator, reaching 50% at its maximum contribution. Thereafter the amount of back scatter decreases as the energy of the primary beam increases, because there is a reduction in the amount of scatter produced and more photons are scattered in the forward direction. At mega-voltage energies there is less scattered radiation outside the beam edge and less variation of central axis dose with field size, because the scatter is mainly in the forward direction and its contribution reduced.

This may again be observed through comparison of isodose curves for orthovoltage and megavoltage beams. The isodose curves for orthovoltage are more rounded due to the higher probability of scatter being produced at large angles at these lower energies. Indeed, the scatter contribution at these energies causes the 10% and 20% isodose curves to lie outside the geometrical edge of the beam (see Chapter 10).

The partial mass attenuation coefficient for Compton scatter decreases with energy approximately inversely proportional to the $keV^3$. However, the relative importance of Compton scatter in the interactional processes increases with increasing energy due to the partial mass attenuation coefficient for the photoelectric process being more dramatically dependent on the beam energy, e.g. inversely proportional to $keV^3$. It is dependent on both the physical density and the electron density of the medium traversed but is independent of the atomic number because the interaction process only involves 'free electrons'.

## Practical relevance of Compton scatter to radiotherapy

When employing custom-made blocks to irradiate tissue in an irregularly shaped field or to shield particular structures, it is important to acknowledge that the area directly beneath the shielding block will still receive some dose due to partial transmission through the block and, more importantly, due to the contribution of scatter from tissues outside the shielded area. This increases when the shielded area is central to the path of the beam. In addition, large amounts of shielding may actually reduce the expected scatter component to those tissues that require irradiation. In these instances a revised equivalent square is vital for accurate dose calculations.

Without digital enhancement, verification portal radiographs taken at megavoltage energies exhibit a poor contrast ratio between bone and soft tissue compared with those taken using kilovoltage X-rays. At megavoltage energies, the image is produced as a result of differential absorption due to Compton scatter. Unlike the photoelectric interaction, the partial mass attenuation coefficient for Compton scatter is independent of atomic number and, therefore, there is very little difference in absorption between bone and soft tissue. However, the difference in actual densities of structures in the path of the X-ray beam contributes to the image produced. For example, areas containing air (density $0.3 \, g \, cm^{-3}$) attenuate the beam less than soft tissue (density $1.0 \, g \, cm^{-3}$) or bone (density $1.8 \, g \, cm^{-3}$), therefore allowing more X-rays to be transmitted to the film. In addition, any differences in electron density enhance this effect, e.g. hydrogen contains twofold the average value for electron density and, as soft tissue contains a high proportion of hydrogen, the Compton effect is often greater.

A consideration when using megavoltage X-rays to treat target volumes in the thoracic region is the increased transmission through lung as a result of the decreased attenuation in air caused by the lower density. The soft tissues beyond the lung subsequently receive a greater dose than is initially expected and an inhomogeneity factor is usually used in the planning process to account for this. The presence of malignant lung tissue further complicates the planning process because the density can be considered similar to that of soft tissue and not of air. However, this complexity is not usually taken into account when planning radical radiation treatment to lung tumours due to the inherent difficulties in accurately localising and immobilising all malignant tissue.

A further practical relevance is again highlighted in the choice of materials used in the radiation protection of imaging and treatment rooms (see below).

## Pair production

Pair production can be considered a two-stage process, although it will become evident that the title is gained from the first stage of the process, which results in the production of two particles. This interaction process provides an excellent example of Einstein's theory of the equivalence and transposition of mass ($m$) and energy ($E$) as quantitatively represented by the equation:

$$E = mc^2$$

where $c$ = velocity of light ($m\,s^{-1}$).

### Stage 1: creation of mass from energy
- The protons in the nucleus of the atoms of the attenuating medium carry a positive charge, resulting in an electric field around the nucleus.
- A high-energy incident photon passes close to the nucleus of an atom in the attenuating medium and interacts with the electric field.
- The incident photon spontaneously 'disappears', transposing all its associated energy in the formation of two particles, each having a mass equal to that of an electron but carrying opposite negative and positive charges. These particles are usually referred to as a *negatron* (−) and a *positron* (+) (Figure 4.5).

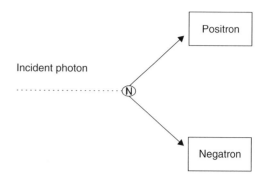

**Figure 4.5** Pair production stage 1: creation of mass from energy.

- The total charge in the interaction therefore remains at zero.
- The positron and negatron move through the attenuating medium.

This is an illustration of the creation of matter from energy. By substituting the mass of an electron ($9.1 \times 10^{-31}\,kg$) and the value for the velocity of light ($3 \times 10^8\,m\,s^{-1}$) into Einstein's equation, and using the conversion of $1.6 \times 10^{-19}\,J$, being equivalent to $1\,eV$, it is calculated that the energy equivalent to the rest mass of one electron is $0.511\,MeV$. As previously stated, during this first stage of the attenuation process, two 'electron' particles are produced, the negatron and positron, and therefore a threshold value for this stage to occur exists and must exceed the rest masses of both particles, i.e. $1.022\,MeV$. Thus, the pair production process is relevant only at megavoltage energies above $1.022\,MeV$.

Excess energy of the incident photon above the threshold value of $1.022\,MeV$ is divided between the negatron and positron as kinetic energy. This may or may not be divided in equal amounts between the two particles, resulting in the production of a possible range of particle energies. The particles are gradually brought to rest as they pass through the attenuating material, causing particle interactions as their kinetic energy is dissipated in the medium.

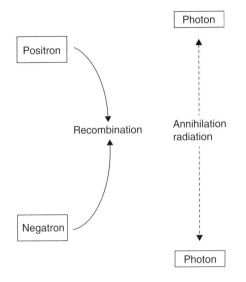

**Figure 4.6** Pair production stage 2: creation of energy from mass.

## Stage 2: creation of energy from mass
- The positron and negatron are brought to rest.
- The positron is very unstable and recombines with a negatron.
- The positron and negatron are annihilated and energy is created from mass according to Einstein's equation.
- Two photons, referred to as *annihilation radiation*, are produced travelling in opposite directions (Figure 4.6).
- Each photon has energy of 0.511 MeV.

The pair production process is of particular note in the interaction processes discussed in this chapter, because the probability of the process occurring actually increases with increasing incident photon energy once the threshold value of 1.022 MeV has been reached. As described earlier, the probability of the photoelectric process and Compton scatter occurring decreases with increasing incident photon energy.

The electric field of the nucleus of an atom is dependent on the number of protons contained within that nucleus. A higher number of protons, i.e. a higher atomic number, produce a greater magnitude of electric field with which the incident photon can interact. Therefore, it follows that the probability of pair production occurring is proportional to the atomic number of the attenuating material. A practical relevance of this is highlighted in the slight contrast between soft tissue and bone exhibited on a portal radiograph taken using X-rays interacting by the process of pair production.

In summary, attenuation of the X-ray beam by the process of pair production is possible only at megavoltage energies above the threshold value of 1.022 MeV. Even at the most common megavoltage energies used in radiotherapy (4–20 MeV), the predominant process is that of Compton scatter. Indeed, due to the dependence of pair production on the atomic number of the medium transversed by the X-ray beam, this process is of little relevance in soft tissue at the energies stated.

## Electron interactions and ranges

Common to each interaction process is the production of a high-speed electron that is able to travel through the medium and produce chemical and biological changes within the atoms. It is unable to pass directly through the medium and follows a tortuous path as a consequence of the induced repulsion caused by the electron cloud surrounding each nucleus and by the induced attraction caused by the positive nucleus. This therefore reduces the actual depth to which the electron is able to travel through the medium.

As it travels, the electron may interact with the atoms themselves causing excitation or ionisation, with an associated rise in temperature, depending on the amount of energy transferred to the atom. An 'excited' atom may be chemically reactive or may re-radiate the energy given to it by the photoelectron in the emission of ultraviolet or visible light. Ionisation, due to the ejection of an electron, may cause disruptive chemical changes within the atoms because it is the outer electrons that play a major role in the formation of chemical compounds. There will also be an associated emission of characteristic radiation.

If no chemical changes occur due to ionisation and excitation, recombination of the electron with a positive ion rapidly follows and characteristic radiation is emitted. In theory it would be possible for photons to be produced as a result of the electrons being decelerated by the proximity of the electric field of the nucleus, i.e. bremsstrahlung production, as described in Chapter 2, but this is unusual because soft tissue has a low atomic number. Bremsstrahlung production is dependent on the atomic number of the medium and therefore there is a greater possibility of this occurring in materials of higher atomic number.

Although it has been noted that a range of secondary electron energies is produced as a result of the various interaction processes, it is important to be able to indicate the average range of electrons produced by specific photon energies. In practice, this range increases dramatically from lower photon energies to megavoltage photon energies. Photons used in the orthovoltage range produce electrons with a range of <0.1 cm, insignificant when compared with the average range (in centimetres) for megavoltage energies (approximately one-quarter that of the photon energy [MV]). This partially explains the use of megavoltage X-rays for treatment of tumours at depth within the body. Lower-energy photons that produce electrons with an extremely small range are unable to penetrate deeply, making them suitable for treating superficial lesions only.

A further significant factor is that the electron interactions do not occur evenly throughout the range of the electron. A higher-energy electron produces fewer ionisations per unit length than an electron possessing lower energy. Therefore, the effects of electrons with a low energy and subsequent short range are seen close to their point of origin in comparison to the effects of high-energy electrons which are observed towards the end of the range when they are travelling

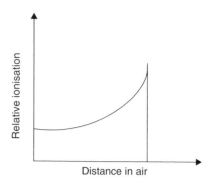

**Figure 4.7** Bragg ionisation effect.

more slowly. This is represented by the *Bragg ionisation effect* graph (Figure 4.7).

This phenomenon partially explains the dose build-up region and subsequent 'skin-sparing effect' seen with megavoltage energies, approximately equal to the range of the electrons. This is not seen for orthovoltage beams because the energy deposited by the short-range electrons occurs very close to the point of origin, e.g. close to the surface of the patient. In addition to this there is the significant effect of the back scatter mentioned previously.

## Further practical relevance of the interaction processes

Materials used in radiation protection measures must take into account the energies of the X-rays that they are designed to shield. In general, all radiation protection materials have a high atomic number, density and electron density, making them suitable to attenuate the beam efficiently by all the interaction processes discussed and, therefore, at all energies used in the radiotherapy department. Although lead is an ideal choice ($Z = 82$, density = 11 350 kg m$^{-3}$) at lower X-ray energies, it is considered impractical at megavoltage energies due to the large thickness required for adequate shielding. Solid concrete (density = 2350 kg m$^{-3}$), usefully used in the actual construction of rooms housing megavoltage equipment, offers a practical and less expensive alternative. The effectiveness of any barrier may be related to the alternative thickness of lead required to provide a similar degree of protection and is stated in millimetres of lead (Pb) equivalent, accompanied by the photon energy of the X-ray beam. A review of radiation protection materials can be found in Chapter 14.

Tissue-equivalent materials known as phantoms are used in radiotherapy when simulating the X-ray interaction in the human body for the purposes of radiation measurements. Phantom materials include water, Perspex and mix D (paraffin wax, polyethylene and other materials). All possess an atomic number, electron density and physical density similar to those of soft tissue and may represent the interaction of X-rays in the body by the photoelectric, Compton scatter and pair production processes. Other tissue equivalent materials known as bolus may used to fill tissue deficiencies such that the X-ray beam does not enter an oblique body surface. Materials such as paraffin wax or 'Lincolnshire bolus' fill any 'gaps' and similarly attenuate the X-ray beam and generate the same scatter radiation and dose distribution as that produced by soft tissue. Bolus material placed over the skin surface eliminates the skin sparing effect of megavoltage radiation treatment, ensuring that the maximum dose is at the skin surface. This may be useful when treating scar regions but does increase the skin reaction.

## Self-test questions

1. Define the term 'intensity' of an X-ray beam.
2. What is meant by the term 'attenuation'?
3. What is meant by the term 'absorption'?
4. What is meant by the term 'scattering'?
5. List two effects of transmission X-rays.
6. An attenuator of thickness $y$ is placed in the path of a homogeneous X-ray beam. The intensity is reduced by 50%. If an attenuator of $3y$ is used, what is the percentage reduction in intensity?
7. What are the SI units of (a) linear attenuation coefficient and (b) mass attenuation coefficient?
8. State the relationship between HVL and linear attenuation coefficient.
9. List the three main interaction processes that occur at radiotherapy energies.
10. At what energies does the process of photoelectric absorption occur?
11. Briefly summarise the photoelectric process.
12. What is the atomic number of (a) iodine and (b) barium?
13. How does the probability of photoelectric absorption occurring relate to the atomic number of the attenuating medium?
14. Where is the maximum dose to be found for an orthovoltage X-ray beam?
15. Which two particles undergo a collision interaction during the Compton process?
16. How does the probability of Compton scatter occurring relate to the atomic number of the attenuating medium?
17. What is the equation that represents Einstein's theory of equivalence and transposition of mass and energy?
18. At what energy does the pair production process become relevant?
19. Briefly summarise the pair production interaction.
20. List two materials used in radiation protection.

## Further reading

Bomford CK, Kunkler IH, Sherriff S. *Walter and Miller's Textbook of Radiotherapy*, 6th edn. Edinburgh: Churchill Livingstone, 2003.

Graham DT, Cloke P. *Principles of Radiological Physics*, 4th edn. Edinburgh: Churchill Livingstone, 2003.

Meredith WJ, Massey JB. *Fundamental Physics of Radiology*, 3rd edn. Chichester: John Wright & Sons, 1977.

Williams JR, Thwaites DI. *Radiotherapy Physics in Practice*, 2nd edn. Oxford: Oxford University Press, 2000.

## Chapter 5

# PRE-TREATMENT IMAGING

## Caroline Wright, Jonathan McConnell and Katheryn Churcher

### Aims and objectives

By the end of this chapter you should be able to:
- describe the principles of conventional and digital image production
- identify the key features of digital imaging systems and describe the applications in the pre-treatment process
- discuss the effect of kV and mAs on the appearance of an image
- describe how digital images are displayed and manipulated
- describe the physical principles and key features of CT, MRI, US and PET equipment
- describe the application of each modality in the pre-treatment process
- describe the basic principles of image fusion and registration.

## Introduction

This chapter presents an overview of pre-treatment imaging. It describes the physical principles of image formation for the range of imaging modalities used in radiotherapy pre-treatment imaging (conventional and digital radiography, computed tomography [CT], magnetic resonance imaging [MRI], ultrasonography [US] and positron emission tomography [PET]). An overview of the key features of the equipment and techniques used to acquire optimal images for each

of these modalities is outlined. The clinical application of each modality in the pre-treatment process is discussed with the associated advantages and disadvantages. A brief overview of how the modalities can be used independently and in combination with one another is presented together with considerations for future applications of the modalities.

## Production of a radiographic image

Although the properties and interaction of X-rays with matter remains the same, the technology associated with production of the images has changed significantly over recent decades. Conventional methods of imaging and image processing (film based systems) are becoming less prevalent in the clinical environment. It is important that these are considered in this chapter because they form the basis upon which current practice has developed. Before each of the contemporary pre-treatment imaging modalities is reviewed, it is necessary to take a 'step back' and look at the properties of X-rays and how they enable us to visualise anatomy.

## Properties of X-rays

X-rays were discovered in 1895 by Roentgen and they possess the properties that are noted in other forms of electromagnetic radiation. It is these properties that make X-rays unique in that they allow for 'non-invasive' visualisation of internal body structures.

### Fluorescence

This is one of the properties of X-rays. It occurs in certain chemical salts such as calcium tungstate or gadolinium oxybromide. Both these substances are used to create intensifying screens that were components of the radiographic process before the advent of digital imaging.

### The photographic effect

This is a unique process and is similar to that which occurs with light in the ordinary photographic negative. X-rays produce a *latent image* on photographic film that is revealed when processed. The direct effect of X-rays on film may also be employed in personnel dosimetry as a method of radiation monitoring. Most plain imaging is now generated electronically via a *photostimulable phosphor* (PSP) *imaging plate* which is held in a cassette or amorphous silicon phosphor or amorphous selenium photoconductor.

### Penetration

This occurs in substances that are opaque to visible light. During this process the X-rays are absorbed to a greater extent the further they travel through the tissue. The amount of absorption is dependent on the atomic number of the tissues as well as the energy of the X-ray photons. Diagnostic radiography relies upon processes that control the amount of radiation that is absorbed by the different tissues and organs in the body. This is dependent on the kilovoltage (kV) used to generate the X-ray beam.

### Ionisation and excitation

These occur in the atoms and molecules through which the X-rays traverse. It is the amount of ionisation produced by the X-rays that provides a basis for measuring exposure.

### Chemical changes

These occur when X-rays impart energy to substances. This is particularly important when considering the effect of ionising radiation on body tissues.

### Biological changes

These are observed after X-rays have imparted energy to cellular substances, resulting in some of these cells undergoing changes in their structure.

It is the combination of these X-ray effects that allows them to be used in imaging, the pre-treatment process and radiation treatment.

We now look at how X-ray images are produced in radiography. This process relates to methods of image production in the conventional radiotherapy simulator and also provides the basis for an understanding of contemporary image generation and visualisation.

Conventional radiographic imaging has been used for many years in the diagnosis and localisation of cancer. As technology has developed, conventional imaging has been largely superseded by computed and digital imaging. However, regardless of which system is used, the steps taken to acquire an image are similar, starting with X-ray production and resulting in the formation of a radiation map, which is converted into a visible image (Figure 5.1).

## Production of the X-ray beam

Photons/X-rays are produced by the X-ray tube (see Chapter 2) and have energies in the kilovoltage (kV) range (between 25 kV and 150 kV).

The method of X-ray production for the newer *computed radiography* (CR) and *digital radiography* (DR) techniques is consistent with conventional/plain film radiographic imaging. In recent years, it is the way in which the radiation map is generated, converted into the visible image, recorded and then displayed that has advanced.

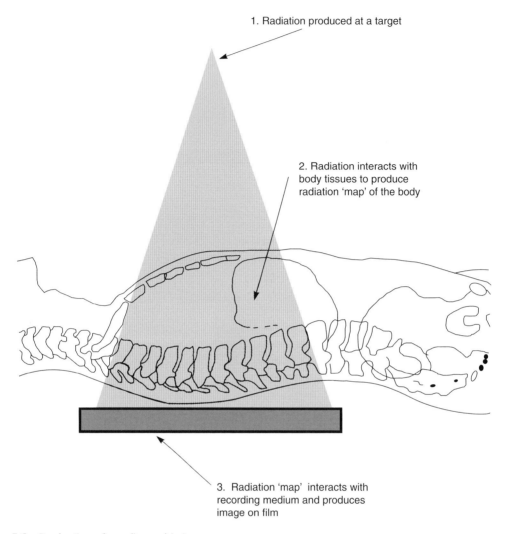

1. Radiation produced at a target

2. Radiation interacts with body tissues to produce radiation 'map' of the body

3. Radiation 'map' interacts with recording medium and produces image on film

**Figure 5.1** Production of a radiographic image.

## Interaction with tissues

Once X-rays have been produced and are directed towards the body they travel through the body tissues, being absorbed, scattered or transmitted (see Chapter 4). In addition, the X-rays will interact with the materials that the imaging machinery is made from (Figure 5.2). Absorption (*attenuation*) creates a variation in the X-ray pattern that emerges from the patient. This means that there is a reduction in the quantity of the beam and what is left has changed its energy or quality. The type and thickness of the tissue through which the beam passes determine the quantity and quality of the emerging beam. As might be expected, the portion of beam passing through a high-density material such as bone will be much reduced in quantity compared with radiation that has encountered only soft tissues such as fat. The emerging *photons* form what is known as a 'map' or 'shadow image'. Production of the map/shadow image was previously achieved using an *image capture device* (ICD) such as a film cassette. However, with the advent

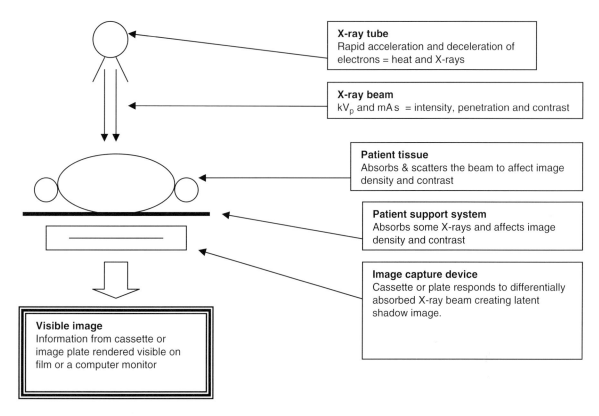

**X-ray tube**
Rapid acceleration and deceleration of electrons = heat and X-rays

**X-ray beam**
$kV_p$ and mAs = intensity, penetration and contrast

**Patient tissue**
Absorbs & scatters the beam to affect image density and contrast

**Patient support system**
Absorbs some X-rays and affects image density and contrast

**Image capture device**
Cassette or plate responds to differentially absorbed X-ray beam creating latent shadow image.

**Visible image**
Information from cassette or image plate rendered visible on film or a computer monitor

**Figure 5.2**  Passage of X-rays through the body to produce an image.

of CR and DR, the images are now produced on an image plate in a cassette or on a *direct digital radiography* (DDR) plate.

*Scattering* of the X-rays alters the beam direction and velocity, which in turn affects the energy being transmitted to the tissues. As a result, the number of X-rays emerging from the patient and reaching the ICD is reduced. This means that the beam is directed at other areas in the body that we do not need to image (a situation that we would particularly like to avoid from the point of view of protecting the patient from over-exposure to radiation). These scattered photons travel in a direction that will not add to the image. Instead, they will hit the ICD, resulting in a loss of contrast and creation of un-sharpness in the image. Scattering may take place more than once until all the energy that the X-ray

beam possesses is dissipated and the photon is absorbed. The X-ray beam that is directed at the patient is called the primary beam, whereas scattered radiation is termed secondary radiation.

## Image contrast and density

When producing images using conventional radiography, it is important that the quality and quantity of the radiation delivered to the patient are of the appropriate levels. This enables the emerging radiation to create a good image with respect to contrast and density.

The quantity of the beam is controlled by altering the milliampere seconds (mAs). This relates to the number of X-rays that are produced in a given time. The quality of the beam or 'penetrative power' is controlled by altering

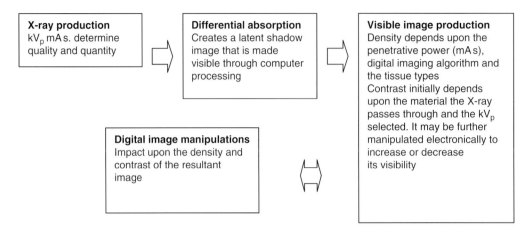

**Figure 5.3** Summary of X-ray interaction and contemporary image processing.

the kilovoltage in kV (voltage/potential differ-ence) that is applied across the X-ray tube. The X-ray beam energy (its penetrative power) is an important factor in terms of the contrast and density produced in an image. Figure 5.3 demonstrates the interaction process and contemporary image processing. The following descriptions and Figure 5.4a-e illustrate the effect of kV and mA s on an image.

In Figure 5.4a exposure factors were selected such that bone, fat and soft tissue organs are visualised on the image. (Precise exposure factors used are not quoted because they depend on the type of equipment being used. Instead, they are simply called 'standard exposure values'.) This means that the beam has some photons of sufficient energy to penetrate the thinner, less dense portions of bone, and thus reach the film and make the detail of 'spongy' bone visible. At the same time, the beam has sufficient low-energy photons, which are absorbed by fatty tissues, to make a difference to the amount of radiation passing through fat and air, enabling distinction between the two tissue types. In Figure 5.4a, the compact bone is the whitest shade, air is the darkest and there is a slight but distinctly visible difference between liver and kidney, although the tumour in the liver (represented by a circle) is the same shade as the liver and cannot be seen.

The grey scale ranges from white through to black, but the difference between adjacent grey levels is small, so the image contrast is not high.

In Figure 5.4b, the mA s remains the same but the kV has been raised above the 'standard' value. Therefore, the beam has more energy and more of it penetrates all tissues, increasing the amount of blackening overall. The fat is black similar to the air and therefore cannot be seen. The black cannot get any blacker in appearance (to the naked eye), but all the other shades become darker. The grey scale now ranges from pale grey to black, so the contrast is reduced. The differences in grey shades between the liver and kidney are much reduced and it is difficult to differentiate between them.

In Figure 5.4c, the mA s has been reduced below the 'standard' value in an attempt to compensate for the increase in kV. Although the bony tissue is now paler, the increased energy in the beam means that even the densest bone has been penetrated by some radiation, so there are no completely white areas. The black is still as black as can be resolved by the naked eye and the shades of grey in the image still range from pale grey to black. However, the palest grey is lighter than that seen in Figure 5.4b. Therefore, *contrast is increased* compared with Figure 5.4b but reduced compared with Figure 5.4a.

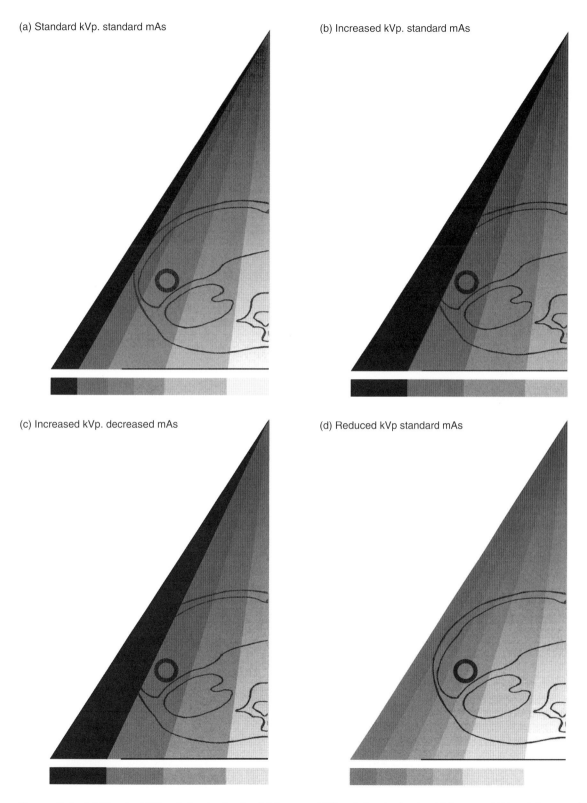

(a) Standard kVp. standard mAs

(b) Increased kVp. standard mAs

(c) Increased kVp. decreased mAs

(d) Reduced kVp standard mAs

**Figure 5.4** (a) Standard kV and standard mAs; (b) increased kV and standard mAs; (c) increased kV and decreased mAs; (d) reduced kV and standard mAs; (e) reduced kV and increased mAs.

(e) Reduced kVp increased mAs

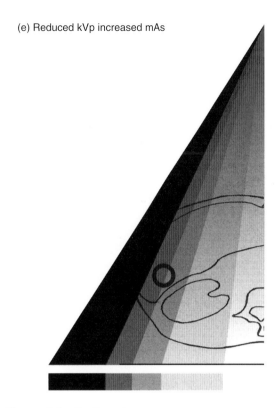

**Figure 5.4** Continued

In Figure 5.4d, the 'standard' value of mAs has been selected, but the kV is below the 'standard' value. There is insufficient penetration through bone to affect the film so it is completely white. There is less penetration through fat and air, so those areas are also paler than on the original image. The small differences between the tumour and liver tissue may *just* be visible. The grey scale ranges from white to dark grey so *contrast* is *reduced* compared with Figure 5.4a.

In Figure 5.4e, the mAs has been increased to compensate for the reduction in kV. As the energy of the beam is too low to penetrate the bone, there is still no effect on the film in that area, regardless of how much the mAs increases, so the bony areas remain white on the film. However, the beam still has enough energy to penetrate the fat/air and the quantity of the radiation can be increased to whatever is required to make the

film black in those areas. Thus, detail has been lost within the bone – it is all white – and the fat can no longer be seen because it is completely black similar to the air. The grey scale ranges from white to black as in Figure 5.4a, but the *contrast of adjacent tissues* has been increased and the boundary of liver, tumour and kidney can be seen clearly, so the overall *radiographic contrast* has been *increased*. In Figure 5.4e, the high contrast enables visualisation of liver pathology and so is helpful, but high contrast does not necessarily always equate with good contrast, e.g. high contrast would not allow the detection of a bony metastasis because the bony detail would not be seen. In fact, higher contrast usually means less overall information, although the narrower range of information available is usually visualised better due to the enhanced contrast between areas of similar tissue composition.

The following descriptions and accompanying diagrams in Table 5.1 compare the effect of kV and mAs on contrast and density with respect to plain film and DR.

**Contrast**
- If the X-ray beam energy is too low then all the energy will be absorbed by the patient and no photons will reach the imaging device. Thus, there will be no density differences to create contrast between adjacent body tissues.
- If the X-ray beam energy is too high and the mAs remains the same as for the previous examination, the image will be too dark with poor contrast.
- Where the beam energy is too great, but the mAs is correct, large amounts of scattering occur. This scatter reaches the imaging device background, causing fogging, which reduces the contrast differences rendered on the image produced and lowers the contrast between adjacent parts in the image. Secondary scatter grids that absorb photons not travelling in a direction perpendicular to the imaging device can improve this problem. The use of these

**Table 5.1** The impact of exposure factors and image rendition between film and digital

| Film-based responses | | |
| --- | --- | --- |
| **mAs too low but kV correct** | **mAs and kV correct** | **mAs too high but kV correct** |
| | | |

| Digital imaging-based responses | | |
| --- | --- | --- |
| **mAs too low but kV correct** | **mAs and kV correct** | **mAs too high but kV correct** |
| | | |
| Note the speckled appearance from insufficient signal to generate image. Here not enough mAs and possibly kV was employed | Good quality image as part penetrated with appropriate density | Although over-exposed on film the image algorithms in digital enable the image to be presented as acceptable image quality |

grids stops the scattered photons degrading the image. Thus, they do not reach the imaging device and therefore the contrast between adjacent tissues is enhanced.

It was stated earlier that the mAs of an X-ray beam (intensity or quantity) was important in terms of the density produced in the resultant image. We can consider this in a few ways using film as our image capture medium.

## Density

- If the mAs is too low but the kV is correct, the image produced is 'noisy' or 'light'. In this case it is difficult to differentiate between tissues of similar density on the image.
- If, however, the mAs and kV are correct, the image produced should have good density and contrast with optimal noise characteristics.
- If the mAs is too high but kV is correct, the image density will be too great. In digital images this is not a problem because the computer image can be manipulated, but the dose delivered to the patient remains excessive. In film-based radiography the image would be too dark, giving an indication that an excessive dose was used.

## Plain radiography image generation: conventional, computed and digital radiography systems

The radiation map that is produced represents the internal structure of the patient. At this stage the image is not yet visible. The map from the patient interacts with the recording system, which converts it to light. The more radiation reaching the recording system, the more light is produced and the greater the degree of blackening on the recording system. Thus, the radiation map of the body is translated into a visible monochrome (grey scale) image.

## Conventional image formation

In conventional film-based radiography the image is generated from exposed crystals of *silver halides*. These crystals are then 'processed' by electron donation from a developing liquid. This stage is 'stopped' by a 'fixing liquid' that prevents over development. The film is then washed and dried for storage. The size of the silver halide crystals determines the speed of the reaction. The films are seen to respond characteristically, which means that only part of their response is linear with exposure (equal amounts of radiation reaching the film causing equal amounts of density change (Figure 5.5). The predictability of exposure in conventional radiography is not as reliable in digital systems.

## Digital image formation

The detail that we see in the digital image is controlled by the size of the matrix used to generate the image. This can be explained by using the analogy of a 'chess board'. The squares seen within the image are termed 'picture elements' or *pixels*. Digital image detail is controlled by the number of pixels in the chess board. The greater the number of squares, the easier it is to visualise small objects. Thus, as matrices increase in size they can reveal more information (Table 5.2).

## Pixel manipulation

Each pixel in the matrix represents one 'colour'. This is usually a shade of grey between black and white. It is a numerical allocation using 'binary coding' to represent a shade of grey. This matches the amount of radiation hitting that point of the ICD. Magnification of the image using a digital system is achieved by 'stretching' the pixels on the screen. The term 'pixellated' is used when this pixel is large enough that its perimeter is visible. The more pixels in a matrix means that we can stretch the pixel to make smaller items visible but reduce the chance of creating a

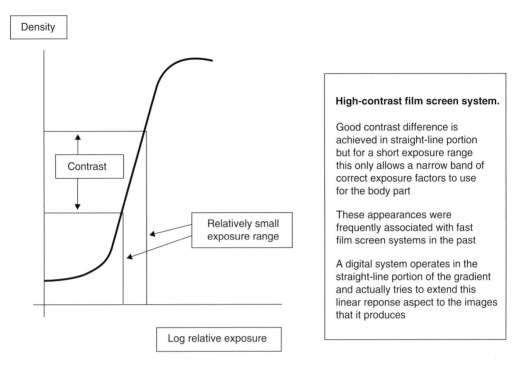

**Figure 5.5** A characteristic curve of response as seen in film-based systems.

pixellated image (Figure 5.6). The white to black spectrum is stretched across this grey scale and we can alter the image by raising or lowering the gradient to change contrast. We can also apply 'look-up tables' (LUTs) that enable us to see the useful greys and apply software filters that enhance the edges of objects. It is also possible to manipulate the brightness and contrast levels for easier visualisation, which allows a poor exposure to reveal information without re-exposing the patient.

## Computed and direct digital radiography image capture explained

Computed radiography (CR) was rapidly followed by the development of direct digital radiography (DDR) technology in the ability to produce the digital image. The key differences between CR and DR can be seen in Table 5.3. Essentially both systems capture the latent/ shadow image and project them onto a viewing monitor.

The excitation of the photostimulable phosphor (PSP) in CR releases retained electronic energy, which is matched with a monitor scanning sequence (raster) to project pixels of a given grey value and build a recognisable image. By comparison, DR uses either an amorphous silicon or selenium full-field detection photoconductor (see comparative diagrams for construction and operation – Table 5.3). Essentially CR must be sprayed with a laser to release the energy whereas the DR system downloads energy changes through electron-based switches created via the thin film transistor (TFT) that rests in close contact with the amorphous field detector.

## Visualising the image

In recent times there has been a transition in the way that images are viewed. In the past, images

**Table 5.2**   Matrix size

A simple shape is spread on a matrix

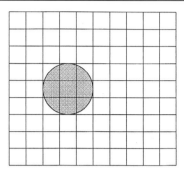

If we plot those squares, where the shape takes proportionately most of the area to generate information, we may represent the circle as above

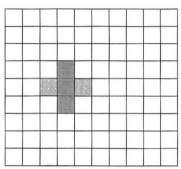

A larger matrix (smaller boxes/pixels) means more shape can be defined in the image. Far more squares would be required to give an anatomical object the amount of detail required. Film can do this best due to the small crystals of emulsion that are activated by light or X-rays that have been differentially absorbed and respond to the amount of radiation falling on them

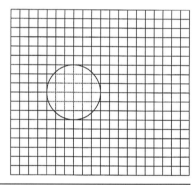

were produced as hard copies and viewed with light boxes. Today, electronic methods of image display are common using computers and monitors to create and display the images and compact disks for storage of the image data sets.

### The cathode ray tube

Most conventional imaging systems use cathode ray tube (CRT) monitors to display their images. The CRT is an electron gun, situated in an evac-uated glass tube, which sprays an accelerated electron beam, steered by a magnetic coil, onto a phosphor output. The effect of the electrons falling onto a portion of the screen causes fluo-rescence and a visible image to be generated. Colour monitors are more complex because these have three electron guns that spray electrons on to a red, blue or green phosphor; when combined together these generate the colour image. Although relatively inexpensive for static systems, these units tend to be large and heavy and have

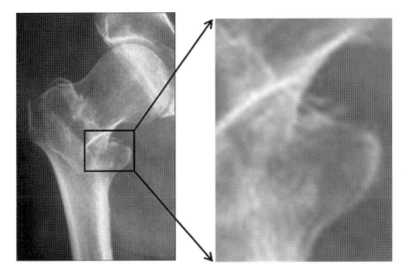

**Figure 5.6**   Pixel enlargement to aid visualisation of a small area.

**Table 5.3**   Construction of computed radiography (CR) and digital radiography (DR) image capture devices

| Computed radiography | Direct digital radiography |
|---|---|
| The plate | Amorphous selenium detector |

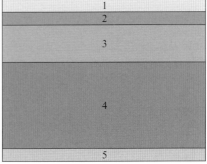

**Computed radiography:**

1 = protective overcoat
2 = photostimulable phosphor (PSP) layer
3 = adhesive layer
4 = antihalo (non reflective) layer
5 + 6 = support layers

**Direct digital radiography:**

1 = face electrode
2 = dielectric
3 = selenium semiconductor
4 = electronics and signal collecting system
5 = glass plate support

| Computed radiography | Direct digital radiography |
|---|---|
| Image plate drawn through 'reader' and sprayed with laser energy | X-rays that have been differentially absorbed fall onto selenium (or silicon) plate and convert this energy to an electrical signal used by the TFT |
| Energy is released by 'spraying' with laser light to enable light photons to be generated | A matrix of TFTs aligns with the selenium layer. Each TFT covers a width of about 0:15 mm, and so controls pixel number and size. Mammography plates can achieve a pixel size representing 0.08 mm |

**Table 5.3** Continued

| Computed radiography | Direct digital radiography |
|---|---|
| Light is directed to photomultiplier tube (PMT) by fibreoptics<br><br>Light is amplified as analogue signal through PMT | Although a thick layer of selenium enhances the electron capture and hence signal noise the selenium thickness is limited to about 1 mm as a larger voltage (over 10 kV) is needed to extract the electrons from the system |
| Signal matches TV raster and pixels to generate digital image | When electrons from the capture layer are released, these activate the TFTs |
| Image stored and manipulated via computer | TFT matrix positions are calculated via the computer to enable the image to be constructed from the signal |
| Image plate sprayed with light to clean old information<br><br>Plate is reinserted for use into cassette | Direct digital plates are therefore cleaner at detecting the signal and do not require the same number of interim stages seen in the CR plate |
| Representative diagram of PSP reader | Representative diagram of TFT digital plate |

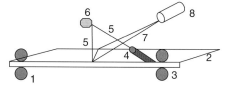

1 = transport roller    5 = path of laser light
2 = PSP plate    6 = rotating mirror – for laser path across PSP
3 = transport roller    7 = emitted light guided to PMT
4 = laser    8 = PMT (creates electrical signal from light)

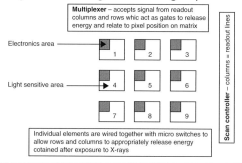

high energy consumption, resulting in heat generation that may be problematic.

## Flat screen systems

The earliest systems were termed 'gas plasma displays'. These were able to produce only monochrome outputs, essentially consisting of bubbles of neon gas trapped between two electrodes to act as a pixel surface. When the electrodes were turned on, the gas glowed to display the image.

## Liquid crystal displays

These work by making use of the change in shape of crystals when an electric current is passed. The change in shape allows light to pass through. Development has allowed this technology to permit fractional changes and so create a differential transmission of light; this allows shades of grey and colour to be demonstrated. There are two types of liquid crystal display (LCD) screen, namely passive and active.

*Passive screens* use a system that reflects a fluorescent light through the crystals to project the image out of the screen. As a monitor these suffer from a reduced brightness and a degree of lag in responding to the changing image, and also have a low viewing angle (similar to viewing a lap top screen). *Active screens* use a light-emitting diode (LED) approach to displaying an image. The light from these monitors is much brighter and, even though there are manufacturing issues, they rival CRTs by way of contrast and resolution and are closer by way of the viewing angle compared with 'normal' TV monitors.

## Screen resolution

The resolution of screens is described by the number of dots per inch or the *dot pitch* (DPI). Pitch is measured by the distance between successive colours, thus making monochrome screens inherently sharper. The monitor's resolution of a picture may be described by the number of pixels in the image matrix.

In summary, monitors are smaller, able to resolve better and have faster refresh rates and a wider ability to adjust to the viewer. They also generate less heat but require a special interface to enable a TV signal to be converted for use on this type of equipment.

## Electronic access to images

The use of monitors to view images is now commonplace in radiotherapy departments. Further advances in technology enable these images to be viewed remotely and transferred electronically to other remote centres. A system known as *picture archiving and communication system* (PACS) is used to do this. The PACS store all the patient data. It can then be electronically transferred around a hospital when requested by anyone who wishes to view images. For the transfer of images between hospitals, there needs to be standardisation of the image format. This is achieved using *digital imaging and communication in medicine* (DICOM – see Chapter 6). If hard copy images are still required they can be printed using a laser printer. The laser receives the electronic signal from PACS.

## Image storage

Apart from the ready access to images discussed in PACS, digital imaging systems can readily store many more images in a smaller space than the days of image libraries which took up significant amounts of space. The images can be stored on CD or DVD (digital versatile disk). Information is usually added to CDs/DVDs via the hard drive of the computer.

By comparison the computer hard drive uses magnetic material impregnated with polished aluminium to enable more information to be stored. Information stored to the hard drive is safe even when there is no power to the system, unlike random access memory (RAM), and loses the stored information only when you deliberately remove or change it. When material is stored to a disk this is logged and a code is provided to enable the machine to select information from the appropriate disk when information is requested from the system. Usually departments will employ a 'juke box' system whereby multiple large optical disks are stored together as a library. As data banks grow more 'juke boxes' are connected to the system to enable storage capacity to increase.

## Processing and manipulating the digital image

The use of digital images provides an opportunity to extract more information or correct for problems in the original data generated by the exposure. When an image is generated, a vast array of grey values is represented in the DR panel. This is known as the system 'fidelity'. It is a requirement of the system that this is as faithful as possible. This material is stored as *raw* data and forms the basis from which the image can be manipulated. Several approaches such as histogram analysis and exposure control may be adopted to achieve this, with the view to improving image rendition for the human viewer and to ensure maximum information is retrieved from the examination.

## Computed tomography

Computed tomography (CT) is an imaging modality that uses X-rays to produce image slices through selected planes of the body. This means that the images are cross-sectional in nature and may be oriented along any of the standard anatomical planes throughout the body. Through advanced computer technology, CT scanners can now reconstruct images in any direction. The use of CT in the pre-treatment process is currently the radiotherapy standard, with many radiotherapy departments having their own dedicated CT scanner as well as, or in place of, a conventional simulator. The data from CT scans can be transferred directly to radiotherapy planning systems, where the electron density information from the scan can be computed (using algorithms) and translated into dose distribution data. Anatomical data from the CT scan is used to produce *digitally reconstructed radiographs* (DRRs) which are used in treatment verification and image matching.

## The evolution of CT

Godfrey Hounsfield is credited with the invention of CT in 1972. The first scanner took several hours to collect the raw data, which was used to generate a single image slice. It took several days to reconstruct the image into the form that is so familiar to us today. Several types (generations) of scanner have been developed over the years with the X-ray beam and detector configurations being the elements which have changed in each new generation of scanner.

### First-generation CT scanners
These had a single (pencil) X-ray beam that was projected on to a single detector. It took the early scanners 20 minutes for each slice to be produced, but this eventually reduced to about 5 minutes.

### Second-generation CT scanners
Rather than using the pencil beam, these scanners used a fan beam and several detectors (Figure 5.7). This meant that a larger area could be imaged in a shorter amount of time. In the case of these machines, scan times were reduced to 20 seconds per slice. The advent of computer technology significantly improved the time that it took for images to be reconstructed.

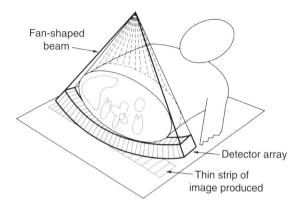

**Figure 5.7**  Fan beam of radiation in a CT scanner.

### Third-generation CT scanners and beyond
These scanners are the most common in use today where both the X-ray tube and the detector array rotate around a gantry. There are also *fourth-generation scanners* that have a fixed detector ring in which the tube rotates across with a fan beam and *fifth-generation scanners* that enable helical slices to be produced.

In the older scanners, the slices of the body that were imaged were thicker than those that can be achieved today. Slice thickness related to the detector type being used and, as a result, from a visualisation point of view, anatomical detail was limited. Technological developments in the positioning and array of detectors have enabled thinner slice thicknesses to be acquired. This enhances image capture from a resolution perspective (enhanced detail) and also speeds up the image acquisition process. This is of importance in planning where visualisation of surrounding anatomy is crucial to ensure that organs at risk are not irradiated and involved lymph nodes are included in the fields.

The speed of image acquisition is important in the localisation process because patients have to be placed in the treatment position for the duration of the scan and this is sometimes difficult for them to maintain for long periods of time. It would have been a challenge for patients to achieve this using the early scanners, as a

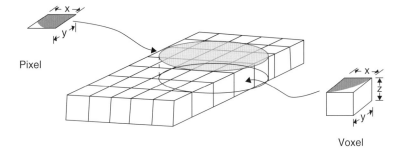

**Figure 5.8** Differences between a pixel and voxel in a CT image.

result of the extended time taken to acquire an image.

## Image formation

The images that are generated from third- and fourth-generation scanners take a standard digital format of picture elements or pixels. As each slice has a finite thickness, each pixel also represents a depth or thickness of image slice and this is termed a 'volume element' or *voxel* (Figure 5.8). Each voxel is projected as a grey shade on the monitor. The spatial resolution of the voxels varies according to the slice thickness and the number of them in an image matrix. This essentially means that the best representation of anatomical information gained from a patient is with a thin slice thickness and a greater number of voxels per image.

## Windowing

When a CT image is produced it has a range of grey shades that represent different tissue types and their respective densities. The actual scope of the grey shades acquired is far beyond the range of the human eye. To counteract this, a technique termed 'windowing' is used to manipulate the image. Windowing allows tissues to be represented across a range of grey values that are discernible to the human eye.

The grey scale matches what is known as the *hounsfield unit* (HU) or *CT number* for specific tissues. These are a set of nominal values that represent different materials. Water is given an HU or CT number of zero and the value for gas = −1000. The value for bone = +1000 and these values represent the transition from black through the various shades of grey to white (i.e. from air to water and then to bone). Thus, where there are a number of subtle differences between tissues, setting a window on a particular level allows the viewer to show those tissues within that range. This then enables the visualisation of soft tissues or delineation of the detail in a high-density object, such as bone, so that greater information is represented through high contrast resolution.

This property of CT images means that there is excellent contrast resolution. However, due to the limitations in slice thickness discussed earlier, CT images are also considered to have poor spatial resolution. Furthermore, the use of electronic reconstruction techniques means that the newest machines can reliably define structures to under 0.5 mm, which is particularly advantageous in radiotherapy planning.

## Scanner components

A CT scanner consists of a table and a gantry that houses an X-ray tube, a series of detectors with X-ray filters, and collimators between the source and detectors. A large computer is employed to reconstruct the image. Where required, a hard copy-imaging device will be available similar to the system described in the digital image section, although many departments are now opting for a PACS network. These systems have also allowed for the emergence of image fusion and co-registration, where the properties of all imaging modalities can be exploited for radiotherapy planning purposes. The CT image can be combined (fused) with that of MRI or even PET to enhance visualisation and assist in volume delineation during planning.

## Image display

### Window width and level

The windowing technique allows for the visualisation of tissues within a certain range on the grey scale. In CT, we are concerned with the window width (WW) and window level (WL). The WW is the range of hounsfield units displayed on a projected image. The width selects how many hounsfield units are displayed and the level selects which ones are presented. Wide windows (ranging between 400 and 2000) are used when tissues in the image vary greatly in density (e.g. the thorax where the parenchyma in the lungs has a low density and the vasculature of the region is of a much greater density). Narrow window widths (ranging between 50 and 400) are used when tissues of similar densities are to be displayed (e.g. when imaging the brain it is necessary to achieve greater differentiation between the tissues, because fewer HU numbers are assigned to each shade of grey). If we were to widen the window this would result in the suppression of 'noise' in the image, so increasing the window width can improve the image appearance for obese patients or, e.g. when metal artefacts are present such as dental fillings or prosthetic limbs. The disadvantage is, however, that the end result provides less discrimination between tissues that have similar densities.

In contrast, using a narrow window width can result in over-interpretation of tissues in certain areas, where the contrast of the 'noise' in the image can be enhanced and therefore produce unrealistic and confusing tissue edges and shading.

The WL is set in the mid-point for the range selected by WW. An example may be WW400 at a level of 100. This would mean 200 HU/CT numbers are displayed above and below that point, so that actual HU/CT values of −100 to +300 would be visible in the image. The optimal WW and WL vary enormously from one patient to another depending on the size and composition of the body. There is a large degree of variance in areas such as the abdomen, with less variance when imaging areas such as the brain; therefore there is no definitive WW and WL for all situations. Rather the WW and WL require some level of modification between individual patients. It is important also to note that different CT scanners can require different WW and WL settings in order to provide comparable images (Table 5.4 illustrates the effect of WW and WL on an image).

### Enlarging the image

In some cases it may be necessary to visualise large areas and therefore not possible to view all of the information clearly on the monitor at one time. In this case, one of two approaches can be taken to facilitate viewing:

1. Magnification: this effectively stretches the information from one point across the whole screen. Image clarity is, however, lost using this technique because the number of pixels covering the initial scan area is stretched across a larger image.
2. All of the scan information of a small area can be transferred as a whole into the matrix. This is possible because each voxel and subsequent pixel are made up of many thousands of data points, which contribute to the pixel at those coordinates in the image. Thus, a greater amount of information is available to spread across the 'new' pixels.

**Table 5.4** Window width and level in action

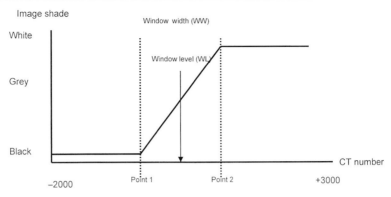

The level is the CT number that marks the centre of the window of a given width. Narrow windows give high contrast as CT numbers inside the window width are spread across the black-to-white continuum seen on the y axis of the graph. Conversely a wide window at a given level creates a shallow gradient. The interplay between level and widow enable a range of contrasts to be seen so more information is extracted from the image as seen below

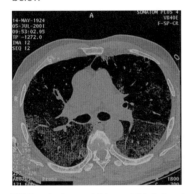

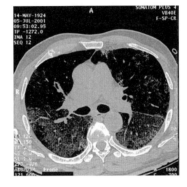

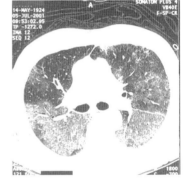

Wide window width and high level allows bone to be seen but does not give a good soft tissue image:
WW = 2950
WL = 1100

Mid-range window width and level gives good contrast (especially when contrast media is used in CT), so the mediastinum and vessels are clearly visible:
WW = 650
WL = −100

A lower level and narrow width will enable high contrasts to be seen. Where large tissue differences evident, e.g. lung alveoli and branching bronchi this is good:
WW = 750
WL = −700

## Other features of CT scanners

### Identifying the tissue composition of a given point

When we are uncertain about the content of a point within the image, we can apply a cursor that is a directed segment over the area of interest. This is called the *region of interest* (ROI). It allows us to obtain a finite measurement for that specific area so that definitive CT numbers can be established. In doing so, a clearer representation of the image is formulated so that we can be certain of the tissue type at a certain point.

It is important to note that, once a patient's name or scan sequence is assigned to a scan dataset, this information is fixed and cannot be changed. That said, it is possible to add labels and from the scout/pilot image the reference point can also be projected into the image frame. This means that the actual slice is apparent relative to a 'standard' radiographic lateral or anterio-posterior (AP) projection. Thus, the viewer can quickly orientate him- or herself with the exact position of the scan slice, start or end point in a sequence, or identify any angle set on the gantry to produce that image.

All CT scanners display a measurement scale on the image to allow the viewer to estimate the size of an object. A cursor can be overlaid to give definitive dimensions and even used to outline an object so that, with multiple slices, its volume can be estimated. However, 'system geometry' means that, as the distance from the centre of the gantry increases, the greater the distortion of an image, making measurements less accurate.

## CT image formation

### Pencil and fan beam CT

To understand how images are formed, the simplest type of CT scanner is considered (first-generation scanner). The construction of a first-generation scanner is such that it produces what is known as a pencil X-ray beam (Figure 5.9).

This is transmitted through the patient towards a single detector. The X-ray tube and detector move transversely over the patient and the amount of X-ray energy transmitted through the patient changes according to the tissues that it crosses. This sideways movement is called *translation* and the beam energy change is termed its 'profile'. So, an image is formed by a series of translations in line with rotations of the X-ray tube for a particular view. This is known as a *translate–rotate sequence*. The gantry then rotates through 1° and the process begins again for at least 180° to create a series of views that are reconstructed into a CT slice. This would take 4–6 minutes to generate the raw data for reconstruction into an image.

The speed of this process was increased in second-generation scanners which housed an array of several detectors parallel to the beam (Figure 5.10). With these scanners, as the number of detectors increases, the time taken to translate across the patient is reduced. In these scanners the pencil beam is replaced by a fanned X-ray beam. With the use of a fanned beam, the rotation of the X-ray tube and detectors is in larger increments (approximately 3–5° per translate–rotate sequence) which reduces the scan time to between 20 seconds and 3.5 minutes per slice.

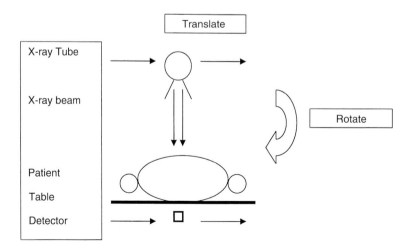

**Figure 5.9**  The pencil beam and translate–rotate system of first-generation scanners.

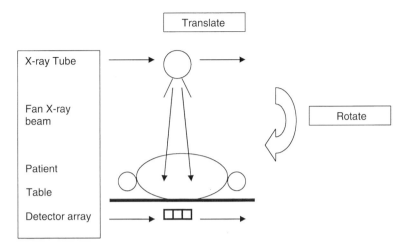

**Figure 5.10** Single slice detector array and fan beam configuration of translate: rotate system of second-generation scanners.

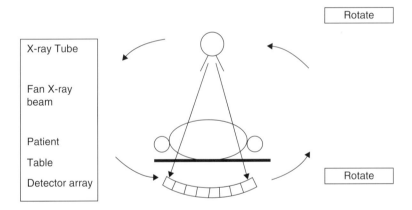

**Figure 5.11** The third-generation rotate–rotate system with a fan beam and curved array of detectors that both rotate around the patient.

Third-generation scanners have an arched bank of detectors opposite the X-ray tube. These rotate at the same time through a connection in the CT scanner gantry. This means that both the X-ray tube and detectors rotate around the patient during an exposure, which allows the scan data to be collected according to the speed at which the gantry system rotates (Figure 5.11). There is a drawback involving the cables in the gantry. As the system rotates, it would result in crossing of the cables, which means that the unit has to 'unwind' itself by performing each scan slice in an opposite direction. However, the system enables scans to be generated in just a few seconds per slice for data acquisition.

Fourth-generation scanners have a stationary ring of detectors in a complete ring around the patient. The X-ray tube rotates around the patient within the ring of detectors, so the distance from tube to skin surface is shorter and geometric un-sharpness potentially greater. As there are a greater number of detectors, the failure of one may have a less noticeable result on the image.

Spiral or helical scanners use slip rings, rather than cables, to provide the coupling between power supply and control/data transfer. These allow for continual rotation of the X-ray tube and detectors while the patient is moved through the beam. (In the previous types, the couplings were cables so the tube could rotate only so far before it had to 'unwind' in the opposite direction.) This technology allows the tube and detectors to rotate as the table moves continuously, to corkscrew through the area of interest and speed the whole acquisition process. Not only does helical scanning allow faster scanning, but also the dataset acquired relates to a large volume of tissue, giving greater reconstruction possibilities.

*Multi-slice CT* is the most recent development in CT scanning technology. It incorporates multiple rows of detectors that enable several slices to be imaged at the same time. It is possible for these detectors to be either the same size or a variety of sizes. It is the size of the detector that affects the slice thickness, so, for those scanners with detectors that are thin in width, the slice thickness can be increased by merging information from these. Ultimately, the beam width and number of detectors will control the time taken for a scan and the spatial resolution achievable.

## Image reconstruction

To construct an image it is necessary to have several views or projections (at $180°$ of rotation). Within each view, we obtain a series of values equivalent to total absorption of an X-ray beam along a path at a given angle relative to the rotation of the X-ray tube and detectors around an object. This value is the *ray sum* and we need as many ray sums as possible to enable the computer to create an image that represents all the structures inside the object. Reconstruction of this information into an image uses various algorithms. These are rules that produce a specific output from a given input. Once the algorithm

has reconstructed the image, it can be viewed and used for delineation of the tumour and organs at risk.

## Magnetic resonance imaging

The MR scan is similar to a CT scan in that it provides visualisation of the body in slices. It uses the magnetic properties of hydrogen atoms (the most commonly occurring element in the body, contained in water and fat) to generate images. Thus, a great advantage of this modality is that patients are not exposed to ionising radiations as is the case with plain radiography and CT. The use of MRI in the pre-treatment process is becoming increasingly prevalent. It is particularly valuable when the target volume includes a number of adjacent soft tissues that are of low and similar density to each other (such as those of the central nervous system, particularly the posterior fossa and brain stem, head and neck, abdomen or pelvis). MR images are also of use in the planning of brachytherapy (pelvis and thorax) and stereotactic treatments (brain).

### Physical principles of MRI

#### The spinning nucleus

It has already been established that hydrogen atoms are responsible for producing MR images. So, how does this occur? If one considers the structure of atomic nuclei, there are either isotopes of elements with an even number of protons and neutrons in the nucleus such as carbon ($^{12}C$) or oxygen ($^{16}O$) or those with an uneven number of protons and neutrons such as hydrogen ($^1H$) or sodium ($^{23}Na$). Both protons and neutrons have the ability to spin. When there are the same number of protons and neutrons in the nucleus, the spins cancel each other out, so the net effect is zero nuclear spin. A *net spin* therefore occurs only in isotopes that have uneven numbers of protons and neutrons. As hydrogen nuclei consist of one proton only, there is a net spin. As the

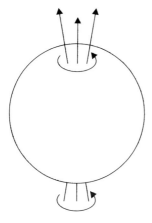

**Figure 5.12** Precession of hydrogen atoms about an axis.

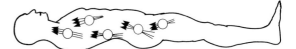

**Figure 5.13** Protons in longitudinal alignment within patient.

hydrogen nuclei spins it also wobbles a little (*precesses*) about its axis of spin, rather like a spinning top (Figure 5.12). The velocity of spin of the hydrogen nucleus always remains the same, as does the precessional frequency (number of rotations in a given period about the precessional axis) also termed the 'Lamor frequency'; however, the direction of axis of the spin can change. Just as with any charged particle that has an uneven number of protons and neutrons, the spin of the moving proton in hydrogen generates a magnetic field. So, how can we relate this to imaging of the human body?

## Magnetism in the body

The human body is composed of 98% water ($H_2O$) and as such it is rich in hydrogen atoms. Hydrogen atoms possess the simplest nucleus of all atoms and have the strongest magnetic signal of all the elements. This is because they have a single positive charge. Thus, hydrogen is the best atom to use in the generation of MR images, which are dependent on magnetic spin. Imagine that each proton in every hydrogen atom is like a small bar magnet that has a magnetic north pole and a magnetic south pole. The term 'spin magnet' is used to describe them because they are in constant motion (spin magnets have different

characteristics to bar magnets). Even though each of the individual protons is spinning and creating a magnetic field of its own, there is no net magnetisation in the body. This is because, in their 'normal' state, the axes of the protons are aligned randomly in different directions to result in the total magnetic effect being cancelled out. Therefore, rather than using the effect of individual protons spinning and creating their own magnetic fields in a given volume (voxel) of tissue, MRI utilises the total combined magnetic effect of the group of protons in the voxel to create an image.

## Introduction of the body into a magnetic field

The randomly aligned, spinning protons have the ability to alter their direction in the presence of a magnetic field. When the patient is placed in the magnetic field of the MR scanner, the protons align in one direction. This results in a small net magnetisation (paramagnetism) in the long axis of the patient (Figure 5.13). The precessing spin magnets emit radiofrequency (RF) waves/signals that are specific to each isotope of an element. This signal in the body is not as strong as it might be because the direction of field of each proton is slightly different due to its *precession*.

## Introduction of a radiofrequency pulse during magnetisation

If we want to change the orientation of the spin magnets (which are not truly unidirectional because of their non-synchronous precessions) when the hydrogen atoms are in their magnetised state, an RF pulse can be introduced. This RF pulse is introduced perpendicular to the long axis of the magnet and the patient so that it 'cuts through' the magnetic field. This results in an interruption of the magnetisation effect. If this RF pulse is the same *resonant frequency* (equivalent to the Lamor frequency) as the $^1$H protons, 42.6 MHz per tesla (SI unit of strength of magnetic flux density), they change direction. This change in direction occurs because they absorb the energy from the RF pulse. The effect of this is that the spin magnets flip through 90°, which in turn causes two distinct and separate effects:

1. Enough hydrogen protons flip through 90° to reduce the net magnetisation in the longitudinal direction to zero and to cause some magnetism to be established in a transverse direction.
2. The pulse that flips them through 90° has the effect of starting them all off from the same point of spin and for an instant (a few milliseconds) they *resonate*, i.e. they precess in synchrony (in phase) with each other. This causes the transverse magnetic signal to be relatively strong and a 'true' unidirectional field is created.

It is this process which allows the MR signal to be produced. Upon the introduction of a conductor (*the coil*) into the constantly changing magnetic field an electromagnetic effect is produced (refer to Faraday and Lenz laws). This means that a current of a specific voltage is created and runs through the coil. When the RF pulse ceases, the two effects also cease, in the following way:

1. The energised protons lose the energy that they had gained from the RF pulse and relax back to the 'more-or-less' longitudinal alignment. This causes the transverse component of the magnetism to decay. As a result, the longitudinal component of the magnetisation is re-established (Figure 5.14). The effect is exponential with time and the time constant for the return of the longitudinal magnetism is known as T1.

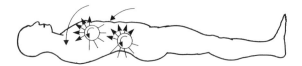

**Figure 5.14** Longitudinal alignment re-establishing.

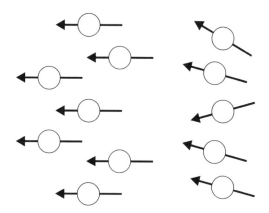

**Figure 5.15** Illustration of one group of protons in phase and one out of phase, showing perfectly versus imperfectly aligned magnetism.

2. The protons precessing in phase (Figure 5.15) experience interference from other protons in the vicinity (spin–spin interactions) and rapidly lose the synchronisation. This results in the *magnitude* of the transverse magnetic component rapidly decaying. At this point the orientation of the protons once again becomes more generalised within the patient (as they were before the RF pulse was applied). In a perfectly homogeneous magnetic field this is also exponential with time and the time constant is known as T2.

**Utilisation of T1 and T2 relaxation in scanning**
The term relaxation relates to the magnetic effect returning from a state of non-equilibrium to a state of equilibrium. As we have just discovered, the relaxation process has two components, which are exploited when scanning different tissues.

The recovery rate for realignment in the longitudinal direction (T1) occurs more slowly than the decay rate of the magnetic field created in the transverse direction (T2) (i.e. transverse magnetism is lost more rapidly than it takes for reinstatement of longitudinal magnetism). In the case of T1 relaxation this is exponential in that at the start of the process the longitudinal realignment occurs rapidly. However, as time progresses and the closer all the spin magnets get to the point of realignment, the longer it takes to reach the end point. In the case of T2, the decay of the transverse magnetisation is rapid at the start (when the RF pulse is removed) and it then slows down towards the point at which zero transverse magnetisation occurs. The amplitude of the voltage signal which is created as a result of electromagnetic induction in the coil depends on the T1 and T2 times. These times vary for different tissues for example T1 and T2 for fat is shorter compared with water (this will be further explained).

The variation in T1 times for different tissues is related to molecular motion. As molecules move, tiny magnetic fields are created in local field area (fluctuations of this local field in the range of the Lamor frequency have the strongest effect). The larger, slower moving molecules such as fat feel the 'pull' of these tiny magnetic fields more readily than water. Thus, their protons realign more rapidly. The relaxation times for T1 are in the order of seconds. White matter is the fastest to return to longitudinal alignment, grey matter being next and cerebral spinal fluid (CSF) taking the longest time. It is this difference in T1 times of tissues that affords the sharp contrast in MRI. For the purpose of radiotherapy imaging, it is the water content of tumours and different tissues that gives them different T1 times, which results in the difference in contrast and thus different appearance on MR images.

At the time of T2 relaxation, the spin magnets that were aligned and spinning in synchrony in the transverse direction begin to spin 'out of phase' with each other. They then revert back to their initial state, which was observed before the RF pulse (spinning individually). The flow of current in the coil is temporarily suspended for this short period of time and thus there is no MR signal. The T2 times are much faster than those of T1 and are in the order of tens of milliseconds. CSF has the longest relaxation time and white matter the shortest. It is the interaction of the 'spin–spin' between the protons and the process of the longitudinal relaxation that allows more rapid decay. The alteration in spin also changes the local field, which affects the precessional frequency. This means that the spin magnets are out of synchrony with each other. As each body tissue has a different T2 relaxation, these can be seen as MR image contrast.

### Pulsed RF to create an image

The image cannot be produced by the application of a single RF pulse, however. A series of pulses, known as a *pulse sequence*, is required. Pulse sequences used in clinical practice vary in sophistication, but two of the simplest are mentioned here.

A *saturation recovery sequence* consists of a series of 90° pulses and the time between pulses is known as the *repetition time* (TR). It has already been said that tissues have different T1 times. For the same TR, tissues with shorter T1 times will give larger signals than tissues with longer T1 times. If the TR is kept short (about 500 ms) relative to the T1 under investigation, there will be insufficient time for the longitudinal component of the magnetism to be re-established between pulses, and so fewer protons will be tipped through 90° by the next pulse. This is particularly so for tissues with a long T1 time and the TR effectively emphasises differences between the tissues with different T1s. These images are known as *T1-weighted images*. In a T1-weighted image, white matter has the brightest shade and CSF the darkest (Figure 5.16a). *A spin-echo sequence* may consist of a 90° RF pulse followed by a 180° RF pulse (Figure 5.17). As the protons relax back into the longitudinal alignment, and have begun to de-phase (lose

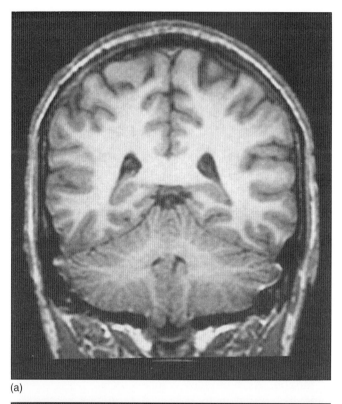

(a)

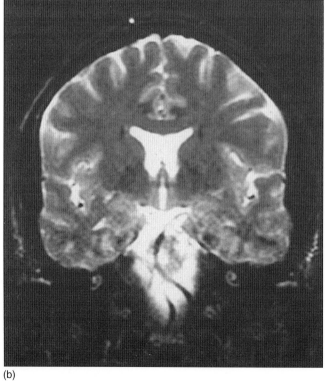

(b)

**Figure 5.16**   (a) T1- and (b) T2-weighted scans.

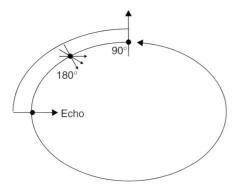

**Figure 5.17** Relaxation plane with protons after 90° and 180° pulse.

their synchronisation), they are flipped through 180°. Thus, they continue to precess in the same plane but in the opposite direction. This brings them into line again so that for another brief instant they precess in phase again, giving rise to a second strong signal, called an echo. The interval between the 90° and 180° pulses is called the *echo time* (TE). A series of 90° and 180° pulses constitute the pulse sequence, and the time between each *pair* of pulses is the TR. Again each tissue has its own unique TR due to this process. If both the TE and TR are kept relatively long, the differences between tissues with different T2 values are enhanced. This results in a T2-weighted image in which CSF appears as the brightest grey level on the image and white matter as the darkest (Figure 5.16b).

As there is a choice of relaxation processes, the patient contrast (differences between body tissues) is not fixed as it is in imaging using radiation. In addition, the pulse sequences can be varied enormously to suit the clinical requirements of an individual investigation. It is this flexibility that gives MRI a major advantage over other imaging modalities.

**Variation of body section imaged**

To be energised, protons must experience an RF pulse that is at their resonant frequency (42.6 MHz/T), and therefore the strength of the

magnetic field affects the frequency of the RF pulse required. If the magnetic field is graduated along its length, there will be only one specific section or 'slice' of the patient's body in which the protons will be energised by the pulse, so only that slice will be imaged. The field *gradient* can be varied to alter the slice imaged. Other field gradients are employed that affect the frequencies of the signals *across* the selected slice and the phases of signals vertically *along* the slice so that the signals from each voxel can be separately identified and represented in the final MR image.

We have already seen that with 'plain radiography' and CT soft tissue contrast is poor and this is where MRI excels. With MRI, superior soft tissue contrast and image resolution are seen and excellent quality images can be produced in any plane throughout the body (transverse, sagittal, coronal and oblique), whereas in the case of CT (which is dependent on tissue electron density), sagittal and coronal image planes have to be reconstructed from the series of axial slices. In the radiotherapy planning process MRI provides an excellent means of enhancing visualisation of the interfaces between adjacent tissues themselves and between tissues and tumours. The images also prove useful in gross tumour volume (GTV) margin delineation and in contouring organs at risk, particularly in the craniocaudal plane.

**Functional MRI**

Functional MRI, or MRI dependent blood oxygen level, allows for visualisation of blood flow in regions of the brain. When an area of the brain is active, the blood flow increases through the capillaries in order for oxygen and glucose to be deposited there and metabolised by the neurons. This increased metabolic activity and resultant oxygen uptake of the active neurones are markedly different to that of inactive neurones. The small magnetic difference between oxyhaemoglobin (which is diamagnetic) and deoxyhaemoglobin can be detected as changes in MR signals. It is this difference between magnetic effects of oxyhaemoglobin and deoxyhaemo-globin that allows for cortical activity to be captured. This technique is useful in visualising tumours of the CNS and the surrounding active brain tissue. It is anticipated that in the future many more uses of physiological and biochemical MRI imaging (see Chapter 15) will be developed.

A technique known as *diffusion-weighted MRI* (DW-MRI) is one of the newest procedures for tumour imaging. Its mechanism of action is related to the diffusion of water across cell membranes, which is different in normal and tumour cells. The most common use of DW-MRI is for the identification of brain tumours. However, it is also used to detect the response of brain tumours to radiotherapy and predict treatment outcome.

There are limitations with the use of MRI in the pre-treatment process, such as resource issues associated with the availability of scanners. There is also the suboptimal ability of MRI to image bone and high-density tissues/structures. This is because it does not depend on the electron density of tissues (as is the case with CT). This property of MRI results in challenges associated with achieving accurate dosimetry, because planning algorithms depend on the interface with bone and soft tissue to formulate isodose distributions in a target volume. In addition, MRI does not provide accurate visualisation of the external contour of the patient, which is again vital for planning purposes. For these reasons the scope of MRI as a sole imaging method for planning purposes is limited. It is therefore more likely for MRI to be used together with CT. This affords exploitation of the advantageous aspects of both imaging modalities, in accurate volume delineation, as a result of using MRI and superior dosimetric calculation resulting from the properties of CT. The process of using a combination of modalities (also including PET when necessary) is termed 'image fusion/registration' (explained later in the chapter).

## Safety

It is important to note the issues related to safety of patients and personnel when using MR scanners. The magnetic field of the MR scanner has to remain constant in order to ensure image accuracy. This means that patients and personnel should ensure they that they do not have any magnetic materials/objects within them (e.g. pacemakers). It is also necessary to ensure that any metallic objects such as hairpins and watches are not worn because this can result in serious injury and damage to the equipment. A rigorous routine should therefore be employed by staff to ensure that anyone entering the vicinity of the scanner conforms to the safety regulations. In the case of planning, the immobilisation devices used must be checked to ensure that they do not contain any magnetic substances.

## Ultrasonography

Ultrasonography uses high-frequency sound waves to produce an image. The frequencies used lie in the 1–20-MHz range, well beyond the range of normal human hearing. These sound waves are used to image body organs and thus provide information about the structure and function of tissues. This is a popular choice of imaging investigation because it is painless, non-invasive and does not have the hazards commonly associated with ionising radiation.

Ultrasonography has been used for a number of years in the diagnosis of cancer and is the modality of choice when differentiation between cystic/benign and malignant lesions is needed. One advantage of ultrasound (US) imaging over conventional radiography is that the internal structure of a lesion can be demonstrated. It is of particular use in imaging organs such as the uterus, ovary, prostate, liver, kidney and breast. In breast cancer it is used together with mammography to differentiate between cystic lesions, which are visualised as homogeneous fluid, and malignant lesions, which appear solid. US is also used in the staging of malignant disease and allows differential diagnosis of cervical node lymphadenopathy.

More recently US imaging has been employed in the pre-treatment process for localisation of the prostate gland, with follow-up daily US at every subsequent treatment for verification purposes. It has been used in the past with limited success for evaluating the size of the surgical cavity post-lumpectomy, to facilitate the decision whether to use electron boost dose or not it also plays a role in brachytherapy.

## Physical principles of US

### Vibrating particles

There are a number of different interactions that occur when sound waves come into contact with body tissues. In a similar way to light, US can be absorbed, reflected and refracted in a medium. The principal difference between US and light is that US waves and the resultant particle motion are propagated in the longitudinal direction. This is different to light particle motion (electromagnetic radiation), which is directed in the transverse direction, at right angles to light wave motion. Thus, sound waves travel through tissues by vibrating in the longitudinal direction. As a sound wave enters a tissue it starts a 'chain reaction' of vibrations as it travels through. As each particle vibrates it comes into contact with the next, which then starts to vibrate; this effect moves (propagates) through the tissue. As the tissues in the body differ, so do the acoustic properties of each tissue; it is this property that is exploited with US.

### The production of US images

When a US examination is undertaken, a uniquely designed hand-held probe (*transducer*) which houses a special crystal made of *piezoelectric material* (Figure 5.18) is placed next to the patient's skin. This probe has the ability to convert an electrical signal into ultrasonic energy

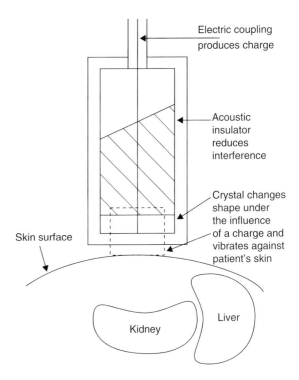

**Figure 5.18** Ultrasound probe.

which then propagates through tissues. As the waves of sound are travelling through the tissues an *echo effect* is generated from some of these interactions. The echo reflects the sound waves back in the direction from which they were initially generated towards the transducer. As well as generating the electrical pulse that converts to sound, the transducer can also convert the echo of sound that travels back through the tissues into electrical energy. It is possible to record the time between the initial pulse of the US and the resultant echo. This time indicates the distance between the transducer and the tissue (depth of the tissue in the body) that created the echo, which in turn can be used to generate an image.

### Piezoelectric crystals

The piezoelectric layer of *lead zirconate titanate* (PZT) crystals is located near the face of the transducer. These crystals have special properties in that when a voltage is applied to them (via an

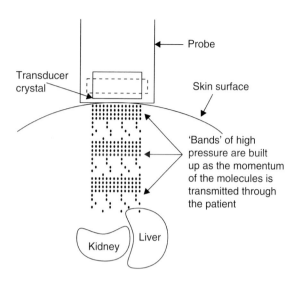

**Figure 5.19** Transmission of an ultrasound pulse through the patient.

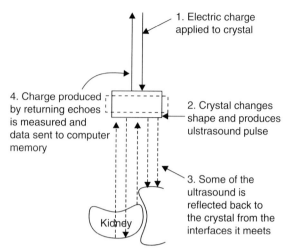

**Figure 5.20** Generation and detection of an ultrasound pulse.

electrical power source) they change shape. Depending on the polarity of the charge applied, the crystal either contracts or expands. If the current changes direction regularly (an alternating current is generated) the crystals contract and expand according to the changes in the direction of the applied current. The net effect of this contraction and expansion of the crystals is that the surface in contact with the patient effectively delivers a tiny 'punch', in the form of a mild vibration, to the patient's skin. This 'punch' causes the molecules in that area to be compressed, so there is a localised increase in pressure within the medium. The momentum of those molecules is passed on in the same way that a line of carriages run into the back of each other when one is hit by a shunting engine, so the pressure wave is transmitted though the patient (Figure 5.19).

### Transmission and reflection

When the wave strikes an interface between two types of tissue, some of the wave continues through the new medium (*transmission*) and some is reflected back towards the probe (*echo*) (Figure 5.20). The returning pressure wave impacts on the face of the piezoelectric crystal

and the mechanical force causes an electric charge to be produced on the surface. A short pulse of US is generated and the returning waves, or echoes, are detected and measured before the next pulse is applied. This is known as the *pulse-echo technique*. The transducer has an insulator (*backing block*) inside it that allows the vibrations to be absorbed in time for the returning echo to be detected.

### Acoustic impedance

The amount of sound which is either transmitted through the tissue or reflected back to the transducer depends on the properties of the two tissues that are adjacent to each other. The acoustic impedance (Z) of tissues is a function of the density of the tissues and the speed of sound within them. If there is a large difference in Z between two adjacent tissues more of the sound will be reflected rather than transmitted; thus, US does not provide good images of bone or air-filled spaces. Consider an interface of air and water; the density and Z of the water are greater than those of the air. Thus, most of the sound waves get reflected back to the transducer as an echo and only a few propagate through water and are transmitted. There is also a differential in the $Z$ of air and skin that provides a challenge when attempting to use US to produce images of the body because is necessary to have a small gap between the face of the transducer and the skin surface. This means that, when a sound wave is emitted from the crystals and directed towards the skin, most of the waves would be reflected back to the transducer without entering the body. To counter this effect, a medium that is of similar $Z$ to the crystal and the skin has to be introduced in order to 'bridge' the air gap. This is termed the 'coupling medium' which usually consists of a gel-like substance that is applied on the skin over the area that is to be scanned. Once this is applied to the skin, a continuous more homogeneous medium (crystal > gel > skin) is created through which the US wave can move.

### US echo and creation of the image

Different tissues reflect signals to different degrees, so strong signals denote one tissue type and weak signals another. The US image is an electronic map of the data generated from a series of returning echoes. These are displayed as different grey levels on the monitor, and thus the contrast is built up. The ultrasound wave travels at a known speed, so the time that it takes for an echo to be detected must indicate the distance that it has travelled (speed × time = distance). Therefore, the depth of the interface causing the beam to reflect back can be calculated. It is half the total distance because the pulse travels there and back, and its image is displayed in the correct spatial position. Thus far, the spatial information is only in one dimension. The beam can detect the anterior and posterior boundaries of, for example, the kidney, so its thickness can be determined and the depth of the kidney/liver boundary recognised. Spatial information in the second dimension is achieved in one of two ways:

1. A row of stationary crystals is used and the information from each crystal is processed to provide an image

2. The crystal is moved so that it scans a section of the patient.

### Types of ultrasound probe

There are two types of *transducer probe*: the *linear array probe* and the *mechanical movement probe*. The linear array is an example of the static type of probe. It has several hundred tiny crystals, and each crystal has its own electrical connection for the detection and measurement of the echo. The information from each crystal can be updated many times per second to give the appearance of movement. This is termed 'real-time' scanning. The crystal array may be a straight line (Figure 5.21a) or arranged in a curve (Figure 5.21b) to afford a wider field of view as the US waves diverge.

The mechanical movement transducer has a motor drive that causes the crystal either to oscillate (Figure 5.21c) or to rotate (Figure 5.21d). The returning echoes are processed in conjunction with information indicating the direction of the transducer at that instant, so the image is displayed in the correct spatial orientation.

## Doppler ultrasonography

Doppler ultrasonography uses the same principles as the pulse-echo technique, but the interface causing the reflection of the wave is moving, for example, in the case of red blood cells. The pulses are generated at a known frequency, but if the blood cell is moving away from the transducer, the returned frequency is lower than the frequency originally generated. The difference between them represents the *Doppler shift*. If, however, the blood cell is moving towards the transducer, the frequency of the returning echoes is higher. In either case, the change in frequency provides information about the speed of movement of the blood cells. This can be displayed in the following ways:

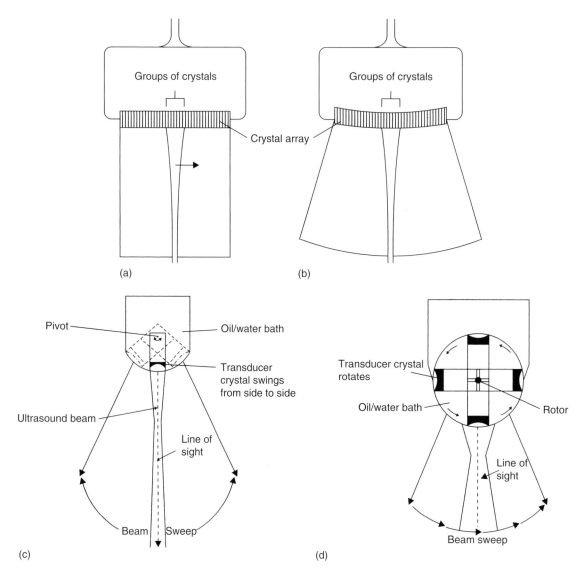

**Figure 5.21** Ultrasound probes: (a) Linear array probe; (b) curvilinear array probe; (c) oscillating probe; and (d) rotating probe.

- As a colour image, in which, for example, blood flowing towards the transducer is demonstrated in shades of red and blood flowing away from the transducer in shades of blue. The density of the colour indicates the speed of flow. This has the appearance of an angiogram but has the advantage of being noninvasive and does not require the administration of a contrast medium.

- As a spectral graph, in which the range of velocities of blood cells in a given area is displayed over a given period of time. The appearance of the graph will vary with the type of blood vessel imaged, e.g. the blood in an artery will experience short bursts of high velocity as the heart contracts, whereas the blood in a vein will move at a more constant speed (Figure 5.22).

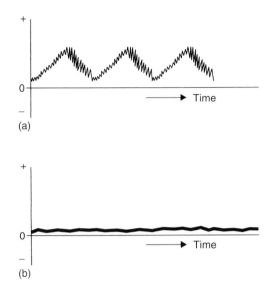

**Figure 5.22** Spectral Doppler for: (a) arterial blood, velocity changing with heart beat; (b) venous blood, constant velocity.

## Safety

Very high intensity US has been found to produce physical effects in tissue through which it passes. This higher intensity that is sometimes used for therapeutic purposes causes effects such as a temperature rise in the tissues and mechanical stress. It can also result in formation of tiny bubbles (cavitation), so complete safety cannot be assumed. However, the intensities and pressure levels employed in diagnostic US are constantly monitored for safety and these effects have not been observed at these power levels.

## Positron emission tomography

In contrast to CT, MRI and US, which provide anatomical imaging information, nuclear medicine investigations offer information about physiological function. *Positron emission tomography* (PET) is one such modality that offers great value in oncological management. PET is based on the emission of positrons from radioactive isotopes that have been administered to the patient (see

Chapter 15). Typically the radiopharmaceutical is combined with a metabolically active molecule, such as glucose, that is readily consumed by living cells. Neoplastic tissue can be discerned from healthy tissues in PET due to the unregulated growth of malignant cells and higher glucose consumption.

PET has valuable applications in the field of clinical oncology, offering the potential for earlier diagnosis and improved staging of primary disease, nodal involvement and the identification of distant metastases. In addition, the visualisation of active malignant tissues, often before any visible evidence of structural anatomical change, is possible.

### Positron emission

As the radiopharmaceutical undergoes decay, it emits a positron. The emitted positron will travel a short distance, often in the submillimetre range, before interacting with a negatively charged electron to produce two 511-keV annihilation photons that travel in opposite directions. It is these annihilation photon pairs that are detected by scintillation crystals housed within ring detectors of the PET scanner. As the two photons travel at almost 180° to each other, a photon pair is identified when two photons hit opposing detectors within the same time frame. It is then possible to identify the origin of the two photons, and thus the location of the emitted positron, by tracing a straight line of coincidence, often referred to as the line of response.

### Image reconstruction

Photon pairs recorded by the ring detectors can each be considered to represent a line in space, connecting two detectors along which the positron emission occurred (Figure 5.23). From each photon pair that is recorded, a map of metabolic activity may be generated. This process is similar to the method used in CT scanners, where scintillation crystals absorb the emitted photons and convert them to light. Each crystalline detector is connected to either a photomultiplier tube or

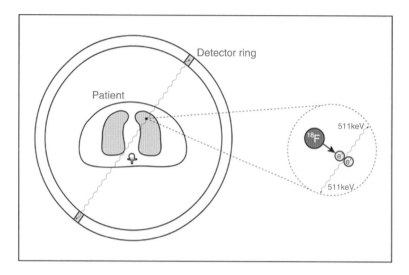

**Figure 5.23**  Registration of annihilation photon pairs from positron emission by a ring of scintillation detectors.

silicon avalanche photodiode (Si-APD), which creates and amplifies electrical signals in response to the light pulse received from the crystals. The amplitude of the electrical signal is proportional to the intensity of light detected, which in turn is proportional to the radiation absorbed by the crystal.

It should be noted that this technique is dependent upon the simultaneous or coincident detection of a photon pair, i.e. photons that are detected more than a few nanoseconds apart are assumed not to form a pair and are therefore disregarded. Image processing algorithms are then used to convert the electrical signals into tomographic images. This description has greatly simplified the image reconstruction process for ease of understanding. However, it should be understood that in practice considerable data processing is necessary to distinguish and correct for a variety of factors such as random photon detection, scatter, differences in tissue attenuation and detector dead time.

## Radiopharmaceutical used in PET

The radiopharmaceutical used for PET scanning depends on the tissue function being investigated.

However, the most commonly used radiopharmaceutical is *[¹⁸F] fluorodeoxyglucose* (FDG), a sugar that is readily taken up by metabolising cells. High FDG uptake measured with PET indicates a high level of metabolic activity within the cells of the tissues being imaged. Differing regions of metabolic activity will be displayed in the PET image by discrete regions of varying intensity, i.e. highly active regions will have a greater intensity compared with regions of low metabolic activity.

One disadvantage of PET is the lack of anatomical detail provided, making it difficult to correlate functional data to structural anatomy. However, this disadvantage has been addressed with the emergence of *hybrid imaging*, in which independent imaging modalities are combined into one unit assembly such as in the case of PET-CT, where a CT scanner is merged with a PET scanner. In these hybrid units the coordinate system is shared between both modalities and image acquisition can be undertaken in direct sequence. As the PET images correspond to the CT images, they can be reconstructed together to provide accurate co-registration of structural and functional data.

At the treatment planning stage, definition of the tumour and healthy tissue is based on CT and frequently supplemented with other imaging modalities such as MRI and/or PET. These other imaging modalities can be registered to the planning CT scan to enhance tumour definition and facilitate accurate and appropriate tumour delineation/contouring.

Accurate image registration is an important requirement for treatment planning; hence image-registration methods that align multimodality images are an inherent feature of most treatment planning systems. In most cases, multimodality image registration is challenging due to the varying patient position at each individual imaging stage, as well as differences in internal organ position due to organ motion. Hybrid PET-CT scanners minimise this inconsistency by acquiring imaging data in the same session, facilitating image fusion without any differences in patient position. In some circumstances it is possible to use the CT data from the hybrid unit instead of an additional planning scan. Considerations such as modification to the couch, installation of a laser alignment system and commissioning of the treatment planning system to accommodate the CT data may be required.

The use of FDG-PET for the diagnosis and localisation of malignancies has resulted in a large number of PET-CT scanners being installed over the last few years.[1] In particular, PET-CT studies have demonstrated enormous benefits in the imaging of lymphomas, head and neck, thorax and abdominal cancers, changing clinical management in around 30% of patients.[2] The ability to improve the accuracy of radiotherapy treatment planning has been significant. Tumour volumes and nodal disease are often more appropriately contoured on the basis of both anatomical and molecular/functional information compared with just anatomical information alone. In addition, this information can determine the amount of normal tissue included or excluded from planning target volumes.

The advent of new technological innovations is changing the world of radiotherapy. Develop-

ments in pre-treatment imaging modalities have made it possible for treatment planning to be more individualised and patient specific than ever before. This process is set to continue, with the introduction of alternative imaging methods that will further influence radiotherapy planning in the future such as functional magnetic resonance imaging (fMRI) and single photon emission computed tomography (SPECT).

## Image fusion/registration

Image registration is the process of superimposing two or more images from different imaging modalities, into one single image with just one coordinate $(x, y, z)$ system. The original image is often referred to as the 'reference image' and the second image as the 'target image'.

It is valuable in radiotherapy treatment planning because it allows the strengths of different imaging modalities to be exploited for further improvement of the accuracy of tumour volume and critical organ delineation. Specially designed computer algorithms are used for the registration of multimodality images, most working on the principle of mutual information recognition, i.e. the algorithm looks for points of similarity between the two images. To give an example, if attempting to fuse a CT planning scan (reference image) with that of an MR image (target image), the coordinates of the MR image data are distorted by the registration algorithm until the mutual information between it and the reference CT image are maximized.

Despite the high specificity of these registration algorithms, it is important to recognise that the amount of distortion applied to the target image in order to co-register the images may at times be inappropriate. Thus, any automatic registration process should always be manually verified for alignment accuracy before accepting the registration and proceeding to treatment planning.

## Self-test questions

1. List the seven effects that are generated by X-rays.
2. What would be the resultant effect if the penetrating power of an X-ray beam was too low?
3. Identify three different methods that are used to display digital images for viewing.
4. Describe what a CT number/hounsfield unit represents and identify the CT numbers for water, bone and gas.
5. Define the term ROI and describe its function.
6. Describe the construction of a third-generation CT scanner.
7. Describe the function of slip rings in CT scanners.
8. Why are hydrogen atoms the most appropriate for MRI?
9. Why does MRI have to be fused with CT for radiotherapy planning?
10. Which part of the body is fMRI used to image?
11. What special patient safety checks have to be undertaken before performing MRI?
12. In which direction do US waves and echoes travel?
13. In relation to US, what special characteristic does the material *lead zirconate titanate* exhibit?
14. Define the term 'acoustic impedance'.
15. Identify one investigation that utilises Doppler US.
16. Identify the particles that are involved in annihilation during the process of PET.
17. Name the radiopharmaceutical usually used in PET imaging.
18. How can neoplastic tissue be discerned from health tissue using PET?
19. Define the term 'image registration'.
20. Why is it necessary to manually check images that have been co-registered?

## References

1. Wood KA, Hoskin PJ, Saunders MI. Positron emission tomography in oncology: a review. *Clin Oncol* 2007; **19**: 237–55.
2. Gambhir SS, Czernin J, Schwimmer J, Silverman DH, Coleman RE, Phelps ME. A tabulated summary of the FDG PET literature. *J Nucl Med* 2001; **42**: 1S–93S.

## Further reading

Bushberg JT, Seibert JA, Leidholdt EM, Boone JM. *The Essential Physics of Medical Imaging*, 2nd edn. Philadelphia: Lippincott Williams & Wilkins, 2002: 1–15, 327–31.

Hedrick W. *Ultrasound Physics and Instrumentation*, 4th edn. St Louis, MO: Mosby, 2005.

Heggie JCP, Liddell NA, Maher KP. Computed tomography. In: *Applied Imaging Technology*, 4th edn. Melbourne: St Vincent's Hospital, 2001: 269–81.

Herzog H. Methods and applications of positron-based medical imaging. *Radiat Physics Chem* 2007; **76**: 337–42.

Kremkau F. *Diagnostic Ultrasound Principles and Instruments*, 7th edn. St Louis, MO: Elsevier Saunders, 2006.

Kuperman V. *Magnetic Resonance Imaging: Physical principles and applications*. San Diego, CA: Academic Press, 2000.

Oakley J, ed. *Digital Imaging: A primer for radiographers, radiologists and health care professionals*. London: Greenwich Medical Media, 2003.

Seeram E. Computed tomography. In: *Computed Tomography: Physical principles, clinical applications, and quality control*, 2nd edn. Philadelphia: WB Saunders, 2001: 2–19.

Sprawls P. Magnetic resonance image characteristics. In: *Magnetic Resonance Imaging*. Madison, CT: Medical Physics Publishing, 2000: 1–11.

## Chapter 6
# SIMULATION EQUIPMENT

Alan Needham

### Aims and objectives

The aim of this chapter is to provide an overview of the equipment employed within pre-treatment imaging.
    After studying this chapter the reader should:
- have a good understanding of the equipment available for pre-treatment imaging purposes and the use of DICOM and PACS systems
- be able to describe the design of the basic conventional radiotherapy simulator equipment
- have a good understanding of computed radiography, SIM-CT and CT simulation.

## Introduction

Recent technological development and the adoption of volumetric treatment planning has transformed the equipment required and processes employed within the pre-treatment section of the radiotherapy department. Nevertheless, in a period characterised by the declining use of conventional radiotherapy simulators and their replacement with equipment capable of acquiring CT data, the principles of localisation and verification remain at the core of the radiotherapy process. When selecting simulation equipment the user may choose from several modalities, each capable of fulfilling part or all of the localisation and verification function. These are:

- the conventional simulator
- the conventional simulator with CT acquisition capability (SIM-CT)
- the CT simulator (CT + laser system + virtual simulation application).

Before describing these options in detail, it is worthwhile considering factors that may inform selection of modality.

**The size of the department and simulator suite**
Decisions taken by a department replacing its sole simulator may differ from those where there is freedom to mix modalities. Taking an 'all or nothing' approach through removal of a conventional simulator may necessitate major changes in process and techniques to accommodate that choice.

**Technique complexity**
Departments undertaking or developing complex methods of treatment delivery, such as intensity-modulated radiotherapy (IMRT) or image-guided radiotherapy (IGRT), may derive no benefit from use of a conventional simulator for localisation, or even verification.

**Verification methods**
Use of radiographic film or electronic portal imaging device (EPID) images and verification through registration of two-dimensional (2D)

anatomy, requires high-resolution digitally reconstructed radiographs (DRRs) that may be produced from either conventional or CT simulation. However, should Cone Beam CT be available for three-dimensional (3D) verification at point of treatment delivery, the need for any simulator verification at all can be reduced.

### Workstream issues

Departments must consider where, when and by whom verification and isocentre marking will be performed before first fraction delivery. Since on-line verification can increase pressure on linac slots, it may be preferred to retain a pre-treatment unit to perform this function.

### Imaging medium

Despite the adoption of picture archiving and communication system (PACS) and filmless working, hard copy images are often required to supplement soft copy images viewed on a workstation or PC. Questions of how images will be viewed, stored and archived are fundamental to the selection of equipment and, in cases where traditional film format is required, use of computed radiography (CR) offers a chemical-free digital alternative.

## DICOM and the radiotherapy department

Whenever simulation devices are introduced, attention must be paid to the means by which its data, increasingly in digital format, is produced, manipulated, exchanged and stored, and to how the equipment will fit within an existing local network. This requires a basic understanding of the digital imaging and communication in medicine (DICOM) protocol, adopted as the universal standard for handling radiotherapy images and associated data.

Before DICOM, introduction of new equipment often required the writing of additional software to facilitate exchange of information with existing devices that utilised different data formats. Increased computing power and networking demands, however, created pressure for development of an interface standard that would address issues of connectivity between devices, and be reliable, robust, secure and at the same time accessible.[1] The result was the DICOM standard, jointly developed in the 1980s by the National Electronic Manufacturers' Association (NEMA) and the American College of Radiology (ACR). The standard is now in its third version (DICOM-3) and although unlikely to be superseded it remains under review and revision with new elements added and old ones retired each year. Through a system of rules the standard provides a level playing field for manufacturers, supporting imaging modalities as diverse as CR, CT, MR, nuclear medicine, ultrasonography and angiography.

The standard consists of 16 parts, although devices are required to conform to only those parts necessary to perform its assigned tasks. The 16 parts contained in the profile can be reviewed further in Oosterwijk.[2]

### DICOM functions

DICOM uses concepts common to object-oriented programming, defining information as *objects* and considering them in terms of the functions that can be performed on them (such as storing, moving, finding or printing them). These operations are described as *service classes* and, when defined for a device, inform the user what the device can and cannot do in relation to other devices. This information is contained within the *conformance statement* described below. Some commonly used examples of service classes include image storage, query/retrieve, print management and modality worklist (enabling retrieval of patient demographic information)

Each device can exist as either (or both) a *service class user* (SCU) or *a service class provider* (SCP) for a given service and object. DICOM always operates between an SCP and

SCU that together are known as a *service object pair* (SOP). *SOP classes* link a particular service class with a particular object and are assigned a unique identifier (UID) by DICOM. For DICOM communication to occur, the UIDs of both devices must exactly match.

## The DICOM conformance statement

When considering introducing an imaging or radiotherapy device the DICOM conformance statement supplied by the manufacturer is crucially important, because this document informs which parts of the standard are supported and for which modality or services. The statement is therefore used to assess whether two devices could transfer information, the device sending the data implementing as a service class user while that receiving implements as a service class provider.

## DICOM RT

This is an extension of the protocol handling the radiotherapy modality that has a working group overseeing its development. DICOM RT specifies five radiotherapy (RT) objects:

- RT image: concerned with DRRs, portal and simulator images.
- RT plan (RTP): contains geometric and dosimetric data for external beam RT and brachytherapy. An RTP is usually linked to an associated RT structure set.
- RT structure set (RTSS): contains information relating to patient anatomy, e.g. structures, markers and isocentres that are usually defined on treatment planning system (TPS) or VSim workstations.
- RT dose: concerned with dose data such as dose distributions, dose volume histograms, isodose curves and dose matrices.
- RT treatment record: contains data obtained from treatment sessions, historical records of the treatment.

A practical example demonstrates how DICOM might function within the RT process:

> When a patient is scanned a DICOM **CT image** study is produced
> The VSim application query/retrieves the image study
> Virtual simulation is performed, producing **RTSS**, **RTP** and DRRs as **RT image** objects
> The TPS query/retrieves the **CT image**, **RTSS** and **RTP** and calculates a dose plan. New **RTSS**, **RTP** and **RT images** may be produced at this stage
> The R&V query/retrieves the **RTP data**, initialising a treatment
> The EPID system creates its own **RT images** for verification
> During treatment **RT treatment records** are produced for each session

## Some DICOM issues

### The conformance statement
The DICOM conformance statement provides information concerning the ability of devices to establish connections and exchange data. It does not, however, guarantee that a device will be able to process and manipulate that data as required. A distinction must therefore be made between *DICOM connectivity* and *application operability*, which can be proved only through rigorous testing in a clinical setting. Purchasers of equipment must bear this in mind.

### Integration with PACS
Introduction of PACS, entailing central archiving and record sharing, presents specific difficulties for the radiotherapy process. As these systems were developed for radiology they offer limited support for handling the complex mix of DICOM RT images and associated objects. PACS models are designed to integrate primarily with *Radiology Information Systems* (RIS), which create and schedule patient orders for an image study. This order allocates a unique accession

number, sending messages to the PACS and imaging modalities that update and maintain the accuracy of patient demographic details. A problem arises because accession numbers are not a key field in the DICOM standard and have no meaning in an RT context. One solution is to introduce an independent DICOM RT archive, able to store and distribute data and that can assemble RT objects ready to send to the PACS (using HL7 messaging), allocating accession numbers in the process.

## HL7

Health Level 7 (HL7) aims to provide a standard interface for exchange of clinical and administrative data such as patient demographics and reports. It is used for communication between *hospital information systems* (HIS) and the RIS. HL7 ensures that textual information is encoded in a way that allows other computers to correctly read and decipher strings of text. Some parts of HL7 have been used as the basis for textual information storage in the DICOM standard.[1]

## The conventional simulator

The basic design of the conventional radiotherapy simulator, as an isocentrically mounted X-ray tube and detector, capable of mimicking the movements of a treatment unit, has remained unaltered for many years, consisting of the following elements:

- Gantry mounting
- Gantry head consisting of X-ray tube and collimation/diaphragm systems
- X-ray generator
- Imager
- Couch
- Additional attachments.

The gantry acts as mechanical support for opposing head and imager mechanisms. It must be firmly mounted with high levels of mechanical accuracy within the range of normal movements. Movements of the gantry, floor and collimator head must be accurate within 0.5° of the isocentre (Figure 6.1).

The gantry's motorised movements are controlled by thumbwheels and switches contained on a central remote console, or from additional hand pendants within the simulator room or attached to the couch mechanism. All movements should be available at variable speeds to enable precision in operation, with a maximum permissible gantry rotation time of 1 minute for a 360° rotation.

Many simulators allow movement of gantry, collimator and couch to preset positions as selected on the simulator workstation interface. Positions of all components are indicated by a combination of mechanical and digital readouts, visible in simulator room and control areas.

The ability to raise or lower the gantry head to accommodate a range of focus–axis distances (FADs) and to allow simulation at extended source to skin distances (SSDs) should be possible.

The simulator incorporates a range of safety features to prevent or reduce the impact of collisions during use. These include *motion enable bars* that prevent accidental movement, touch-guards sited on the gantry head, collimator, imager and base of gantry, *emergency stop* buttons throughout simulator and control areas and *anti-collision software* (described below).

### Gantry head

#### X-ray tube

The simulator tube (Figure 6.2) is mounted above the collimator within the gantry head and is supplied and controlled by the generator. The tube consists of:

- *The cathode*, a negative terminal comprised of filament, focusing cup, cathode support and connecting wires. When heated by an electric

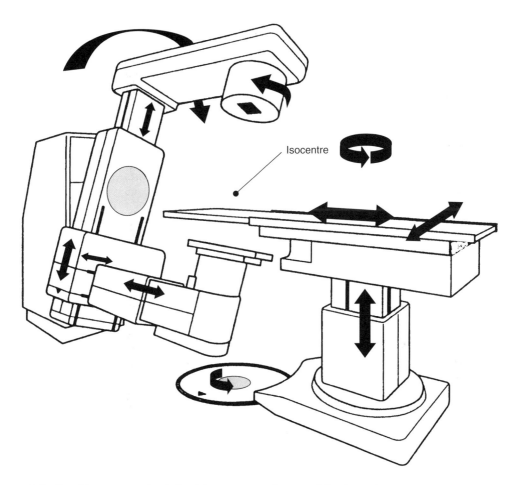

**Figure 6.1** Possible movements of simulator components around the isocentre.

current, electrons are produced by thermionic emission from a tungsten filament. This *filament* is composed of two spirals capable of producing two foci of electrons on the target. A *fine focus* (0.4–0.6 mm), the usual choice offering minimal geometric unsharpness, and a *broad focus* (0.8–1.2 mm), used when increased tube output is required. Electrons produced by the filament are focused on to the positively charged anode, consisting of a target mounted on a rotating anode disc.

• The *target* is manufactured from a 90% Tungsten/10% Rhenium alloy with a high melting point and high specific heat capacity to prevent vaporisation. Because of its high

atomic number it is efficient at X-ray production. Typically the anode has a heat storage capacity of 350 000–600 000 heat units (HU) and is able to rapidly dissipate heat at around 140 000 HU/min. The target is mounted at an angle of 11–14°, providing an effective focal spot smaller than actual focal spot size, improving heat dissipation and reducing beam penumbra.

• The *anode disc*, made from a tungsten track and molybdenum disc is connected through a *stem* to the induction motor. Similar to the target, this device must sustain temperatures in excess of 1000°C to prevent heat conduction damaging the motor and its bearings; it

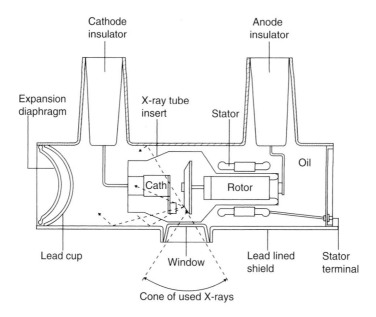

**Figure 6.2** A rotating anode X-ray tube insert and housing.

combines small cross-sectional area with poor thermal conductivity. The disc must rotate, without wobble at speeds of up to 10000 rpm (revolutions per minute).

- To prevent particle interference both anode and cathode are sealed within an evacuated heat resistant *borosilicate glass envelope* capable of expansion without breakage of the seal.
- A *tube casing*, lead lined to absorb leakage radiation, surrounds the glass insert with a protective layer of mineral oil, facilitating heat dissipation during operation. The casing contains an expansion diaphragm linked to a micro switch, which prevents further exposure until tube has cooled sufficiently.

*Collimation/diaphragm systems* The collimation systems limit beam output to a defined area and enable visualisation and marking of treatment fields. Motorised control is from either a pendant or control console and should be allowed at variable speed.

*Radiation field collimators* Radiation field collimators are also known as blades; they consist of independent lead leaves that limit the extent of the radiation field. The field light is produced by a halogen lamp reflected on to a radiolucent mirror of silvered plastic. It is important that this lamp can be changed without requiring realignment or calibration of the optical device.

*Field-defining wires* Treatment fields are defined by orthogonal sets of parallel thin wires capable of independent movement which are projected on to the patient and radiographic image. For increased accuracy these should be positioned as far from the focal spot as possible.

*Optical range finder* A projected scale, this intersects the beam central axis and identifies the SSD. This function may also be provided by mechanical front pointers attached to the gantry head.

The lower end of the collimator consists of a clear plastic sheet containing the reticule –

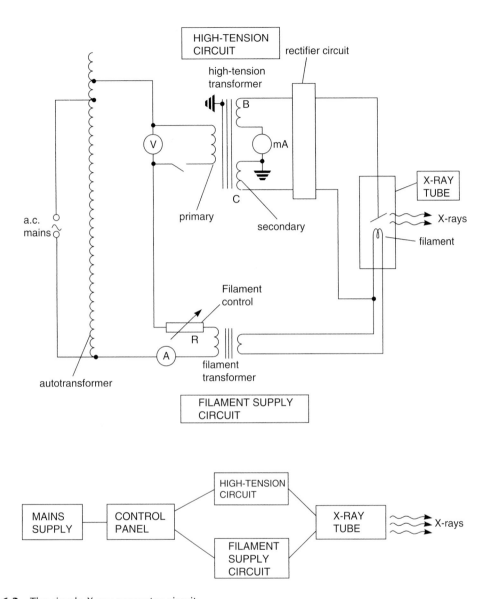

**Figure 6.3** The simple X-ray generator circuit.

intersecting black lines indicating beam central axis. An optional graticule inserted into the gantry head provides a magnifying scale within the radiographic image.

### X-ray generator

The X-ray generator controls the electrical current and potential difference across the tube and other elements of the simulator (Figure 6.3). It consists of a control panel, transformer assembly and timer circuit.

*Control panel* Allows operator to select values of $kV_p$, mA and exposure time. Exposure is a two-stage process, the first stage preparing the tube for exposure by heating the anode and rotating it to a speed of approximately 9000 rpm, whereas the second initiates X-ray exposure until terminated by the timer.

*Transformer assembly* An earthed metal box containing a *low-voltage transformer* which supplies the filament circuit and a *high-voltage transformer* supplying potential difference across the tube. The surrounding oil acts as an insulator, preventing electrical breakdown between components at the high voltages required.

The *filament circuit* regulates filament current, requiring 10 V of power supply and a small current of 3–5 A, provided by a step-down transformer. As filament heating must be precisely controlled, the circuit contains a number of stabilising components.

The *high-voltage circuit* contains an autotransformer acting as a $kV_p$ selector over a range of 40–150 $kV_p$ and a step-up transformer which increases voltage by a factor of 600, producing potential differences up to 150 $kV_p$ across the tube. This circuit contains $kV_p$ and mA meters

A *transformer* contains two wire coils. The first (primary circuit) connects to the mains supply and is insulated from the second (secondary circuit). The windings of each coil are made from turns of copper wire and it is the ratio of turns between primary and secondary circuit that determines whether the transformer steps voltage up or down. The output voltage relates to input through the following equation:

Voltage of secondary (output)/voltage of primary (input) = no. of turns of secondary/no. of turns of primary

The transformer core is composed from insulated layers of a metal alloy with a high inherent electrical resistance, designed to reduce eddy currents induced in the core, which waste energy.

Transformers make use of the laws of *electromagnetic induction* whereby:

- A change in magnetic flux linking with a conductor induces an electron-motivating force (EMF).
- EMF magnitude is proportional to the rate of change.
- The induced current in a conductor caused by a changing magnetic flux is opposed to the change that caused it.

Current flowing through the primary coil creates a magnetic field within the core, which consequently induces a current in the secondary. As this is an alternating current the increase and decrease in magnetic flux induce an alternating current in the second circuit.

Mains supply to the generator is through a three-phase alternating current, which is rectified into a cyclical current in constant direction, thereby ensuring that the cathode remains at negative potential. This uneven voltage wave form is further smoothed out by *capacitors*, providing a constant potential for X-ray production.

### Effects of tube voltage

A beams-penetrating power or *quality* is proportional to the kinetic energy of the electrons striking the target, resulting from applied tube kilovoltage. Similarly its *intensity*, measured as the rate of flow of photon energy through a unit area, is also proportional to this kinetic energy, since higher energy electrons interact with more target atoms. Increasing tube kilovoltage therefore affects both quality and intensity of a beam, although *image contrast* will decline due to an increase in Compton scattering at higher energies.

*Control of kV* is through an *autotransformer* positioned between mains input and the step-up transformer. Consisting of a single winding around a laminated core, the autotransformer works by the principle of self-induction. The AC mains current induces a magnetic flux around the core, which in turn induces an (equal) voltage within each transformer winding. By tapping off at various points along the transformer a varia-

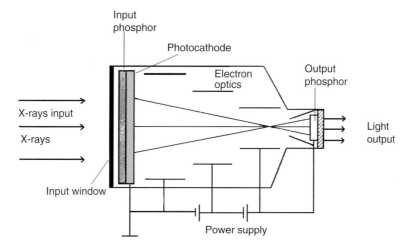

**Figure 6.4** Image intensifier tube design.

ble output voltage proportional to the number of windings can be selected. A $kV_p$ meter is therefore positioned between the two devices enabling selection from typically 40–150 $kV_p$ in 1-kV steps.

The *tube current*, measured as flow of electrons from filament to anode, requires precise control. Through a process known as saturation, whereby the rate at which electrons traverse the tube equals the rate at which they are supplied by the filament, current is made independent of tube kilovoltage and is controlled by filament temperature. A step-down transformer provides the low potential difference required, with mA controlled by resistors that raise or lower the voltage across the transformers primary windings. This may comprise a bank of resistors – allowing pre-set mA values to be applied or through a variable resistor as used during fluoroscopy.[3]

*Tube rating* measures the maximum load in terms of $kV_p$, mA and exposure time that may be applied to a tube and is a function of the heat energy produced during exposure. As temperatures above 3000 °C cause vaporisation of the anode, the generator incorporates hardware and software safety devices that prevent tube from overheating.

## Imaging system

Two imaging devices are available for the simulator.

### Image intensifier

The image intensifier (Figure 6.4), coupled with closed circuit television (CCTV), remains the traditional device for acquiring fluoroscopic images. It is an evacuated cylindrical device composed of several components:

- input screen
- photocathode
- focusing and accelerating electrodes
- output screen

After passing through an aluminium or titanium input window, X-rays strike the *input screen* made from a phosphor material such as caesium iodide. These collisions produce *scintillation* whereby electrons in the valence band of the phosphor are temporarily excited and moved to a higher energy level. Returning to their normal state, excess energy is released in the form of a light photon that is guided through the crystal until striking the adjoining *photocathode*.

The photocathode, an antimony/caesium alloy, absorbs these emitted light photons and through photoelectric effect converts them into photo-electrons that enter the evacuated tube. Within the tube these are accelerated and focused by an array of positively charged electrodes towards the smaller phosphor-coated output screen, producing light in an inverted image of the original X-ray pattern. Through acceleration and consequent production of a larger number of light photons at the output phosphor, image intensification occurs, although the image is reduced in size. This intensity increase may be 2500 times that of the original, although contrast and resolution are not inherently improved. Magnification of the image can be modified by varying the voltage across the tube.

As a result of the electronic focusing requirements the diameter of the input window is a determining factor in the physical height and size of the intensifier mechanism. As the assembly can restrict simulator movement a compromise between image and assembly size is often necessary.

To view the image produced on the output screen, image processing is required, traditionally achieved through CCTV linked to a TV monitor, although charge-coupled device cameras are currently employed.

### Charge-coupled devices

A charge-coupled device (CCD) is a light-sensitive integrated circuit that displays pixel data through storage of electric charge proportional to the intensity of the incident light. These devices have advantages in terms of geometrical accuracy, signal uniformity and size. The CCD can be coupled to the output screen through several methods (Figure 6.5). *Lens coupling* uses a lens and mirror system that has the advantage of separating the CCD from the imager (allowing easy replacement), but which provides a low light throughput due to levels of stray light within the system. *Fibreoptic coupling* increases light throughput to the CCD by around 60%, demon-

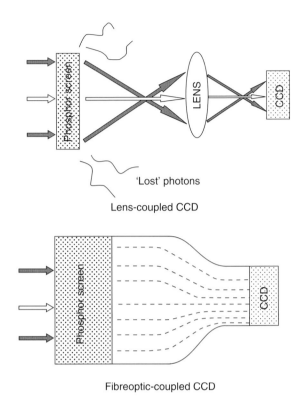

**Figure 6.5** Methods of CCD coupling.

strating better signal-to-noise ratio, but represents a permanent coupling within the imager.

### Conversion into a digital image

Modern simulators invariably convert the analogue output from the intensifier into a digital image capable of manipulation, transfer and storage. So that such images can be used for verification it is necessary that the geometric distortion of the image be corrected. Despite intensifier design reducing distortion through curved input and output phosphor screens (ensuring photoelectron paths of equal lengths), this is never entirely resolved. Therefore, when the fluoroscopic image is retained through an image hold facility, distortion correction and scaling are automatically applied by the system software.

Another problem relates to image size, limited to the physical dimensions of the input screen and therefore far smaller than a standard film format. Image processing software may therefore allow for two to four digital fluoroscopic images to be merged into a composite DRR of comparable size.

## Flat panel detector

The imager provided with modern simulators is the flat panel detector (FPD), a device capable of acquiring real time and radiographic images and which is also utilized for cone beam CT acquisition.

The flat panel detector consists of a 2D array of amorphous silica photodiodes, combined with thin film transistor switches (TFTs) and embedded electronic circuitry. They function through the ability of the photodiode to accumulate electric charge upon absorption of X-rays. This charge is retained within each photodiode (corresponding to a pixel), its flow regulated by the switch mechanism to provide an output used to construct a digital image.

There are two processes by which detectors can convert X-rays into a detectable charge. *Intrinsic* or *direct conversion* uses X-ray photons to create hole–electron pairs directly in the amorphous silicon diode. For practical reasons this is not used in medical detectors as the low X-ray absorption of silicon requires such panels to be 10–20 mm thick. The *indirect conversion* method is a two-step process whereby X-ray photons are first turned into visible light by a *scintillator* and the consequent light photons are themselves converted into charge within the photodiode. The ideal properties of a scintillator require high atomic number, good X-ray absorption and a yield of many light photons for each incoming X-ray photon. Two types of phosphor materials may be used as scintillators:[3]

- Rare earth oxysulphide scintillators use gadolinium or lanthanum, doped with terbium.

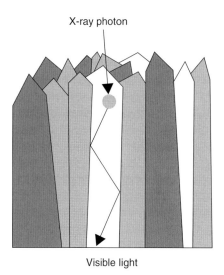

X-ray photon

Visible light

**Figure 6.6** Movement of light photon through a caesium iodide crystal.

These are granular compounds with grain size affecting resolution and brightness. A disadvantage is the high level of light scatter produced in the thick layers required to attenuate higher-energy X-rays.

- Caesium iodide scintillator: most radiotherapy detectors use crystalline caesium iodide (Figure 6.6), grown into fine needles of 5–10 μm diameter. These needles channel the light photons in a forward direction, reducing scatter and allowing thick layers to be used. Doping CsI with thallium means that light emitted from the scintillator is at the peak spectral sensitivity of amorphous silicon – a combination providing high *detective quantum efficiency* with minimum image degradation.

### Image production

As described, scintillators are compounds that absorb X-ray photons and convert them into light photons, a property exploited in X-ray cassettes by use of a screen adjacent to the film. Within the FPD the scintillator adjoins the array of amorphous silicon photodiodes to produce an electronic X-ray detector (Figure 6.7).

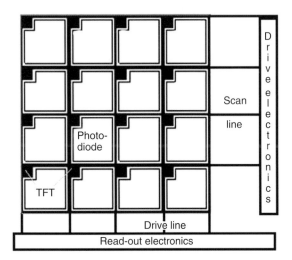

**Figure 6.7** Schematic design of a photodiode array.

Each individual photodiode (pixel) has a controlling TFT switch, maintained by a voltage applied through integrated electronic circuitry comprising horizontal and vertical row and data lines. Light photons reaching the photodiode reduce the charge stored within in proportion to the amount of light received. When the TFT switches, controlled by a *row line*, are switched on, the charge required to recharge each photodiode is read through the orthogonal *data lines* and assigned a digital value. The next (and subsequent) row lines are then activated and their readings measured. In this way a grey-scale value is assigned for each photodiode (pixel) and is used to construct an image over the whole panel.

The amount of time in which charge is allowed to accumulate before being discharged is known as the frame period and the frequency with which the process is repeated during continual exposure described as the frame rate per second (fps). Fluoroscopy using this method requires a frame rate of 15–30 fps and uses a reconstruction matrix in the order of 1024 × 768. If a larger matrix is required, the increase in data that must be processed necessitates a reduction in frame rate. Only half the time frame is used to read the pixels, the remaining half being used to irradiate the sensor. A pulsed irradiation source means that during the read-out phase the X-ray beam is not interfering with that part of the process.

Pixel size is determined by photodiode size, usually in the order of 130–200 μm. It is important that the photodiodes comprise as high a proportion of the panel as possible (known as fill factor), reducing the amount of light wasted. An FPD requires its low noise electronics to be positioned out of the path of direct beam.

The advantages of a flat panel detector in comparison with image intensifier are:

- Increased imaging size of up to 40 × 40 cm.
- Less bulky than the intensifier, which has large size relative to imaging area
- Sampling and pixel quantification carried out at point of detection and not the end of the imaging chain
- Use of amorphous silicon crystals increases resolution by reduction of optical scattering
- No distortions due to the spherical input surface and orientation with the earth's magnetic field
- Same panel may be used for CBCT.

## Computed radiography

If hard copy simulator images are required and a laser image printer unavailable, CR offers a digital alternative to chemically processed radiographs.

*CR cassettes* (Figure 6.8) have identical dimensions to traditional cassettes and are usable in any standard cassette holder; their design features include:[4]

- Thin aluminium sheet at rear of the cassette to absorb X-rays
- Felt sheet protecting the imaging plate and preventing static electricity build-up
- An *imaging plate* replacing film and screen, comprising several layers
- Protective plastic layer
- *Photostimulable phosphor*

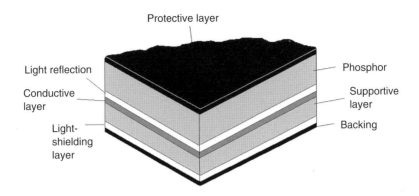

**Figure 6.8** Components of a CR phosphor plate.

- Reflective layer that sends light forward in the cassette
- Conductive layer to absorb static electricity
- Support layer for rigidity
- Backing layer to protect the back of the cassette.

To produce an image the patient is exposed using $kV_p$/mAs values similar to those employed for standard cassettes. The phosphor material within the plate consists of barium fluorohalide crystals doped with euphorium, which on exposure to X-rays is ionised. The electrons liberated are raised to the conduction band, travelling freely in this band until they become trapped in a metastable state with energy levels between valence and conductive levels. The number of electrons trapped in this manner are proportional to the X-ray absorption.

To read the latent image stored on the plate the cassette is fed into a CR reader and scanned by a narrow helium–neon laser beam. This laser stimulates the trapped electrons, raising them back up to the conduction band. An equal number of electrons consequently fall back to the valence band releasing energy in the process, in the form of visible blue or green light.

Using a filter to absorb the red light that initiated the excitation, the emitted light is detected and fed into a photomultiplier tube for conversion to an electrical signal. This signal is then digitised to produce an image matrix, with individual pixels allocated grey-scale values proportional to the light emitted from a corresponding dot on the plate.

When the cassette is read not all 'stored' electrons return to their lower energy state, so most systems have an erasure mode that floods the plate with light to remove remaining trapped electrons. This should be carried out periodically on any cassette not frequently used.

### Simulator couch

Whenever possible simulator couches should be of identical design and dimensions to the treatment units that they support. Invariably this means that they are produced from durable carbon fibre, with low transmission of <1.5 mm Al equivalent. Weight-bearing capacity should be 200–250 kg distributed evenly, although this capacity is reduced at the extremities. Stability of the couch when extended is essential for maintaining isocentre accuracy during simulation.

The couch should be capable of isocentric rotation of at least ±95°, with eccentric rotation independent of the isocentre to assist patient loading. A method of manual offload independent of power supply is advisable. Longitudinal, lateral and vertical couch movement is through local and remote control, operating at a range of speeds and sensitivity. A free float (non-motorised) movement is desirable. With the couch rotated through 90°, a gantry rotation of up to 30° from the vertical without collision of the image intensifier should be achievable.

In addition to an ability to fix a range of immobilization devices, most couches now incorporate rows of pegs separated by a standard distance of 14 cm, which allows indexing of treatment position between simulator and treatment unit. A head extension, allowing patient positioning further towards the gantry, may increase the effective couch length.

## Accessory equipment

This includes:

- *Block supporting trays* which match the source to tray distances of supported linacs and can accommodate Perspex trays to hold either templates or mounted shielding blocks.
- *Electron end-frame adaptor* mounted into the gantry head that allows direct simulation of electron fields using actual electron applicators.
- *Mechanical front pointers* that provide alternative to the optical display image and can be used during quality assurance (QA) procedures.

## Features of the modern simulator

### Digital simulation

As modern simulators produce output data in digital format, integration of the simulator into the radiotherapy network is essential, DICOM interfaces permitting:

- Import of demographic information from a PACS, RIS or HIS (using DICOM modality work list)
- Import of plan data from the TPS, reducing need for manual input of parameters

- Import of DRRs from VSim or TPS for use during verification, image registration and isocentre adjustment
- Export of simulated field parameters to a TPS or R&V system
- Export of simulated images to TPS or R&V system for comparison or registration with EPID or machine check films
- DICOM printing of image and plan data.

The digital simulator includes several workstations or monitors responsible for controlling the individual elements of the simulator process, such as control of movements, the X-ray generator and the management of plan and demographic data.

Digital or electronic simulation enables simulation to be performed directly upon the digital image acquired by the detector, mouse control being used for target delineation and adjustment of field parameters, couch position and multi-leaf collimator (MLC) leaf positions. Upon completion of this task, image-controlled simulation will move the simulator to its required position for acquisition of updated images without the need to reposition under fluoroscopy. Acquired plan data can then be exported to either TPS or directly to the R&V system.

Imaging workstations may also permit 2D image registration between imported orthogonal reference DRRs (generated on a TPS) and corresponding images produced on the simulator, enabling isocentre correction if required. Registration may be a manual or automatic process.

If hard copy images are needed, a 'virtual' display of the relative positions of blades and field wires in relation to the imager or film cassette can be useful for ensuring correct cassette positioning, preventing the incidence of repeat images

A device described as a *digital shape projector*, contained within the collimator mechanism, uses liquid crystal (LCD) technology to provide an alternative light source, enabling conformal field shapes, defined using MLCs or blocks, to be projected directly onto the patient. A mirror mechanism switches between this mode and the conventional light source. Such systems require daily QA and calibration.

Images may be acquired from the detector either as digital fluoroscopy images or using a higher-quality digital radiography mode. A merge function will enable several acquired images to be combined into a single larger image for use in treatment verification. If CR or conventional films are required the simulator may incorporate *automatic exposure control* whereby exposure time is controlled automatically, with kV and mA settings evaluated from data produced under fluoroscopy.

## Preset protocols/automatic set-up

This function allows predetermined, frequently used parameters or imported plan data (including MLC apertures) to be uploaded to the simulator through an automatic set-up function. A mirror function will produce an exactly opposed beam for use in plan production.

Ideally simulator display and output of its data should be in the same format as the treatment unit simulated for. The simulator software should therefore allow creation of a library of all departmental linacs, each configured to display data in either machine or IEC 1217 convention, and which will include any restrictions in movement, such as individual diaphragm range or the ability to cross central axis.

### Tracking modes
*Pair mode* preserves a predetermined distance between the blades and field wires during operation, reducing patient dose and improving image quality through reduction of scatter.

*Track mode* reduces the blade settings to match the active size and position of the imager during fluoroscopy, also reducing dose by preventing exposure outside the viewable area.

## Anti-collision management

This safety feature comprises hardware components such as motion enabling bars, touch-guards and collision sensors alongside detection and control mechanisms within the simulator software itself. Software control aims to prevent collision of scanner, couch and gantry during operation through pre-programming of the dimensions of the individual simulator components. A virtual safety zone is identified around the patient, the entry of any component into which causes an offending movement to slow down or cease. Options for overriding this function are usually provided at operator risk. These systems are not detection devices and cannot therefore take into account size and position of the patient or ancillary devices, although it may be possible to modify the safety zones to take into account different scenarios.

A *monitor unit calculator* may be included within the application, enabling simple dose calculations when 2D simulation is undertaken, on the basis of information acquired during simulation.

## Simulator quality assurance

A simulator QA programme should be followed that encompasses the radiographic and fluoroscopic functions, mechanical motions and readouts from the imaging system.

Acceptance tests (ensuring the simulator meets specification) and commissioning tests will provide baseline figures against which future QA will be matched.

### Mechanical motions and readouts
Mechanical accuracy must conform to that of the supported linear accelerators. Isocentric rotation of all movements can be checked using a reference front pointer with resulting rotation axes describing less than a 2-mm sphere. Scale readouts should be within 0.5° of actual position. Focus-to-axis distance (FAD) accuracy can be checked by exposing a radiographic film at

known field size and FAD. By increasing the FAD a set amount and re-exposing the same film, field size accuracy and central axis wander can be verified.

Couch lateral and longitudinal movements and their scales can be verified using a ruler against the central axis and should be accurate to within 2 mm. Vertical movement can be checked in the same manner as for FAD.

Light field/X-ray field correspondence is performed by marking field corners on a radiographic film with a pin and comparing against the X-ray image. Verification during fluoroscopy uses a grid marked for different field sizes with ball bearings.

To confirm laser alignment with the isocentre at a range of gantry angles, a cube with a ball-bearing in the centre and central axes marked on all faces can be set up with the light field and viewed under fluoroscopy.

Daily mechanical checks should include accuracy of field size, gantry isocentricity, couch scale, laser system, optical SSD indicator and the light/radiation field alignment.

### Radiographic system/fluoroscopic system/imaging system

Output checks at a range of mA/mAs settings requires use of an ionisation chamber. Beam quality is confirmed through measurement of peak kV using solid-state detectors and filters to calculate half-value thickness. Timer accuracy must also be verified.

Effective focal spot size can be measured using a pinhole technique or star test method. A Leeds Test Object is used to check spatial resolution of the image intensifier and camera system at a range of different contrasts. This contains small discs of increasing diameter and thickness, which can be visualised at different mAs. If an imaging system begins to deteriorate, e.g. due to intensifier saturation or TV monitor deterioration, the number of discs visualised will be reduced.

Checks of auto-exposure control mechanisms are made by comparison of film density with

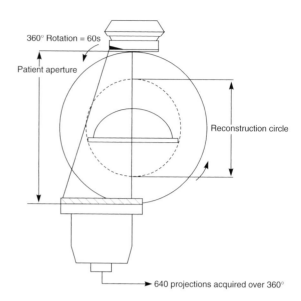

**Figure 6.9**   Simulator – CT.

original measurements obtained under similar exposure conditions.

### SIM-CT

SIM-CT is the term describing production of tomographic images on a conventional simulator. The first units able to provide CT-like images were fitted with image intensifiers (Figure 6.9) and were capable of producing a single slice per rotation. A more recent adaptation uses flat panel detectors, described above to produce volumetric cone beam CT studies (CBCT).

### First-generation simulator-CT

Enabling a traditional simulator to produce tomographic images requires two additions to the system. First, the simulator must be modified to produce and detect a narrow collimated beam of 4–7 mm from which the axial slice will be reconstructed. This is achieved by inserting both a *pre-collimation* device into the assembly head and a *post-collimation* device over the intensifier, replacing the cassette holding mechanism.

Second, the system requires a PC and associated software to assimilate the acquired image data and to convert that data into a CT image.

Slices are produced in a similar manner to standard CT, namely through a detector mechanism opposing an X-ray source that is capable of 360° rotation around the patient. As CT images are acquired at around 125 kV, improved cooling of the anode is required, usually through a fan mechanism. The *detector mechanism* in these systems is an image intensifier and coupled TV camera.

To achieve a field of view comparable to CT, the image intensifier is offset laterally by 15 cm at a distance of 50 cm from the isocentre. By doing this only half the fan beam data is collected and used to reconstruct the image. As high kV is required for operation a shaped compensation filter is inserted on the pre-collimator to prevent saturation of the video signal at the edges of the patient.

### Data acquisition and reconstruction

During the 360° gantry rotation, X-ray data reaching the detector in the form of half profiles is sampled up to 1000 times. Sampling this data, the reconstruction computer mathematically converts received projection data into linear attenuation coefficient data relating to each point in the sampled matrix. As information is acquired at different gantry angles, data is built up in the matrix as the sum of the various tissue attenuation coefficients along it. The diametrically opposed half-profiles are combined and the resulting profiles back-projected into the image matrix. This convolution and back-projection method of reconstruction is alternatively known as the equivalent Fourier technique. Other mathematical algorithms are now applied to enhance spatial resolution and contrast of the image. The reconstructed image is calibrated to Hounsfield units (CT numbers), the resulting image being compared with a previously calibrated phantom image, enabling removal of inherent system artefacts common to both images.

*Image manipulation and store* The final image is usually viewable on a 512 × 512 matrix and is capable of manipulation within the SIM-CT application using standard tools of Pan, Zoom, Window Width and Level adjustment. Images may be transferred or archived within the RT network. It may be possible for 'real-time' simulator beams to be overlaid on the acquired slice data, provided that the CT acquisition devices are immediately removed and the simulator reverted to conventional mode without alteration of patient position.

*Practical aspects*
- To prevent collision, the CT simulator can only scan with intensifier and couch in pre-set positions. The resulting aperture of about 85 cm, while comparable to standard CT, does not guarantee that patients positioned on breast boards or with arm supports can be scanned.
- CT simulators offer FOVs ranging from 25 cm, suitable for head and neck, up to a maximum of 50 cm for other sites.
- Image quality and CT number accuracy close to the aperture edges may be suboptimal.
- Due to long acquisition time, motion artefacts are inevitable on the acquired image, although in a radiotherapy context this is not usually problematic.

### Second-generation SIM-CT: CBCT

Replacement of image intensifier with flat panel detectors has the additional benefit of enabling production of CBCT scan series of comparable lengths to CT studies instead of the limited slice numbers available from earlier SIM-CTs.

Whereas conventional CT scanners (and earlier SIM-CTs) collimate X-rays from the source as a fan beam, CBCT devices use a wide field of view 'cone beam' projected on to the flat panel array, acquiring a series of 2D fluoroscopic images at numerous points during the course of a 360° rotation. This data is subsequently reconstructed

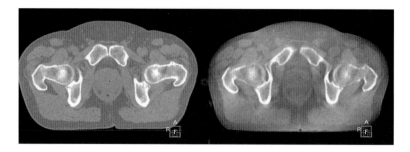

**Figure 6.10**  Comparison of conventional CT (left) and cone beam CT with respect to image quality.

by associated software into volumetric CBCT data, usually in a 1024 × 1024 matrix. Such systems are capable of calculating between 300 and 900 projections per rotation. Reducing the number of projections may result in faster collection and reconstruction, at lower doses, but this will be at the cost of an increase in the contrast to noise ratio.

Cone beam reconstruction uses a *Feldkamp algorithm*, similar to the filtered back-projection algorithm used in fan beam CT but which combats many inherent cone beam artefacts.

A CBCT simulator is capable of providing scan lengths of between 15 and 20 cm during a single rotation and, although this improves on earlier SIM-CTs, is too short to make the modality a viable alternative to CT. This limitation can be overcome through the ability of software to merge two or three contiguous series, producing a composite volume of up to 60 cm length.

CBCT scanners can also increase the field of view, limited by the physical size of the detector, by offsetting the detector and using an asymmetrical, partial fan. In these situations it should be noted that anatomy at the edges may be irradiated only for a fraction of the total rotation compared with the centre.

### Dose and image quality

The inability to modify kV or mA during CBCT means that patient doses received may significantly exceed those of conventional CT scans.

Doses may be reduced through acceptance of reduced image contrast through limitation of sampling. Pelvic scans requiring high contrast result in the highest doses received whereas for head and neck scanning CBCT doses are comparable to conventional CT and may even be lower than those obtained during electronic portal imaging (EPID) acquisition (Figure 6.10). The merging of double and triple scans can result in substantial overlap between the series, substantially increasing total dose received.

CBCT images invariably have higher noise levels than fan beam CT scans, which theoretically may affect the ability to perform image registration. Testing of some systems have additionally found increases in ring artefacts and poor hounsfield unit uniformity.

### Clinical uses

Simulator CBCT scans have primarily been used for 3D *verification* of plans produced from conventionally acquired CT data. There has been a general reluctance to use CBCT data directly for *localisation* during treatment planning due to a perceived reduction in accuracy of density information. Comparison of plans produced from CBCT and CT-SIM scans does, however, suggest that density resolution, temporal stability, contrast resolution, scan uniformity and noise are comparable and that differences in resulting plans may only be in the order of 0.5–1%. This makes SIM-CT a possible alternative to CT for purposes of target delineation, particularly for those departments wishing to maintain a conventional simulator.

When used on the linac, CBCT scans offer the possibility for *adaptive planning* during the course of treatment. CBCT also offers the advantages of an aperture comparable to a wide-bore scanner, for use with larger patients and with restricted techniques.

CBCT has also found wide application within *brachytherapy* for localisation of seeds and implants. The process often carried out under anaesthesia benefits from the large clearance offered and gives the potential for verification CT scans to be carried out before each fraction is delivered.

## CT simulation

CT simulation, the modality that has driven the increased use of 3D data within radiotherapy treatment planning, is made up of three main components located within the simulator suite: a CT scanner, moving laser system and virtual simulation application.

## CT scanner

Acquires the image data that will be reconstructed by the virtual simulation application into a 3D virtual model of the patient. Although CT design and functionality is covered elsewhere it is necessary to identify some features relating specifically to use within radiotherapy.

### Scanner aperture size

Historically, scanners designed for diagnostic operation were employed, often located within radiology departments and temporarily adapted to the radiotherapy process through addition of flat couch overlays, immobilisation devices and an external laser for marking of reference points. Currently it is more usual for a dedicated therapy scanner to be located within the radiotherapy department itself.

Since the traditional 70 cm scanner aperture, with 50 cm maximum field of view (FOV) is too limiting for many radiotherapy techniques, most manufacturers now produce 'large bore' versions of their popular multi-slice scanners, providing apertures up to 85 cm which enable most therapy patients to be scanned in an optimal position. Reconstruction algorithms may also provide a FOV as large as the physical size of the aperture itself, although quality of image data and CT number accuracy within these extend regions means it may be of limited clinical use. Use of wide-bore scanners inevitably results in a slight reduction in high contrast resolution and will increase image noise and dose in comparison to standard scanners, although in the radiotherapy context these factors are not usually considered significant in comparison to the benefits provided.

### Issues relating to 4D-CT

Fast tube rotation times of 0.5–1 second, allowing rapid acquisition of large volumes of data, although advantageous from a diagnostic perspective could be considered undesirable in some therapy scenarios because they generate image data at a rate unrepresentative of the period of radiotherapy delivery. Techniques may be required that acquire scan data over timescales comparable with the breathing cycle (Figure 6.11), through use of low pitch (slowing couch movement) or combining slow tube rotation with thin reconstruction slices.

If *4D-CT* is to be employed, scanner control software should provide the means whereby the breathing cycle demonstrated during scan acquisition can be related to the images reconstructed. Using low pitch and thin slice thickness (around 1 mm) it is possible to divide the study into a number of sub-studies, each relating to an identifiable segment of the respiratory cycle. This data can then be used to either 'gate' treatment delivery on the linac (exposure only occurring within predefined ranges), or alternatively it can used to identify extremes of organ and tumour

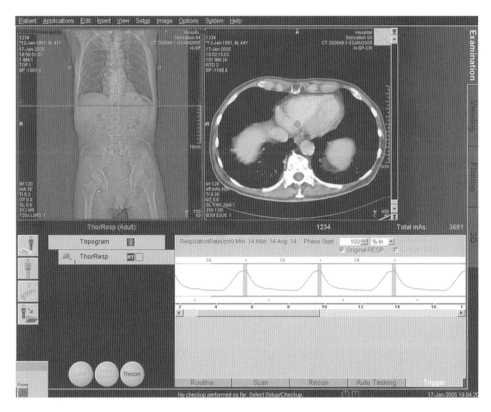

**Figure 6.11** Four-dimensional computed tomography (4D-CT): demonstration of respiratory cycle during image acquisition.

movement, enabling a composite PTV to be produced.

### Scanner couch

Provision of a flat, stable couch is essential for radiotherapy planning and is invariably provided through a commercially produced carbon fibre overlay, most of which can be adapted to fit any scanner cradle. Shared use of the scanner with radiology requires that this can be easily removed and accurately replaced. Couch sag and weight-bearing capacity should be comparable to a linac couch and it must be level and orthogonal in its movements through the scanner aperture, with a maximum deflection of 2 mm along its range. As with conventional simulators, scanner couches should ideally be compatible with the supported treatment units, able to attach in-house or

commercially available immobilisation devices and following similar indexing systems. Many scanner manufacturers offer overlays of identical dimensions to the most common linac couches (Figure 6.12). The design of the couch must be assessed with respect to the production of artefacts through joints, screws, etc.

With increasing complexity of treatment techniques, inclusion of the treatment couch within the planning data could improve dosimetric accuracy. In these circumstances the CT overlay must be consistent with the linac in terms of materials and dimensions, and is required to rest above the cradle (allowing the latter's removal from the dataset). Such an arrangement does, however, decrease the effective size of the aperture. A recent development is the production of a dedicated RT couch in which the cradle itself

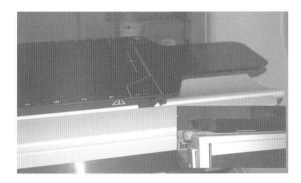

**Figure 6.12** Scanner couch with indexed radiotherapy overlay.

is adapted for therapy use without the need for a separate overlay.

### Use of intravenous contrast during radiotherapy scanning

The timed delivery of intravenous contrast agent, used to assist in the differentiation of blood vessels from surrounding anatomical or pathological structures – a crucial element of diagnostic protocols – is assuming increasing importance within the radiotherapy planning process.

Delivery of contrast is through a remote contrast injector, a medical device that can operate as a stand-alone unit or that may be coupled to the scanner. allowing automatic control of bolus delivery. A typical system consists of:

• A pedestal or ceiling-mounted injector head, containing the contrast-filled syringe, tubes attaching syringe to cannula and a plunger to inject the agent at a pre-programmed rate.
• A control console located adjacent to the scanner (although dual control may be available in the scanner control area) into which the infusion rate is programmed. The console allows termination of the procedure if required and may contain a number of safety features.

Once a loaded syringe is attached and flow rate programmed, a predetermined scan delay, usually 25–60 s is entered into the scan protocol.

Scan and injection are then started concurrently ensuring that image data is acquired while the contrast bolus passes through the blood vessels. The operator overseeing the procedure is responsible for identifying signs of tissue extravasation or adverse reaction, stopping injection and scan if they occur.

### Practical issues

Operation of these devices raises a number of practical issues. First, sufficient staff must be trained to cannulate and oversee the procedure. Once trained, a sufficiently high workload is required to maintain competency and confidence. Staff must also be competent in identification and management of the following:

• Tissue extravasation: many injectors are now capable of automatic detection of extravasation, using RF waves to detect fluid pooling beneath the patients skin.
• Adverse reactions to contrast agent: these range from mild to severe and require that operators are able to identify and evaluate contributing risk factors, and are aware of the signs and symptoms of onset and subsequent actions required. Access to emergency drugs, oxygen and suction and provision of clinical cover during and immediately after administration are mandatory.
• Air injection, arising from loading of an empty syringe, is potentially fatal and consequently injector design provides features to reduce its likelihood, through detection of air in the catheter or use of automatic auto-plunger advance when the empty syringe is fitted.

Modern scanners may also incorporate software that triggers scan commencement when contrast agent is detected within the area of interest.

## Laser systems

### Lasers incorporated within the scanner

All scanners contain an internal laser to identify the scan plane. The relative 'inaccuracy' of this laser means that they are not generally used for marking of scan references. If the scanner provides a second 'external' laser within the gantry casing at a defined distance from the scan plane, these may be used to mark scan references provided that regular QA procedures are followed.

### External room lasers

This system, consisting of wall-mounted and sagittal devices is independent of the scanner, communicating directly with the virtual simulation application.

Within the simulation process they may serve two functions:

1. They are used to mark a reference within the image data from which beam isocentre coordinate(s) are defined.
2. They are used to mark (on the patient) coordinates defined during simulation and that may represent isocentres, field corners or markers.

External lasers can be fixed in position or be capable of movement within their casing. The configuration chosen will impact on the way that the lasers are used post-simulation.

### Wall-mounted lasers

These project at a set distance (usually 500 mm) from the scan plane. If non-moving lasers are provided, these are mounted at a set height in relation to the scan aperture, requiring vertical movement to be effected through adjustment of couch height. If moving lasers are provided the anteroposterior (AP) laser shift can be automatically loaded in relation to the scan reference.

### Overhead sagittal laser

Projecting at the same fixed distance as lateral lasers but orthogonal to the scan plane, these lasers are always capable of lateral movement because the scanner couch may not.

When lasers are positioned at a zero setting, their intersection point is coincident with the centre of the scan plane.

## Virtual simulation application

### The development of CT simulation

The CT or virtual simulation modality as a replacement for conventional simulation is a relatively recent phenomenon, although its theoretical origins date from the early 1980s when Galvin suggested that a CT scanner might be able to perform many of the functions of the simulator. In 1987 the concept of virtual simulation as the 'bilateral communication between scanner, laser positioning system, workstation and treatment planning system (TPS)' was defined.

Although Goltein attempted the reconstruction of digital projection radiographs (beam eye views) as early as 1982, the practical use of digitally reconstructed radiographs (DRRs) that traced 'X-rays from the X-ray source through a three-dimensional (3D) model of the patient made up of voxels determined from CT scans' did not become incorporated within treatment planning systems until the early 1990s.[5]

The development of the dedicated virtual simulation application, able to produce and process DRRs through use of mathematical filters and window/level manipulation, dates from the mid-1990s and was made clinically acceptable by the expansion in computing power and consequent reduction in DRR reconstruction times. Such applications, often perceived as more 'user friendly' than the TPS, offered departments a flexible approach to simulation and facilitated the adoption of a range of techniques within the umbrella of what became known as the virtual simulation process.

### The CT (virtual) simulation process

Although the concept of virtual simulation is a broad one, a core VSim process may be identified to demonstrate its potential use (Figure 6.13):

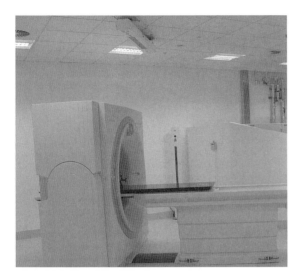

**Figure 6.13** Wide-bore scanner with sagittal and vertical moving laser system.

1. The patient must be adequately immobilised and positioned on the scanner couch so that the area of interest is contained within the scanner FOV.
2. Using external lasers a scan reference is marked on the patient or shell in a position determined by the simulation and treatment techniques to follow. This reference may either represent the final treatment isocentre or be the point from which the isocentre will be shifted. The stability of the reference must be considered and this may require that the external laser is shifted horizontally or vertically. As the reference (and its coordinate) must be identifiable within the TPS or VSim application, it is often necessary to overlay the point(s) with radio-opaque markers.
3. After marking the patient is advanced to the scan plane and the scanner couch set to zero.
4. The CT study is now acquired with consideration given to:
   the *scan length* required to include proposed volume with suitable margin for planning and verification purposes

the reconstruction *slice width*, determining DRR resolution and amount of data that requires processing
*mA* required to ensure optimum noise levels and image quality.
5. On scan completion, slice data is reconstructed within the virtual simulation application into a 3D patient model upon which simulation and other functions can be performed.

If the VSim application (Figure 6.14) is to be used to create treatment beams, their isocentre position(s) will ultimately need to be defined in relation to the previously marked reference. Some systems enable the scan reference to be 'locked' by the user and used as a basis for automatically calculating the magnitude and direction of any shifts required. Alternatively this may require a manual calculation of the difference between reference and isocentre coordinates to be performed.

The final treatment isocentre can be realized in a number of ways:

- The marked scan reference may be used as a treatment isocentre, requiring simulation with independent diaphragms. Although this has the advantage that the isocentre is marked during the scan appointment, it relies on knowledge of anticipated treatment volumes and ability to relate this to surface anatomy.
- Real-time simulation occurs, with the patient remaining on (or returning to) the scanner couch. A combination of couch and laser movement is used to position external lasers at the isocentre position before marking. This represents a time-consuming, often restrictive option.
- The treatment isocentre can be allocated and marked before initial treatment delivery on either conventional simulator or treatment unit.
- The patient undertakes a daily shift from reference cross (as tattooed or marked on the shell) to the treatment isocentre. Use of couch indexing and/or couch zeroing facilities may reduce

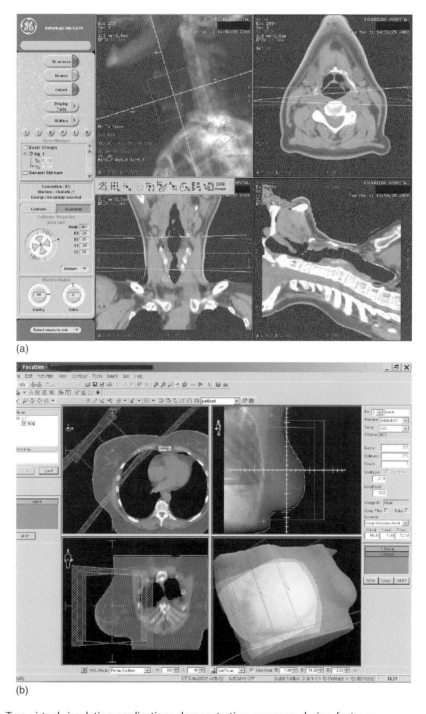

(a)

(b)

**Figure 6.14** Two virtual simulation applications demonstrating common design features.

the risks of daily set-up errors associated with this option.

## Features of the virtual simulation application

### Application platform/network issues

Many early VSim applications operated on a UNIX platform and were located on stand-alone workstations. Although capable of transferring image and plan data within a network, they did not utilise a central server to manage and control their workload. Data transfer involved production of 'copies', meaning that for departments with several workstations problems developed over management of multiple active versions and with issues of back-up and archive. This situation improved through development of PC-based applications and adoption of server–client relationships. With data now stored and saved on a central server, the simulator PC assumes the status of a remote node and dependent on licensing arrangements, the function of simulation could theoretically occur anywhere within the network. The capability also now exists for remote simulation using laptops, with scan data downloaded, simulated upon and subsequently uploaded back to the server.

A related development is the re-integration of VSim applications within Treatment Planning Systems (TPSs) with which they share functionality such as production of DRRs, volumes and structures. Many VSim applications are now available as 'modules'; within a total planning package that employs uniform graphical user interfaces and allows sharing of image and plan data between components that may also include fusion and plan review.

### Simulator graphical user interface

A number of common design features have contributed to a perceived 'user friendliness' of the VSim application, including:

- Provision of a familiar screen layout, consistent with related applications

- Separation of the screen into discrete functional areas, while the use of multiple display formats allows the user to customise the layout or to select alternative combinations of images and functions
- Separation of functions of beam, isocentre and structure management
- Use of icons, tool and menu bars for intuitive function selection by non-experts
- Mouse control of all functions
- Use of context dependent drop-down menus
- Offering of multiple methods for performing common tasks; this might include entry of values into data boxes, click and drag with mouse or selection from a menu
- Ability to maximise, zoom and pan images and to distinguish between active beams (from which the BEV is derived) and secondary beams
- 'Undo' options to reverse unwanted amendments
- View of a 3D patient model demonstrating either a skin render or the relative position of defined structures
- Projection of beam entry (and exit) onto reconstructed skin surface
- Graphical display of the treatment unit.

## Image display

Within the image display area, three image types may be viewed.

### Multiplanar reconstructions

VSim applications provide MPRs in sagittal, coronal and axial planes and possibly user-defined angles. Their role in the simulation process is to:

- Allow visualisation of and navigation through patient anatomy in three dimensions, achieved through mouse control of a cursor or tracking bar
- Enable volumes and structures to be drawn – always possible on the axial slice but some

systems allow contouring on sagittal and coronal views, subsequent interpolation producing a composite 3D volume

• Demonstrate position of beams, aperture or shielding blocks.

### Digitally reconstructed radiograph

Virtual simulation applications generate divergent DRRs for beams created by the user and are able to update them in real time after modification of beam or isocentre (and therefore virtual source position). DRRs serve two functions:

• When contour production is not desired they provide similar methods for viewing or editing fields and isocentres to that of fluoroscopy. Fast processing speeds, dependent on computer hardware, are essential to generate and rapidly update DRRs in the clinical setting.
• They provide gold standard images against which megavoltage images can be compared during verification.

DRR quality is determined by the quality of CT image data from which it is generated, being affected by slice thickness, slice spacing, CT voxel size and reconstruction matrix.

The VSim application also provides tools with which to manipulate DRRs, such as;

• Application of mathematical filters to simulate low- or high-energy images:
• Window width and level manipulation
• Selection of an image quality option (from course to fine)
• Alteration of depth of field, reconstructing the DRR from a use-defined 'slice', removing data that contributes nothing to the verification process
• Use of 'blending', a method that allows two qualitatively different DRRs of the same field to be created independently and merged. Figure 6.15 shows such a DRR demonstrating airways blended with one created to optimize bone structures.

Of increased use are *digital composite reconstructions* allowing visualisation of structures through selection of their CT values. A *maximum intensity projection* (MIP) is one such image used to demonstrate only high-density tissue (Figure 6.16).

### 3D view

A 3D model of patient surface with defined structures is provided and can be used to assist field placement or to gain a visual understanding of the relationship between target structures and organs at risk. Projection of field entry and exit on to patient surface is usually offered, although this may require prior production of an external outline.

The key functions of virtual simulation, beam, isocentre and structure creation are carried out and managed within separate areas of the application

### Beam management

Beam management involves the creation, naming, editing, copying and deletion of beams. Most applications provide for the creation of a library of beam configurations defined by the user and specific to their requirements.

All beams created must be assigned to a treatment unit (either model specific or generic), which requires linac configuration data to be entered during system set-up. This will ensure that parameters are displayed in correct format (e.g. IEC 1217) and that unachievable collimator, gantry and diaphragm positions are restricted.

Modification of beam parameters or MLC positions may be through entry into a data box or from mouse manipulation of the DRR. Irregularly shaped fields are produced through creation of MLC apertures or through addition of user-defined shielding blocks.

As multiple beam arrangements are usually employed, methods are available through which beams may be linked via a shared isocentre. In addition some systems provide an 'equal angle' function which can maintain beams at an

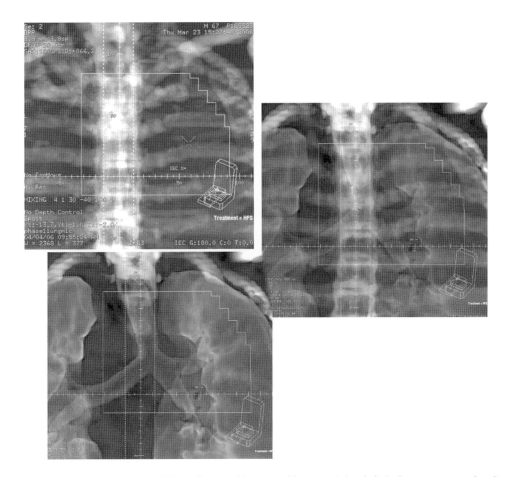

**Figure 6.15** A 'blended' DRR created from fusion of lung- and bone-weighted digitally reconstructed radiographs (DRRs).

'opposed' 180° separation during simulation. The ability to copy parameters between opposed beams offers the opportunity for editing without the need to delete and recreate secondary beams after each modification.

### Interest points and markers

Most applications allow for 'markers', points of geometric or dose importance, to be produced. These may be assigned to the patient (as structures) or to a specific beam (within a RT plan) and can be used in several ways:

- To determine reference or tattoo coordinates
- To enable points of anatomical interest to be viewed on the DRR
- To define points for which dose information is required on the TPS
- To define a coordinate to which the external laser may be sent, e.g. in the marking of field corners as projected onto the skin surface.

### Isocentre management

Applications provide a variety of methods for assigning and editing isocentre positions during

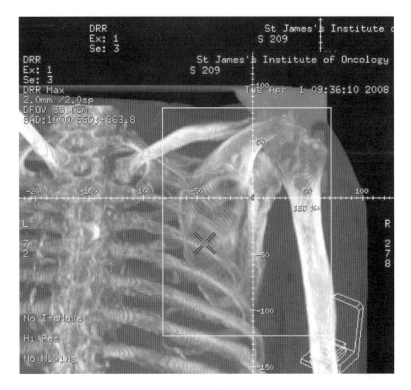

**Figure 6.16** A maximum intensity projection (MIP) digitally reconstructed radiograph (DRR).

simulation. These may include automatic positioning of an isocentre at the geometric centre of an aperture or structure, or mid-plane along the beam axis (thereby equalising SSDs of opposed beams).

Virtual fluoroscopy, mimicking the actions of a conventional simulator, allows the isocentre to be dragged to a specific point or moved to a selected coordinate or marker. To support non-isocentric beam arrangements it will also be possible to directly assign a SSD value to a beam.

### Structure management

The creation, editing and growing of contours are functions traditionally provided by a TPS, but are incorporated into VSim applications where they can be combined with beam and iso-centre allocation. Even if beam creation is not required, the ability to export structures to a TPS means that a VSim offers an alternative platform for undertaking contouring. It is important that the application therefore provides a variety of tools for creation and editing of contours that support individual operator preference. Also required are tools for the interpolation of contours between slices and the ability to add differential margins in all directions, used, for example, when 'growing' a CTV into a PTV. This may include settings to 'avoid' or 'fuse' with other defined structures. Autosegmentation and autocontouring tools that use differences in CT number between adjacent organs may be used to automatically draw contours. Although such tools may be of limited use in abdominal or pelvic regions, they prove useful when defining external patient contours.

A method of removing the scanner couch from the image data or of preventing its use during SSD is required.

## Other features

### DICOM connectivity

Connectivity within the local network allows for the (often bidirectional) transfer of data between VSim and other devices. Examples relevant to the virtual simulation process include:

- Import of image data from CT, MR and PET scanners
- Import and export of RTP and RTSS with the TPS
- Export of RTP data to R&V systems
- Export of RTP data to the laser-marking system
- RTP export to block cutter
- Import and export of RT image DRRs with R&V or EPID systems; some systems support fusion of EPIDs and DRRs for treatment verification
- Import of RT dose data enabling remote evaluation of dose plans and DVHs
- Output of secondary capture DRRs to a printer or laser printer, ideally at a magnification defined by the user (e.g. source to tray distance)
- Output of plan parameters or isocentre information to a printer.

Assessment of connectivity may be made through reference to the DICOM conformance statement provided, but must be tested with own data to ensure interoperability.

### CT/MR fusion
VSim applications provide a platform for fusion of CT with MR or PET studies, allowing contouring to proceed on the merged image data. Fusion may be carried out using manual or auto-matic methods and require users to consider the matching algorithms employed and methods for verifying the quality of any match.

### Linac display
Most applications display a graphical representation of the linac to assist user orientation. It may also be possible to input the physical dimensions of common linac models to assist in determining the achievability of complex beam arrangements during simulation.

### QA of the CT simulator suite
All systems within the treatment planning process require a comprehensive QA programme that incorporates acceptance testing, commissioning and periodic QA. This QA contains several elements carried out on daily, weekly, monthly or yearly basis.

*Scanner QA* Daily QA should test for *systematic uncertainty* through measurement of CT number accuracy ($\pm 5\,$HU) within a water phantom. *Random uncertainty* of the pixel value, known as image noise, is measured as the standard deviation of pixel HU values in a measured region interest (ROI). Noise is sensitive to performance of the scanner. Monthly QA should test the number accuracy of four to five different materials and should also be repeated at variable offset positions within the aperture to mimic radiotherapy conditions. Yearly QA should verify data gathered during commissioning concerning, spatial resolution, contrast resolution and electron density to CT number conversion. The last will ensure that dose distributions are calculated accurately and, as it is scanner dependent, must be repeated for all scanners within the department.

*Couch QA* Professional couch installation is essential, with a regular QA protocol testing that the couch, with and without its overlay, remains level and orthogonal to the imaging plane. One method is to acquire a CT slice of a laser QA phantom when it is positioned both at the top end of the couch and with couch extended as far as possible. The coordinates of two identical points within the phantom can then be compared for accuracy within 2 mm. Horizontal displacement implies that the table top is not level, rotated or rolls during its movement. Further tests of digital indicator accuracy make use of rulers positioned on the couch top with relation to the external laser system.

*Laser system QA*   Accuracy of external lasers is essential when defining reference or simulated coordinates and must be in the order of 1–2 mm over the clinically useful range. They must be set up professionally and vigorously tested during acceptance. It may be possible at this stage to calibrate the lasers to account for couch deflection under an average load.

Regular QA using a laser test phantom is essential to ensure that external lasers identify the scan plane when advanced the pre-set distance, and that wall and overhead lasers are parallel and orthogonal to the imaging plane. A test that laser movement is accurate, linear and reproducible can be made through use of a ruler when shifting the laser a predetermined distance. Accuracy is tested through use of alignment phantom or other tools and should be comparable to accuracy of the linac lasers. Accuracy is tested over a range of laser shifts and with relation to its divergence in horizontal and vertical planes.[6])

## Self-test questions

1. Name four components of the simulator X-ray tube.
2. What is a reticule?
3. What device controls the voltage across the tube?
4. What is tube rating?
5. What does the acronym PACS stand for?

## References

1. Oakley J. *Digital Imaging*, London: Greenwich-Medical, 2003.
2. Oosterwijk H. *DICOM Basics*, 2nd edn. Dallas, TX: O'Tech Inc., 2002.
3. Curry TS, Dowdrey JE, Murry RC. *Christensens's Physics of Diagnostic Radiology*, 4th edn. Philadelphia: Lee & Febiger, 1990.
4. Carter C, Veale B. *Digital Radiography and PACS*. St Louis, MO: Mosby Elsevier, 2008.
5. Aird EGA, Conway J. CT Simulation for Radiotherapy treatment planning. *Br J Radiol* 2002; 75: 937–49.
6. Mutic S, Palta JR, Butler EK et al. Quality assurance for computed-tomography simulators and the computed-tomography-simulation process: Report of the AAPM Radiation Therapy Committee task group No. 66. *Med Phys* 2003; 30: 2762–92.

# Chapter 7

# IMMOBILISATION EQUIPMENT

## Helen White and Nick White

This chapter describes a range of equipment and techniques that may be employed to ensure effective patient immobilisation during radiotherapy treatment planning and delivery. To this end, immobilisation is described by anatomical site. In addition to in-house systems a number of commercially available systems and materials are described in order to provide examples of immobilisation equipment. The reader should note that there are a number of manufacturers in this field and that this chapter cannot do justice to the full range of immobilisation options currently available. The inclusion of equipment suppliers or devices in this chapter does not imply a particular recommendation or endorsement of their use.

### Aims and objectives

These are to overview the range of immobilisation equipment that can be used in the treatment of patients undergoing external beam radiotherapy treatment.

At the end of this chapter, the reader should be able to:
- describe the main forms of immobilisation that are available for use
- discuss the main considerations when deciding on a patient's position and immobilisation technique.

## Introduction

A primary aim of radiotherapy treatment is to optimise the radiation dose to the target volume while reducing the dose to the adjacent normal tissues. By conforming the dose distribution to the target volume and limiting normal tissue doses, there is a potential to achieve dose escalation without excessive normal tissue morbidity. Key to this process is the use of effective patient *immobilisation*. Positioning inaccuracies may be reduced via the use of dedicated immobilisation devices which allow for accurate reproduction of patient position from fraction to fraction. In addition it is important to position radiotherapy patients in ways that ensure comfort and stability. By doing so, the incidence of random positioning errors caused by patient movement may be reduced. Advances and developments in precision techniques such as *intensity-modulated radiotherapy* (IMRT) and *three-dimensional conformal radiotherapy* (3DRT) are achievable only if immobilisation techniques are adequate to ensure the elimination of positioning variability.

The use of suitable immobilisation devices is usually down to individual department choice, and a number of commercially available devices and materials are available. When deciding the patient position and therefore the immobilisation technique that is to be used a number of factors need to be taken into consideration such as:

- Accessibility to the anatomical site for treatment
- General fitness and mobility of the patient
- Treatment intent (radical versus palliative)
- The proposed technique/beam arrangement
- Cost and availability of materials.

It is essential that any positioning or fixation devices are compatible with both the treatment planning equipment (e.g. CT scanner and/or treatment simulator) and the treatment machine, and that they do not create a significant amount of image degradation due to the presence of image artefacts, for example.

## Immobilisation shells

Immobilisation shells are devices that enable the fixation of patients into their treatment position in an effort to limit movement and to obtain treatment reproducibility. Shells are required to be used often for several weeks of treatment, and so must be durable and hard wearing. To be effective they should accurately follow the patient's contour and restrict movement through each of the anatomical axes. For most anatomical sites the immobilisation shell should be semi-rigid, while being smooth against the patient's skin surface to ensure patient comfort. In addition, the practical use of patient shells requires that they accommodate the use of surface markers for treatment set-up such as the position of the isocentre, beam entry points or field edges. Suitable materials for radiotherapy treatment shells should ideally be thin enough to ensure minimal dose, while retaining enough strength to build-up and maintain patient position and withstand recurrent use over several days or weeks of treatment.

## Immobilisation equipment for head and neck treatment

The need for accurate immobilisation in the head and neck region is paramount due to the need to treat target volumes that are often small and located adjacent to radiosensitive structures. The use of highly conformal treatment dose distributions means that patient movement is potentially catastrophic and may result in a geographical miss of the target volume and overdose of critical structures. In practical terms this is minimised by using small set-up tolerances of the order of 1–2 mm in an effort to reduce systematic errors and ensuring a high degree of accuracy; this may be quality assured by the regular use of treatment verification imaging. IMRT and 3D CRT techniques in the head and neck can be attempted only in the knowledge that the proposed immobilisation strategy eliminates unacceptable patient movement. For most radical treatments to the head and neck a comfortable rigid external fixation shell is usually indicated in order to ensure precise positioning. The adoption of 'universal' systems to prevent patient motion is also important where a patient is to undergo a variety of differing imaging procedures, and these facilitate attempts at image fusion.

## Head supports

Before a patient's immobilisation shell is constructed attention should be paid to the choice of headrest. A suitable headrest allows the patient to adopt the required treatment position comfortably at a designated height above the treatment couch. Most radiotherapy departments employ a system that allows a choice from a number of standard head rests, which follow the contour of the patient's head and neck and offer a choice of positioning options to accommodate a range of anatomical variation. For example, during positioning it may be necessary to eliminate excessive neck flexion and reduce curvature of the spinal cord in the anterior direction. Headrests should also ideally limit rotational and lateral movements of the head. This can be ensured by using a headrest that is slightly higher at its edges. A reasonable choice of headrest is important because the head position selected for treatment is dictated by the site and type of the lesion to be treated. Certain treatments may require elevation of the patient's chin and extension of the neck (e.g. during treatment of parotid gland tumours). This can be facilitated by the use of a headrest with a pronounced neck curve and deeper 'head bowl'.

Most headrests are manufactured using materials such as *polyurethane foam* or *thin plastic composites*, although *carbon fibre* options are available. These materials need to be durable because they are for reuse, and should therefore be washable for infection control purposes. Materials used should exhibit minimal beam attenuation properties because it may be necessary to employ treatment beam arrangements that treat through the cushion support (e.g. when using posterior oblique fields). A number of manufacturers now offer custom supports providing individualised head moulds that employ vacuum-cushion technologies or water-activated resins.

### Base plate systems

For accurate treatment it is necessary to fasten the head immobilisation devices to the simulator, scanner and treatment couch top via a dedicated baseplate. The baseplate system should allow easy attachment to the couch and may be indexed such that the patient can be positioned along the longitudinal plane. Most systems also allow for the lateral movement of the headrest so that the patient can be positioned in an offset position towards the edge of the treatment couch. This position may be necessary for the treatment of lateralised volumes and the use of posterior oblique fields without the risk of gantry–couch collisions. The fixation system used should permit a variety of treatment positions, e.g. prone head and neck treatments or supine treatments in the extended, neutral or flexed position. Provision should be made for the angulation of the baseplate in order to ensure the option to select a tilted position as required in flexed 'chin-down'

positioning, e.g. for use during the treatment of pituitary disease.

### Facial masks

For the purpose of irradiation of head and neck tumours facial masks are most frequently used. It is important that the masks used provide suitable immobilisation and retain a degree of rigidity to prevent patient motion. A good shell should closely follow the contours of the patient and should have the following characteristics:[1]

- Permit localisation of the lesion to be accurately determined from surface markers attached to the shell
- Enable an accurate position of the patient to be reproduced from fraction to fraction
- Guarantee an accurate and constant patient contour
- Can be labelled and marked clearly and remove the need to draw marks on the patient
- Offer accurate beam entry and exit points
- Provide a base for the addition of build-up material

Before mask construction it is critical that a suitable amount of attention be paid to the proposed patient position with respect to the position of the head, neck and shoulders. A decision needs to be made as to whether the immobilisation shell is required to encompass just the head (e.g. from skull vertex to chin), or whether a 'full' shell (including shoulder fixation) is necessary, e.g. where lateral fields extending inferiorly are intended.

There are two principal types of shell in use: clear plastic (*polyethylene terephthalate glycol*) (PETG) and *thermoplastics*. PETG plastics are relatively cost-effective and combine both strength and durability. In addition they offer the advantage of good optical properties in that the patient's anatomy can be viewed through the shell. It is important that an assessment is made as to the suitability of fit on a day-to-day basis

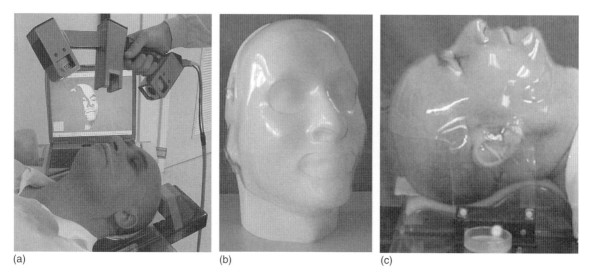

**Figure 7.1** Use of surface laser scanning for the manufacture of immobilisation shell: (a) surface laser scanning; (b) mask vacuum formed onto CNC 'positive'; (c) mask fitting. (Images courtesy of ARANZ Scanning Ltd.)

(a)                                    (b)                                    (c)

due to the risk of problems resulting from patient weight loss, or conversely tissue swelling as a result of treatment side effects. Construction of PETG plastic shells can be an involved process requiring the use of full mould room facilities. The immobilisation material is heated until soft, and then vacuum formed over a positive impression of the patient's anatomy (usually constructed via the use of a plaster of Paris mould). Repeat visits of the patient for the purpose of shell construction and fitting may also be necessary. A full description of the process of shell construction can be found elsewhere.[1] However, there are alternative solutions to the use of plaster of Paris impressions. It is now possible to use laser technologies to replace the need for the construction of a physical impression. Using non-contact laser scanning it is possible to determine the three-dimensional contours of the patient and process the data in order that a positive impression can be milled on a dedicated *computer numerical controlled* (CNC) *milling machine*, or bypassing the machining stage by directly printing a 3D plastic mask. The obvious advantage to this method is that it avoids the need for the patient to undergo

the often claustrophobic process of plaster of Paris impression manufacture (Figure 7.1).

Alternative materials in use include perforated thermoplastics. During construction it is necessary to select a suitable length of the immobilisation material according to need, e.g. a full shell may be required that extends over the shoulders and upper thorax – a consideration for those patients for whom supraclavicular nodal or anterior lower neck irradiation is indicated (Figure 7.2).

Mask construction requires the material first to be softened (usually via the use of a hot water bath) and subsequently draped over the patient's face. While soft, it is necessary to mould the plastic across the patient's contours, ensuring that the material follows the outline of the bony prominences in the head and neck. During subsequent use of the mask it can be accurately sited on these landmarks.

When cooled the material becomes stiff and serves as rigid immobilisation. Slight shrinkage of the material usually ensues, although this does not usually compromise patient fit. One advantage of such materials is that they are relatively

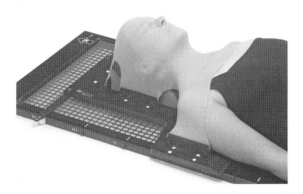

**Figure 7.2** Thermoplastic immobilisation shell extending over shoulders. (Image courtesy of Oncology Systems Ltd, Shrewsbury, UK and CIVCO Medical Solutions, Iowa, USA.)

easy to adjust should a patient gain or lose weight, requiring shell modification to ensure acceptable fit. When reheated the material has a tendency to flatten and return to its original shape – so-called 'plastic memory'. By local heating of the material (e.g. via the use of a heat gun) the mask can be re-formed to accommodate changes to the patient contour.

A reliable fixation mechanism must also be used to attach the shell to the dedicated baseplate system, which allows secure attachment while allowing for easy release of the patient from the device.

Many radiotherapy departments have expanded the use of thermoplastic devices because they preclude the need for full mould room facilities, and there is an increasing evidence base to suggest that they perform favourably compared with other immobilisation systems.[2]

## Bite blocks

For some treatments it may be necessary to treat the patient with the mouth open or to move the tongue away from the target volume during treatment. Despite the external fixation methods outlined previously, there is still scope for treatment position uncertainty due to jaw movements and movement of the tongue. A bite block (or

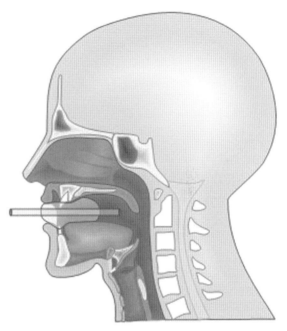

**Figure 7.3** Position of mouth bite *in situ*.

mouth 'gag') provides a means of maintaining the mouth in the open position and ensuring that the tongue remains depressed. Many radiotherapy departments opt to manufacture in-house devices that employ materials used for dental impressions such as specialised *dental wax* or *dental compound*. When used, this material is heat softened and shaped around a suitable plastic tube, which ensures that the patient's airway is not compromised during use. The patient then bites down onto the wax and in doing so an impression of the teeth is obtained. The material is left to harden, and on subsequent use when inserted into the mouth the patient is able to relocate the block into the desired position. The resultant position of the bite block and tongue depressor is illustrated in Figure 7.3. Obviously it is important that the construction of the bite block be undertaken after any remedial dental work has been carried out (e.g. dental extraction), and that it is ready for use before the construction of a facial mask. The use of bite blocks may present some problems for edentulous patients or patients experiencing severe oral mucositis, and for all patients it is usual to disinfect the bite block after each use.

Commercially there are bite blocks available that can also aid head stability, where the bite block attaches to the overlying thermoplastic cast. Rotation and flexion movements may be reduced in addition to suitable tongue displacement.

## Immobilisation equipment for breast treatment

Despite comprising a significant proportion of planned radical work within a typical radiotherapy department, breast irradiation remains challenging due to the complexities of breast planning, given the range of anatomical variation present among this patient group. The breast itself has a complex shape, and has an irregular contour and changing tissue separation along the length of the intended treatment volume.[3] In addition, breast treatment techniques remain involved due to the need for suitable irradiation of the chest wall and overlying tissues while reducing excessive doses to the lung and heart. Rotation of the patient's torso coupled with respiratory motion can compromise treatment accuracy. Patients may also be required to adopt treatment positions that permit supraclavicular and axillary nodal irradiation. For these patients their treatment position is a crucial factor in the determination of accurate field matching with breast tangents, and stability and reproducibility of the patient's position can determine whether there will be overdosing at the match line. The demand for positional accuracy can be frustratingly difficult in patients who present with limited mobility in the upper limb, e.g. after partial mastectomy or axillary lymph node clearance.

### Positioning

Radiotherapy to the breast or chest wall usually requires the patient to be irradiated via the use of glancing tangential fields across the patient's thorax. This can be achieved only if the patient is positioned in a manner such that the arm on the affected side of the body is placed into an abducted position away from the chest wall. It may be appropriate for both arms to be elevated for treatment and positioning may be more reproducible in this position;[4] however, machine restrictions may permit the elevation and support only of the ipsilateral arm. For many patients it is also appropriate to elevate the upper thorax in order to ensure that the sternum is lying horizontally. By doing so the need for collimator angulation on tangential fields is removed, and the irradiated lung volume can be reduced in the caudocephalic direction.[5]

To achieve this treatment position a positioning device is required to maintain thoracic elevation and arm abduction. The device must allow for adjustment of patient position required during the planning process while permitting the adoption of a comfortable treatment position to suit each individual patient. Most frequently radiotherapy departments will make use of a dedicated *breast board*. Modern breast boards employ an ergonomic design that permits the patient to be placed in a suitable position for treatment that is comfortable and stable. It is also necessary for such devices to be compatible with both the CT scanner and the treatment couch. Earlier CT planning techniques were limited to those patients whose position could be accommodated by the width of the CT aperture; however, recently the wider availability and increased use of dedicated radiotherapy 'widebore' scanners (i.e. bore width of 80–90 cm) allows the use of CT planning for most breast patients positioned on a breast board.

### Breast board design

A number of breast board designs are commercially available. Earlier wooden devices have been superseded by the use of acrylic materials and many modern devices are now constructed

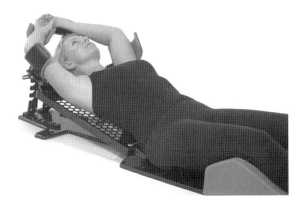

**Figure 7.4** Carbon fibre breast board. (Image courtesy of Oncology Systems Ltd, Shrewsbury, UK and CIVCO Medical Solutions, Iowa, USA.)

from low-density foam within a carbon fibre outer shell. This ensures minimum attenuation of the treatment beam should treatment beams encroach on to the breast board itself. The practical use of such equipment is relatively straightforward and each patient's individual position can be readily reproduced by reliance on an indexing system, allowing the relocation of the arm, elbow, hand and wrist (Figure 7.4). Patient position may vary along the caudocephalic plane; however, this can be addressed by an indexed 'hip-stop' and knee immobilisation to prevent the patient from sliding down the board during treatment. Additional use of vacuum mould immobilisation systems with breast boards may be of use in a few patients for whom comfort is difficult to achieve, although their routine use may not translate as significant elimination of set-up error.[6]

The patient's head position is maintained by a dedicated headrest system that itself can be relocated according to the comfort and anatomy of the patient, while permitting the extension of the chin away from the radiation beams. The headrest system should ideally permit lateral rotation of the head if required, for example, during irradiation of the supraclavicular region.

## Immobilisation for larger breast size

Patients with larger breast size present some particular challenges with respect to immobilisation of the target organ and achieving optimal dosimetry. For these patients the supine position can result in the movement of breast tissue superiorly and laterally, requiring the adjustment of posterior field borders laterally, which can lead to a considerable increase in the volume of irradiated lung. As a consequence it may be appropriate to select a method of immobilising the whole breast and/or selecting the use of a non-standard treatment position.

Most frequently breast immobilisation devices are constructed in house and usually include the manufacture of a custom-made 'treatment brassière' made from thermoplastic or polyurethane-based plastics. Preformed shells may also be available. Their use maintains the position of large or flaccid breasts in a reproducible position while moving the contralateral breast away from the treatment position. They may also be effective at eliminating excessive skinfolds, which can help reduce the likelihood of skin toxicity. However, the use of immobilisation shells for breast immobilisation necessarily reduces the phenomenon of skin sparing. One solution to this is to cut out areas of the immobilisation device, but this can lead to uncertainties in the reliability of the breast position. Modified devices such as a *microshell* have undergone trials, which may go some way to achieving breast support with minimal increases in skin surface dose.[7]

Alternative positioning strategies for this patient group have also been suggested, and include the use of decubitus or prone positions. Use of the prone position for patients with pendulous breasts potentially improves dosimetry, reduces normal tissue irradiation and improves set-up reliability.[8] A number of positioning aids are available that permit customised prone patient positioning, such as *prone breast boards* (Figure 7.5). An important consideration for this

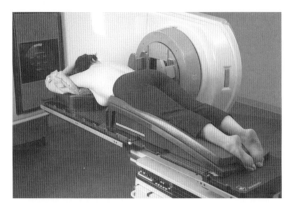

**Figure 7.5** Prone breast board. (Image courtesy of Oncology Systems Ltd, Shrewsbury, UK and CIVCO Medical Solutions, Iowa, USA.)

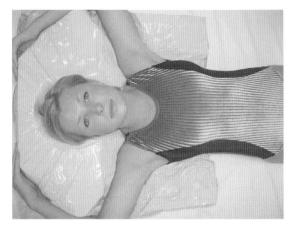

**Figure 7.6** Thoracic positioning mould. (Image courtesy of Smithers Medical Products Inc.)

treatment position is the location of the contralateral breast, which should ideally be rotated away from the treatment beam. A suitable aperture should be present in the prone breast board on the ipsilateral side, which allows the breast to fall under gravity into the required treatment position through an open treatment couch panel. The resultant position of the affected breast permits the use of lateral treatment fields during treatment delivery.

While this prone technique may be effective for some large-breasted patients one important consideration is the position of the presenting primary lesion within the breast. Where the original lesion is in proximity to the chest wall, the prone position may be inappropriate as suitable coverage of the target volume may not be achievable because the lateral treatment fields would collide with the treatment couch.

## Thorax immobilisation

For simple techniques in the thorax it is not necessary to use complex immobilisation devices. For parallel pair techniques to the chest it may be necessary only to select a reproducible position that ensures patient comfort by the use of a standard range of foam wedges and cushions.

For planned volume techniques it is usual to position the patient in an arms-up position in order to accommodate obliquely placed treatment fields while avoiding the patient's arms. This can be achieved by using a *chestboard* which, like breast boards, allows for a range of upper limb positions to be selected but without the use of a thoracic incline. In these patients it is important that the arm receives adequate support and many of these devices feature a dedicated elbow support or characteristic 'wing'. *Vacuum bag systems* or positioning moulds may also be used (Figure 7.6).

## Immobilisation equipment for pelvic treatment

Reproducible positioning of the patient is critical in the pelvis, not least due to the juxtaposition of critical structures and the high-dose treatment zone. Dose escalation may therefore be achieved only if attention is paid to pelvic immobilisation. In addition, interfractional differences in anatomical position of soft tissue structures within the pelvis should be considered, and these themselves can be affected to varying degrees by the positioning of the patient.

For many pelvic treatments the use of simple leg and/or ankle immobilisation is considered appropriate and there is evidence that the use of immobilisation can reduce the incidence of positional errors >5 mm to between 4% and 8% of displacements detected on portal imaging.[9]

For supine treatment positions a variety of foam rubber supports is available that helps maintain stability and aids reproducibility, not least due to the fact that the supports offer additional comfort in the region of the lumbosacral spine for patients lying on a hard treatment couch. There are a number of commercially available devices, and many aim to raise the knees while achieving a suitable treatment position. Ankle positioning devices may also be used where a consistent foot position is desirable during treatment; such devices often take the form of so-called 'ankle stocks' and may extend as far superiorly as the knee joint as 'leg-stocks'. These devices have the beneficial feature that they act to separate the feet while limiting external or internal rotation of the lower limb, which in turn can govern the accuracy of pelvic position.

Alternative methods of pelvis immobilisation can be employed that aim to provide individualised bespoke positioning tailored to the contours of each patient. These can take the form of half-body positioning systems that may extend from hip to ankle. Vacuum bag systems may be used which comprise a reinforced bag containing polystyrene beads positioned beneath the patient. Using a vacuum pump air is extracted and the bag moulds to the contours of the patient. This mould is retained as long as the access port is sealed. This is a relatively easy process and the bags have the potential to be reused once treatment is complete. Care is required to prevent puncturing of the device because any leakage may result in a loss of the rigid patient outline.

Alternatively body moulds can be formed via the use of foaming chemicals within a bag that provides rigid immobilisation. Such systems (e.g. Alpha Cradle, Smithers Medical Products, Inc.)

employ expanded polyurethane foam that is moulded to the contours of the patient. This foam expands and hardens after the mixing of constituent chemicals, and the expansion process takes place with the patient lying on the device within a supporting 'cradle'. During the construction process care is required to eliminate excess air from the bag, and to ensure that the foam is distributed equally across the region of the patient's back, legs and hips. A decision needs to be made whether to use hip-to-ankle or a shorter hip-to-knee mould. Such systems are non-reusable and may constitute some additional storage requirements compared with more simple techniques. In addition one report describes the possibility of difficulties with placing elderly and obese patients into and out of their cast.[10]

Prone treatments present additional positioning challenges. For patients undergoing irradiation of a rectal carcinoma a prone position is frequently favoured due to the need to irradiate posteriorly located treatment volumes, which may necessitate the use of posterior fields encompassing the buttocks. Treating in the prone position enables a degree of separation of the natal cleft, which can help maintain the skin-sparing effect. Immobilisation of prone patients can be inherently problematic, and there are marked difficulties, particularly with elderly patients. The discomfort experienced by patients arises as they attempt to 'balance' their bony pelvis on a hard couch top. Simple immobilisation devices such as ankle pads afford a degree of comfort by allowing slight flexion of the knee joint, avoiding contact of the dorsum of the foot with the couch top. Patients are ordinarily positioned with their arms above their heads; however, care needs to be taken to ensure that the patient's arms and head are comfortable because variation can introduce variability of pelvic skin markings. This can be facilitated via the use of a dedicated positioning aid such as a modified prone pillow. Other confounding factors such as the presence of an abdominal ileostomy pouch can lead to uncertainties as to the accuracy of patient positioning. Prone treatments may also be indicated for other pelvic malignancies such as carcinoma of the prostate gland, although daily set-up variability appears less accurate than supine set-ups, particularly in the absence of immobilisation devices.[11]

In obese patients prone positioning presents additional problems due to the uncertainty and variability of skin marks and patient comfort issues, and that the prone position itself may increase the risk of irradiation of small bowel. Invasive surgical techniques to immobilise the bowel have been attempted such as the use of *omentoplasty* or *intrapelvic prostheses*;[12] however, thankfully the need for surgical immobilisation is rare due to significant developments in imaging and treatment planning. Positioning and immobilisation devices may be used that address the position of abdominal and bowel variability. The use of a 'belly board' or open-couch device may increase comfort and has been highlighted as one method of reducing gastrointestinal toxicities.[13] These devices may be constructed from a variety of materials such as polystyrene, although the use of carbon fibre devices is indicated if the device occludes treatment portals. Each device requires the patient to be supported in a manner in which the belly region can be comfortably accommodated while lying in the prone treatment position (Figure 7.7). Adequate support for the upper legs and symphysis pubis is necessary, as is adequate

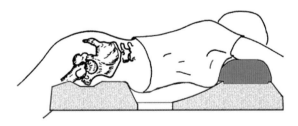

**Figure 7.7** Patient position during use of prone 'belly board'. (Image courtesy of Oncology Systems Ltd, Shrewsbury, UK and CIVCO Medical Solutions, Iowa, USA.)

support for the patient's arms and head. Reproducibility is aided by the use of an indexing system on the device, which enables the isocentre to be located in the longitudinal direction.

Whether supine or prone, consideration should be given as to the use of rigid external immobilisation devices for pelvic irradiation. The use of thermoplastic immobilisation shells may be appropriate for patients with mobile skin marks; however, reported potential gains in the accuracy of positioning[14] may be countered by additional costs and increased set-up complexity. In addition it should be ensured that such external fixation devices are compatible with CT scanners.

## Organ immobilisation

### Rectal catheters

Modern approaches to pelvic treatment delivery require day-to-day reduction in set-up variability in patient position. Translational and rotational movements may be reduced via the use of external fixation devices or the use of patient supports that aid comfort and stability. However, there is a new focus on the notion that the variable position of individual organs themselves should be considered. Uncertainty in the position of the target volume potentially negates improvements in planning accuracy and the use of highly conformal techniques. One of the frustrations of treatment accuracy is that, although it is quite possible to achieve a level of immobilisation of bony elements of the pelvis, there may be a large variability in internal anatomy between successive fractions (interfraction variability) or during each treatment fraction (intrafraction variability). Potential methods that decrease the volume of normal tissue in the high dose region should lead to decreased morbidity, providing scope for dose escalation.[15]

Irradiation of the prostate gland presents some significant challenges due to the often pronounced effect that differential rectal filling and flatus distension have on the position of the prostate gland itself, and the motion of the rectal wall relative to the high-dose region. Reproducibility of the rectal position can be achieved by encouraging the patient to void the rectum before treatment. This relatively simple solution may be unreliable, however, not least due to difficulties in compliance for patients who are required to empty their rectum 'at will', and subjective perceptions of what constitutes an 'empty' bowel by the patient. In addition the rectum position may still be variable when empty.[16] One method in which these variables are reduced is the use of internal immobilisation methods such as the use of an inflated rectal balloon catheter. The catheter is tested for leaks and subsequently covered by a protective sheath before being inserted in to the patient's rectum. Depression of the syringe plunger introduces between 50 and 100 cm$^3$ of air into the balloon (according to patient comfort), which once inflated acts to immobilise the prostate and displace rectal tissue in the posterolateral direction. The procedure is undertaken during planning CT scans and then for each subsequent treatment fraction. Despite this being a potentially distressing invasive procedure, which might otherwise potentially decrease patient comfort, the use of the rectal balloon is reported as being tolerated well by patients.

In addition there may be a dosimetric precedent for the use of an air-filled balloon catheter, since at the interface between the air and tissue there is a slight reduction in dose. This phenomenon appears to affect only a small region of the anterior rectal wall in the region of the interface without compromising dose coverage to the target volume. Research[17] indicates that dose at this point is reduced to approximately 15% less than where a balloon catheter is not used. Potentially this may result in a dose reduction to the anterior rectal wall, which realises lessened acute rectal toxicities.

The use of a rectal balloon significantly reduces prostate motion. An increased degree of immobilisation of soft tissue structures potentially makes planning target volume delineation more reliable and may permit smaller treatment margins to be used. Such precise targeting is essential for 3D-conformal radiotherapy and in particular in the use of IMRT. Obviously the use of a rectal balloon catheter presents an additional treatment procedure that may add to the workload of the radiographer, although routine use and gradual patient compliance would hopefully facilitate the procedure.

## Respiratory movements

Movement due to respiration can be a significant influence in altering the anatomical position of the target volume and may constitute a major cause of intrafraction variability. Chest wall movements may also reduce the reliability of surface reference marks, which can lead to set-up errors. The effects of these movements are obviously important when considering the treatment of intrathoracic disease, but may also exert an influence on organ position at more remote anatomical locations such as the pelvis. Dedicated breathing control systems such as the *active breathing control* (ABC) system[18] provide for regulation of patient breathing via the use of a modified ventilator system that aims to minimise the margins for breathing motion. At a predetermined tidal lung volume inspiratory and expiratory airflow is temporarily blocked, thus immobilising the chest momentarily (nasal air flow is prevented due to the use of an occlusive nasal clip) (Figure 7.8). The system is usually employed in conjunction with thorax immobilisation devices such as vacuum bags or immobilisation frames.[19] This in effect restrains the patient within a breath-held position which has the potential to produce a reproducible position for planning and for use in gated radiotherapy techniques.

ABC devices operate via the use of control valves that close and dictate flow direction at specific points in the breathing cycle. Lung volume detection is critical in the process in

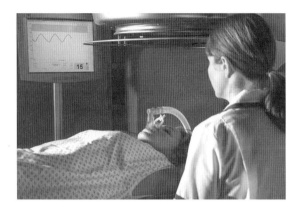

**Figure 7.8** Active breathing coordinator. (Image courtesy of Elekta Ltd.)

order to achieve the predetermined chest position. *Pneumotachograph spirometry* or motion detection imaging may be used together with the use of dedicated computer software to accomplish this. Importantly, ABC systems should also include an abort button that restores airflow in the event of patient distress.

The value of ABC devices is that they reliably hold the patient's thorax at predetermined points in the breathing cycle. This potentially provides positional information of the gross target volume (GTV) throughout the breathing cycle and may also eliminate breathing artefacts during CT imaging procedures.

Despite this it seems likely that the efficacy of the ABC system depends upon the use of patient training before its use; a lack of patient cooperation or compliance may be problematic, particularly where patients present with concurrent respiratory disease, which makes breath-holds problematic. In addition, systems by their very nature may increase treatment times and necessitate additional staff training.

## Immobilisation equipment for treatment of extremities

The irradiation of the extremities requires precise limb positioning, a task that is affected by a high

degree of mobility in the arm and leg. The lower limb position, for example, requires alignment with respect to the normal anatomical range of motion, including rotation, flexion, extension, abduction and adduction. For the limbs, there are also exacerbating considerations such as the need to irradiate long muscle compartments while ensuring the sparing of a strip of tissue in order to reduce the likelihood of oedema. It is usual to consider the immobilisation of the entire affected limb because relatively small deviations in the position of the proximal limb can result in large translational and rotational displacement of the distal structures. Practical immobilisation of the limb also requires due consideration as to whether the proposed treatment position permits treatment through a range of gantry and couch angles. In addition the patient position must ensure avoidance of critical structures and adjacent anatomy. In the case of the leg this means avoidance of the contralateral limb, while immobilisation devices for the upper limb must allow for the arm to be positioned away from the torso. Tumours located in the distal lower limb are often treated with the patient in a 'feet to gantry' position in order for the treatment site to be brought into range of the clinical beam, while permitting the full range of couch movements to be used during set up.

*Limb immobilisation* can be achieved in a variety of ways including the use of vacuum bag systems or positioning moulds (Figure 7.9). Alternatively thermoplastic materials can be employed that can completely immobilise the treated limb. For lesions of the lower limb it is possible to construct an immobilisation 'boot' which anchors the ankle joint and prevents rotational movements. Where used with sagittal skin tattoos a high degree of reproducibility can be afforded. However, it is important to consider immobilising the entire affected limb using an immobilisation shell to prevent movement. In the upper limb similar positioning strategies are used, although it is favourable to choose immobilisation devices that permit the affected limb to be positioned in

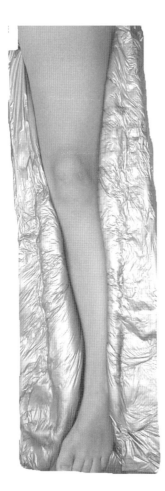

**Figure 7.9** Leg immobilisation using positioning mould. (Image courtesy of Smithers Medical Products Inc.)

the abducted position so as not to inadvertently include the normal tissues of the trunk or axilla. CT planning of limbs can prove to be technically difficult, particularly when there is a need for the elevation of the unaffected limb. In this case there is a need to adapt the position of the contralateral limb during the scanning procedure so that the patient will be clear of the CT aperture.

## Superficial radiotherapy

*Patient immobilisation for the treatment of superficial lesions* tends to be simplistic with patient comfort and stability achievable via the use of foam pads, cushions and immobilisation blocks. Whether using electrons or superficial X-ray photon beams, the aim is to position the patient in a manner in which the affected site is accessible to enable close contact with machine applicators, while being comfortable for the patient.

For superficial skin lesions in the head region the stability of the patient's head position can be maintained by the use of a securing headband or surgical tape, coupled with laterally placed sandbags, which can effectively act to 'chock' the patient's head in position. The treatment technique may also require the use of a custom-made lead cut-out that defines the radiation field and provides shielding to adjacent structures. The lead cut-out is formed so that it follows the contours of the patient's face such that accurate repositioning is achievable. Construction of the lead cut-out requires it to be hammered into shape over a positive pre-formed cast of the patient's face (Figure 7.10). For treatment, the cut-out is positioned over the treatment site so that the treatment field encloses the lesion plus its treatment margin. A suitable applicator size is chosen to cover the treatment site. Very slight movements in the patient's head position should not therefore result in a geographical miss because the lead cut-out may move with the patient's head and the target remains within the treatment beam. For some treatments there is the risk of dosing the radiosensitive mucous membrane lining the nose or inside the lip. In such cases it is possible to use a lead strip inserted into the nasal vestibule or the buccal cavity as additional protection. If treatment involves electron therapy there is a need to line this additional lead shielding, as a means of absorbing any secondary electrons liberated by interaction of the primary beam and the lead.

For superficial treatments elsewhere in the body it may not be necessary to immobilise patients in ways other than to achieve patient comfort with a degree of reproducibility.

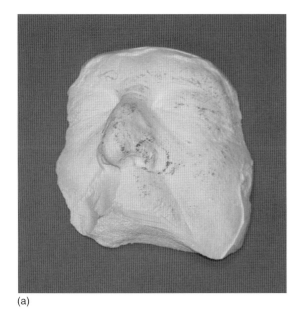

(a)

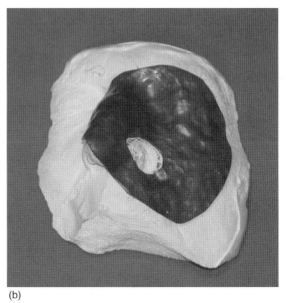

(b)

**Figure 7.10** (a) Impression of patient's face constructed from stone plaster; (b) custom-made lead cut-out in position surrounding lesion.

However, in the use of electrons for phased treatments it is usual to administer these fields with the patient in their associated photon treatment position to prevent an inaccurate junction at any photon–electron match line.

## Immobilisation for less common techniques

There are a number of treatment scenarios for which a conventional supine or prone treatment position is unachievable, or where the patient's position needs to be adapted to facilitate access to the treatments site, e.g. where an electron field is to be employed.

### Seated treatments

For certain emergency cases (e.g. superior vena cava obstruction) or where a patient's immobility prevents the patient from being able to lie down,

it may be necessary to administer treatment with the patient in a seated position. For this purpose a dedicated *treatment chair* can be used. A number of commercially available chairs are available which are either secured on the couch top or can be used as free-standing devices within the treatment room. Once transferred into the treatment chair, the treatment position is maintained by the use of arm supports and a Velcro head strap. Some systems may also use a baseplate system that additionally enables the use of thermoplastic immobilisation masks.

For patients for whom thoracic fields are indicated and for whom a horizontal position is unobtainable, it may be necessary to administer a parallel pair technique with the patient in the treatment chair. This is achieved by administering an unobstructed posterior treatment field via a mesh 'treatment window' in the back support panel. In addition the provision of arm supports permits the use of 'arms-up' or 'arms-down' positions with such devices (Figure 7.11). Accu-

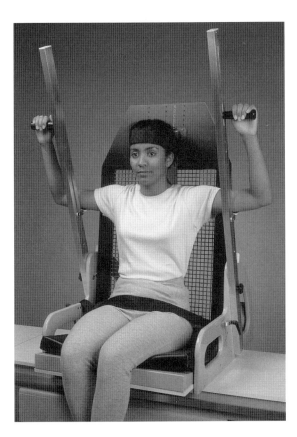

**Figure 7.11** Treatment chair. (Image courtesy of Oncology Systems Ltd, Shrewsbury, UK and CIVCO Medical Solutions, Iowa, USA.)

rate field positioning can be achieved in such systems as the full range of couch and tabletop movements is permissible.

## Unconventional positions

For certain techniques it is necessary for the patient to adopt an unconventional position, e.g. where the anatomical area for treatment is difficult to access. For disease involving the anal margin or perineum it may be necessary to immobilise the patient in a lateral position with the knees drawn upwards. Positioning and immobilisation are facilitated by the use of supports between the patient's knees and under the ankles. An alternative approach is to position the patient

hunched over a supporting pillow in order that the treatment site may be accessed. A relative degree of comfort may be difficult to achieve and it may be necessary for treatment centres to improvise using a combination of pillows and foam rubber immobilisation supports or to develop in-house immobilisation devices.

## Total body irradiation

Individual total body irradiation (TBI) techniques have evolved over time and vary between individual departments. Patient immobilisation and positioning present a number of challenges not least due to the need to undertake extensive in vivo dosimetry at a number of anatomical loci on these patients. TBI techniques ordinarily require treatments at extended treatment distances, and it is not usually practical to achieve such treatments on the usual treatment couch. Many departments utilise a dedicated TBI couch that allows the patient to adopt a semi-recumbent position for treatment, and can be moved easily to the required treatment position and rotated for lateral exposures. For treatment the patient may adopt a position with the arms across the chest to act as compensators, and additional supporting straps may provide the additional support for this purpose. An alternative would be to position the patient such that he or she is lying on the side. Immobilisation can be achieved in this position via the use of an immobilising vacuum bag or bespoke foam support.[20]

Alternatives to the use of a TBI couch may include use of a chair or devices that support the patient in the standing position.

## Radiotherapy treatment of the penis

Irradiation of patients with carcinoma of the penis requires an immobilisation strategy that may also provide a means of achieving a homogeneous dose distribution and ensuring the necessary use of build-up. This is achieved by the use of a Perspex or wax block containing a cylindrical cavity. The position of the penis relative to the block can be maintained by packing the cylinder with paraffin gauze or by the use of a Tubigrip to hold it in position. The treatment block itself is positioned on top of a lead scrotal shield, and it is usually necessary to secure the immobilisation device in place by the simple use of surgical tape or securing straps.

## Stereotactic radiotherapy

Stereotactic radiotherapy involves the use of multiple small conformal beams of radiation that are precisely administered to the patient. This is usually achieved via the use of a three-dimensional external coordinate system that is used to localise the intended treatment site within the patient. Adequate immobilisation is a necessary prerequisite to ensure treatment accuracy, and for treatment sites in the head region the positioning strategy requires elimination of all head motion such that the head is completely restrained: usually achieved via the use of a dedicated head frame that incorporates a three-dimensional referencing system permitting positioning accuracy in the order of 1 mm.

Invasive immobilisation devices were originally used for such purposes, whereby a *stereotactic head frame* such as the Brown–Roberts–Wells device was attached directly to the head via self-tapping cranial screws secured under anaesthesia. This head ring or 'halo' device thus served to fix the patient's head while presenting a reliable set of external stereotactic coordinate points. These are of use in single fraction treatments (stereotactic radiosurgery), e.g. in the delivery of treatment of an arteriovenous malformation (AVM); however, they are generally considered too uncomfortable for protracted radiotherapy treatments over a number of days (stereotactic radiotherapy).

Non-invasive, relocatable, head immobilisation devices are available for use in fractionated techniques. Many of these utilise a custom-made

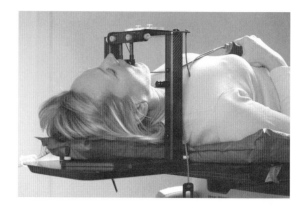

**Figure 7.12** Immobilisation system for stereotactic radiotherapy using bite block and vacuum bag cushion. (Image courtesy of Elekta Ltd.)

bite-block system in which the patient bites down on an integral bespoke bite plate constructed from dental impression material (Figure 7.12). A vacuum cushion may also be used in an effort to reduce lateral deviation and rotation of the head. Additional head support may be offered via the use of head fixation straps, individualised occipital pads or an external fixation device such as a thermoplastic shell.

Stereotactic radiotherapy techniques may also be undertaken at other extracranial locations, e.g. within the thorax, abdomen or pelvis. This is usually achieved using a suitable immobilisation device such as a vacuum bag coupled with an external *stereotactic body frame*, which provides a referencing system for accurate definition of the coordinates of an internal target during CT or MRI planning procedures. Organ motion can compromise the accuracy of target localisation at these sites, however, and it may be necessary to adopt the use of organ stabilisation strategies (e.g. active breathing control) in tandem with stereotactic body immobilisation.

## Conclusion

Although radiotherapy departments vary in their choice of patient immobilisation strategies, the principal of elimination of patient (and organ) movement in an effort to improve accuracy of treatment remains common to all. It is right that, when considering the variety of immobilisation options that may be used, the comfort and safety of the patient remain paramount, not least because a comfortable patient is more likely to

remain still. There may be significant difficulties and challenges where patient immobilisation is indicated, e.g. in the treatment of children or patients who are uncooperative for a number of reasons. For these patients anaesthesia or sedation may be a last-resort strategy to ensure the elimination of excessive movement.

## Self-test questions

1. Why may immobilisation devices be required during external beam radiotherapy treatments?
2. What considerations should be made when deciding on the use of immobilisation devices during CT planning procedures?
3. What considerations may be taken into account when deciding on the use of thermoplastic or PETG as a material for construction of an immobilisation shell?
4. What are the main advantages to the patient in the use of a surface scanning system when constructing a mask of the head and neck region?
5. In creating an immobilisation shell of the head and neck area, specifically which anatomical prominences of the region should be moulded to ensure an easily re-positioned mask?
6. In addition to immobilisation of the patient, what other practical use does the immobilisation mask provide?
7. Why are bite blocks used?
8. When considering patient treatment reactions, what is a disadvantage of using an immobilisation shell for treatment in the head and neck area?
9. How may skin reactions be limited when using an immobilisation shell for treatment in the head and neck region?
10. Why would the breast board generally be set at an incline for treatment of breast patients?
11. When immobilising a larger breasted patient, what difficulties may be encountered using a standard breast board system?
12. Describe an immobilisation strategy that may be used in the treatment of large or flaccid breasts.
13. Which immobilisation technique may be employed during the planning and delivery of planned volume treatments to the thorax?
14. Describe methods of immobilising the patient for treatment to the pelvic region.
15. What advantage does the use of a rectal catheter bring to the treatment of a prostate patient?
16. Describe how respiratory movement may be limited for a patient receiving treatment to the thorax.
17. What practical considerations must be taken into account when immobilising an arm?
18. Describe the immobilisation technique used, when treating a patient with a basal cell carcinoma of the left ala nasi via the use of superficial radiotherapy.
19. Describe the main immobilisation option for a patient who is unable to lie in a supine treatment position for treatment.
20. Describe a non-invasive immobilisation strategy that may be employed during stereotactic radiotherapy to the brain.

## Acknowledgements

The authors of this chapter would like to acknowledge the information provided by various manufacturers mentioned in the text. Particular thanks are also due to Nicola Bartholomew for additional artwork and Becky Hewitt for photography.

## References

1. Bomford CK, Kunkler IH. *Walter and Miller's Textbook of Radiotherapy*, 6th edn. Edinburgh: Churchill Livingstone, 2003.
2. Fuss M, Salter BJ, Cheek D, Sadeghio A, Hevezi JM, Herman TS. Repositioning accuracy of a commercially available thermoplastic mask system. *Radiother Oncol* 2004; 71: 339–45.

3. Winfield EA, Deighton A, Venables K, Hoskin PJ, Aird EGA. Survey of tangential field planning and dose distribution in the UK: background to the introduction of the quality assurance programme for the START trial in early breast cancer. *Br J Radiol* 2003; **76**: 254–9.
4. Winfield EA, Deighton A, Venables K, Hoskin PJ, Aird EGA. Survey of UK breast radiotherapy techniques: Background prior to the introduction of the quality assurance programme for the START (standardisation of radiotherapy) trial in breast cancer. *Clin Oncol* 2002; **14**: 267–21.
5. Griffiths S, Short C. *Radiotherapy: Principles to practice*. Edinburgh: Churchill Livingstone, 1994.
6. Nalder CA, Bidmead AM, Mubata CD, Beardmore C. Influence of a vac-fix immobilization device on the accuracy of patient positioning during routine breast radiotherapy. *Br J Radiol* 2001; **74**: 249–54.
7. Latimer JG, Beckham W, West M, Holloway L, Delaney G. Support of large breast during tangential irradiation using a micro-shell and minimizing the skin dose – a pilot study. *Med Dosimetry* 2005; **30**: 31–5.
8. Algan Ö, Fowble B, McNeeley S, Fein D. Use of the prone position in radiation treatment for women with early stage breast cancer. *Int J Rad Oncol Biol Phys* 1998; **40**: 1137–40.
9. Langmack K, Routsis D. Towards an evidence based treatment technique in prostate radiotherapy. *J Radiother Pract* 2001; **2**: 91–100.
10. Mitine C, Hoornaert M, Dutreix A, Beauduin M. Radiotherapy of pelvic malignancies: impact of two types of rigid immobilisation devices on localisation errors. *Radiother Oncol* 1999; **52**: 19–27.
11. Weber D, Nouet P, Rouzaud M, Miralbell R. Patient positioning in prostate radiotherapy: is prone better than supine? *Int J Rad Oncol Biol Phys* 2000; **47**: 365–71.
12. Logmans A, Trimbon JB, van Lent M. The omentoplasty: a neglected ally in gynaecologic surgery. *Eur J Obstet Gynaecol* 1995; **58**: 167–71.
13. Allal AS, Bischof S, Nouet P. Impact of the 'belly board' device on treatment reproducibility in pre-operative radiotherapy for rectal cancer. *Strahlentherapie Onkologie* 2002; **5**: 259–62.
Malone S, Szanto J, Perry G et al. A prospective comparison of three systems of patient immobilisation for prostate radiotherapy. *Int J Rad Oncol Biol Phys* 2000; **48**: 657–65.
14. Patel R, Orton N, Tomé WA, Chappell R, Ritter MA. Rectal dose sparing with a balloon catheter and ultrasound localization in conformal radiation therapy for prostate cancer. *Radiother Oncol* 2003; **67**: 285–94.
15. Bridge P. A critical evaluation of internal organ immobilisation techniques. *J Radiother Pract* 2004; **4**: 118–25.
16. Teh BS, McGary JE, Dong L et al. The use of rectal balloon during the delivery of intensity modulated radiotherapy (IMRT) for prostate cancer: more than just a prostate gland immobilization device? *Cancer J* 2002; **8**: 476–83.
17. Wong JW, Sharpe MB, Jaffray DA et al. The use of active breathing control (ABC) to reduce margin for breathing motion. *Int J Rad Oncol Biol Phys* 1999; **44**: 911–19.
18. Wilson EM, Williams FJ, Lyn BE, Wong JW, Aird EGA. Validation of active breathing control in patients with non-small-cell lung cancer to be treated with chartwel. *Int J Rad Oncol Biol Phys* 2003; **57**: 864–74.
19. Taylor RE. Principles of paediatric radiation Oncology. In: Hoskin P (ed.), *Radiotherapy in Practice: External beam therapy*. Oxford: Oxford University Press, 2006: 407–37.

## Further reading

Bentel G. (1999) *Patient Positioning and Immobilization in Radiation Oncology*. London: McGraw-Hill.

# Chapter 8
# MEGAVOLTAGE EQUIPMENT

David Flinton and Elizabeth Miles

## Aims and objectives

The production of a photon beam using a conventional X-ray tube permits maximum beam energy only in the kilovoltage region. To produce higher-energy beams a different technology is required. The aim on completion of this chapter is to provide the reader with an overview of this technology, and the mechanisms of production of a clinical beam.

At the end of this chapter the reader will be able to:

- describe the basic components of a cobalt unit and gamma knife unit
- understand the role the components of a linear accelerator play in X-ray production
- describe X-ray production and the changes needed for electron production.

## Cobalt units

Decay of radioactive materials can produce high-energy *gamma rays* that may be used for *teletherapy* treatments. Currently, only one source, cobalt-60, remains in regular use. Cobalt-60 ($^{60}$Co) can be produced by placing cobalt-59 in a strong neutron field, the nucleus absorbing a neutron to form $^{60}$Co. As soon as it is formed $^{60}$Co starts to undergo radioactive decay to nickel-60 with a half-life of 5.26 years. The emissions are a $\beta^-$ particle with an energy of 0.31 MeV$_{(max)}$ and two gamma rays with energies of 1.17 MeV and 1.33 MeV.

The cobalt source is situated in a doubly encapsulated steel container, to prevent any leakage of cobalt; this also acts to filter out the unwanted $\beta^-$ particles. The cobalt is usually in the form of discs 2 mm thick and 17 mm in diameter stacked on top of each other until the desired air kerma rate is reached. Any spare space is filled with blank discs to prevent movement of the discs within the container when the treatment unit moves around the patient.

The unit in which the source is sealed is simple in construction and as such is very reliable. There are two basic types of unit: the *moving source* (a) and *fixed source* (b) (Figure 8.1). In the moving source unit the source moves from a safe position to a position just behind the primary collimator. As the source is continually emitting gamma rays when this movement occurs, the beam effectively switches on. In the fixed source unit the cobalt source is stationary, the primary collimator rotates opening up a passage for gamma rays to emerge.

Over a period of time the number of radioactive $^{60}$Co atoms decrease, and as a result so will the *dose rate*. As a result of this the time needed to treat a patient gradually lengthens and eventually, when the treatment time becomes excessive, the source has to be replaced, which should occur approximately every 3 years.

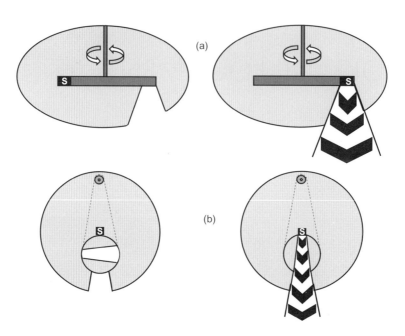

**Figure 8.1** The different types of cobalt unit.

The emerging beam has a $D_{max}$ situated at a depth of approximately 5 mm, which is approximately equivalent to that produced by a 2 MeV linear accelerator. The beam also has a large penumbra compared with beam produced by a linear accelerator. Part of the reason for this is the lower energy and the associated sideways scatter, depositing dose outside of the irradiated area. Another contributing factor is the diameter of the discs (17 mm) which equates to the focal spot size of the unit. This is a large area and can lead to a significant geometric penumbra. To help reduce this, units can be fitted with penumbra trimmers.

## Gamma knife

A more recent development utilising $^{60}$Co is the gamma knife stereotactic radiosurgery unit, essentially a multi-headed cobalt unit. An array of separate cobalt sources produce multiple fine beams of gamma radiation converging in three dimensions to focus precisely on to a small treat-ment volume. To gain the precision needed for treatment the patient is fitted with a stereotactic head frame fixed to the external table of the skull. This allows accurate localisation of the tumour and associated structures in relation to the three-dimensional coordinates of the head frame.

The gamma knife system includes a radiation unit, all components of which are static, and a movable treatment couch that provides the means for patient positioning. The beam geometry of the gamma knife unit can be hemispherical (a) or conical (b) in arrangement (Figure 8.2).

The hemispherical system employs an array of 201 cobalt sources shielded in a cast iron body, each mounted in line with a beam channel. The beam channel consists of a source-bushing assembly, a pre-collimator of tungsten alloy, a primary stationary collimator and a secondary conical collimator located in a helmet. The radiation beams are initially focused through the primary collimator system along the conical channel and through the secondary collimator, which defines the beam diameter at the focus point. There are

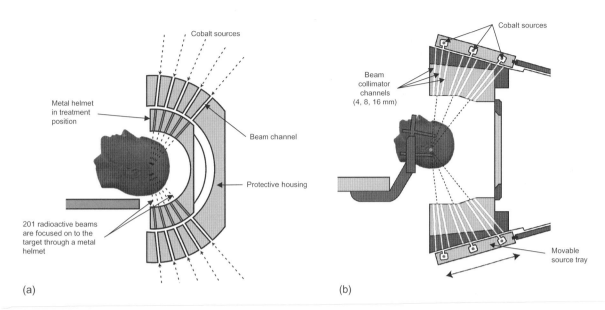

**Figure 8.2**  Hemispherical gamma knife beam geometry. (Images courtesy of Elekta Instrument AB.)

four interchangeable helmets with collimator sizes of 4, 8, 14, and 18 mm. The isodose distribution can be modified by delivering a multiple isocentre treatment using different collimator sizes or by employing beam plugging. The source to focus distance is 400 mm for all sources.

The *cone geometry system* differs significantly from the *hemispherical system*:[1] 192 cobalt sources are positioned in a cone section arranged in 8 sectors. A single sector contains 24 sources and 72 collimators; a single collimator of tungsten replaces the previously described primary and secondary collimator system. No collimator helmet is used; the couch functions as the patient positioning system moving the patient to predefined coordinates. The collimator sizes available are 4, 8 and 16 mm. The sources move longitudinally in a source tray to dock with individual beam collimator channels. Two further docking position are available, sector off effectively blocking a sector or home for when the unit is not in use. The resulting geometry of this unit means that the source-to-focus distance for individual sources ranges from 374 mm to 433 mm.

## Linear accelerators

Linear accelerators are machines that consist of a number of discrete components (Figure 8.3) functioning together to accelerate electrons to a high energy using radiofrequency (RF) waves before the electrons 'hit' a target to produce X-rays. After this the X-ray profile is flattened, shaped (collimated) and measured before clinical use. Linear accelerators are now also capable of producing X-ray beams of different energy (*multi-energy units*) and/or producing both X-rays and electrons (*multimodal units*).

## Production and transport of the RF wave

### RF generators, the magnetron and klystron

To accelerate the electrons to the required energy an RF wave is needed. This can be produced from one of two devices: either a magnetron, typically found in the lower energy units, or a klystron.

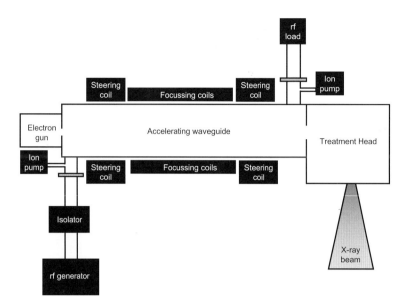

**Figure 8.3** Major components of the linear accelerator.

The magnetron consists of a cathode situated in the middle of a circular chamber which, when heated, releases electrons by *thermionic emission*. Either side of the magnetron is a permanent magnet that produces an axial magnetic field. The magnetic field is perpendicular to the electron's initial radial motion, which causes the electrons to spiral outward in a circular path rather than moving directly to the anode (see later – action of a magnet on an electron beam).

The cloud of electrons, influenced by both the high voltage and the strong magnetic field, form a rotating pattern resembling the spokes of a spinning wheel (Figure 8.4). Spaced around the rim of the circular chamber are cylindrical resonant cavities. As the electron spokes pass the openings of the cavities they cause the free electrons in the metal to spiral around the cavity (like charges repel), first one way then the other; this oscillation induces a resonant, high-frequency radio field in the cavity. An aerial then extracts the RF wave.

A klystron is an RF amplifier. The RF wave is produced by an oscillator. The wave then passes into the main body of the device, which consists of a series of resonant cavities. Electrons produced by an electron gun also enter the main body in phase with the RF wave. The oscillating RF field causes the electrons either to slow down (electrons arriving early in the phase) or to speed up (electrons arriving late in the phase), so causing the electrons to bunch together. When the electron bunches pass over the output cavity they excite a voltage on the output cavity, and the electrons will lose kinetic energy. The excitation of the cavity emits an RF wave that, as the electron bunches were arriving at a time interval equal to one cycle of the RF wave, will be in phase and add its power to the existing RF wave. The RF power then exits the klystron and the electrons, which have lost a significant amount of their energy, are then absorbed in an *electron catcher* or *beam dump*.

## Waveguide

A waveguide is used to transfer the RF wave to the accelerating structure which consists of a

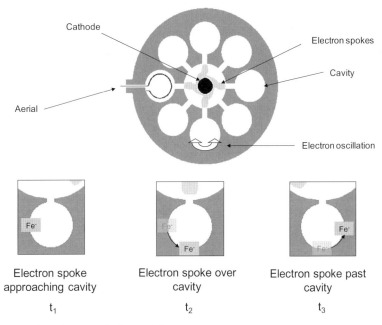

Electron spoke approaching cavity

$t_1$

Electron spoke over cavity

$t_2$

Electron spoke past cavity

$t_3$

$Fe^-$ = free electrons in the metal

**Figure 8.4** Magnetron.

series of hollow tubes. The waveguide contains *sulphur hexafluoride* ($SF_6$), an inert non-toxic gas at approximately two times atmospheric pressure. A gas is present as the transfer of RF waves is more efficient in a medium; however, due to the high energy of the RF wave electric arcing can take place. Sulphur hexafluoride is excellent at quenching the arcing,[2] so stopping excessive loss of power in the transfer of the RF wave to the accelerating structure. At the end of waveguide is an alumina disc ($Al_2O_3$) in a thin copper sleeve that allows the RF wave to pass but isolates the gas-filled RF waveguide from the vacuum in the accelerating waveguide.

Figure 8.3 shows the structure as a straight line, but, because of the position of the RF generator in relation to accelerating waveguide, the RF waveguide has to change directions a number of times; this may cause some reflection of the wave back towards the RF generator. Reflected RF waves passing back into the RF generator can detune the system. To stop this happening an

isolator, a passive device consisting of ferrite slabs, is placed along the RF waveguide which protects the RF power generator by blocking any returning waves.

## Production and acceleration of the electron beam

### Electron gun

Electrons are produced by thermionic emission from a heated cathode; an electrostatic field produced by the *cathode cup* focuses the electrons to a small area of the anode. The *anode*, unlike that in kilovoltage units, contains a hole where the electrons are focused, so rather than hit the anode they pass through the hole and enter the accelerating structure.

Two basic types of electron gun exist: the *diode* and *triode*. In the diode gun the voltage applied to the cathode is pulsed, so producing bunches of electrons rather than a continuous stream. The triode gun obtains discrete bunches of electrons by introducing a third component to the structure – a grid positioned just in front of the anode, between the anode and the cathode. The cathode has a constant potential and the voltage to the grid is pulsed. When the voltage applied to the grid is negative the electrons are stopped from reaching the anode. When the voltage from the grid is removed the electrons accelerate towards the anode. The grid can therefore control the frequency of electron pulses entering the accelerating structure. The pulses to the cathode or grid are controlled by a modulator which is also connected to the RF power generator.

## Accelerating structure

The main function of the accelerating structure is to accelerate the electrons, giving them energy that can then be converted into X-rays.

It is important that the electrons are correctly placed on the wave for maximum acceleration, which occurs in the first part of the accelerating structure, sometimes referred to as the bunching section. If we consider the electron bunches on the RF wave in Figure 8.5, they will all receive energy from the wave, causing them to be accelerated. The electron bunch in position 1 will receive a greater acceleration causing them to catch up with bunch 2. Electron bunch 3 will

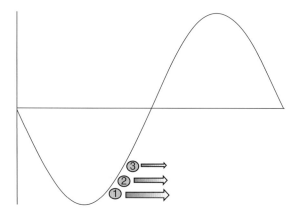

**Figure 8.5** Electron bunching.

receive less acceleration and move backwards on the wave in relation to bunches 1 and 2, until finally all the bunches merge together at the same point on the wave.

The energy given to the electrons is in the form of kinetic energy, but as the velocity of the electrons increase a significant proportion of the energy can be in the form of a gain in mass (see Relativistic changes and acceleration). This is referred to as a 'relativistic change in mass'. As energy and mass are equivalent and interchangeable, $E = mc^2$; this can still be regarded as an increase in energy.

Two different types of waveguide may be used, depending on the type of wave present: the travelling or standing wave.

### Travelling wave waveguide

In the travelling wave waveguide the wave enters at the electron gun end of the waveguide, travels the length of the waveguide, rather like a wave travelling towards the beach, and then exits at the opposite end of the accelerating structure. Once the wave has exited it can be either fed back into the input end of the accelerating structure or alternatively absorbed by an RF load.

The waveguide consists of a hollow tube containing discs of copper that resemble washers with a hole in the centre through which the electrons can travel. Copper is used due to its high electrical conductivity, reducing power loss from the structure. The discs also function to reduce the wave's speed of propagation, allowing the wave and the electrons' velocities to be matched at the start of the waveguide. The discs are spaced less frequently as you move down the waveguide allowing the speed of the wave's propagation to increase.

As the travelling wave moves down the waveguide its electrical field induces a corresponding region of charge in the tube and the copper discs, as shown in Figure 8.6. Electron bunches entering cavities B and F at time $t_1$ will experience acceleration; they will then move through to the next cavity in sequence C and G,

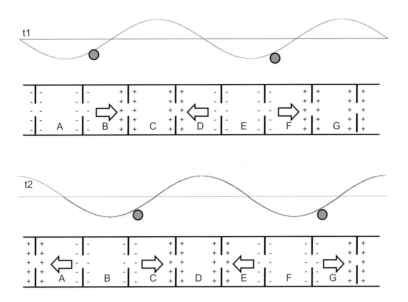

**Figure 8.6** Travelling wave.

which at $t_2$ will have changed polarity due to the wave also moving forward, and again be accelerated. This continues along the length of the accelerating structure until the RF wave is removed.

### Standing waveguide

In the standing waveguide when the travelling wave reaches the end of the waveguide, it is reflected back in the opposite direction by reflective discs. When the original travelling wave and the reflected travelling wave moving in the opposite direction interfere with each other a new wave pattern is formed – a standing wave. The standing wave has fixed points that never undergo any displacement called nodes, which are the result of destructive interference of the two travelling waves, i.e. they cancel each other out. Midway between every consecutive node there are points that undergo maximum displacement called anti-nodes. Anti-nodes are points that oscillate back and forth between a large positive displacement and a large negative displacement. The anti-nodes are the result of a mixture of constructive interference and destructive interference of the two travelling waves and, when the

two waves forming the standing wave are completely in phase, the resulting standing wave has twice the amplitude of the travelling waves. As it is the standing wave that causes the acceleration of the electrons it is not essential for the wave to enter the waveguide at the electron gun end of the accelerating structure.

The theory of operation is basically the same as the travelling waveguide, the wave producing regions of positive and negative charge that will attract and repel the electrons. Figure 8.7 shows a typical standing wave oscillation, the lines showing the amplitude of the wave at different points in time. Those electrons entering a cavity at the optimum point in the wave cycle (cavities C and G at time point 1 and cavities A and E at time point 2) will find themselves accelerated (Figure 8.8). As the standing wave is a composite of two travelling waves the resultant force on the electrons will be greater. Note that because the nodes are always in a fixed place, every other cavity (cavities B, D and F) always has a zero field and so can never contribute to the acceleration of the electron bunch. In practice the cavities that contain the nodes can be moved out to the sides

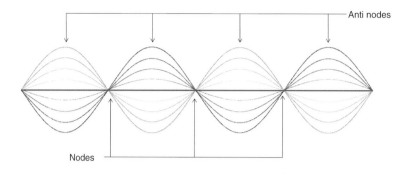

**Figure 8.7** Standing wave.

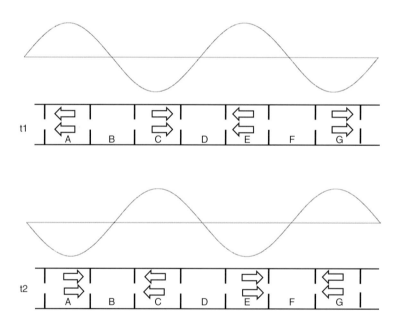

**Figure 8.8** Standing wave acceleration.

of the accelerating structure, making the overall length of the accelerating waveguide much shorter.

## Ancillary equipment

### Cooling system

The accelerating waveguide requires a stable operating temperature. Changes in the temperature will cause a change in the dimensions of the accelerating waveguide, which will affect its efficiency. The RF generator and target also require cooling and a single cooling system usually supplies all these components. A water pump continually circulates water around these structures, which then goes to a heat exchanger.

### Vacuum pumps

A vacuum of approximately $10^{-7}$ torr (see page 145) is maintained within the accelerating structure by *ion pumps*. This high vacuum prevents electrons losing energy through collisions with gas molecules as they traverse the waveguide. Ion pumps only work effectively at vacuums below $10^{-3}$ torr and to get to this pressure a mechanical pump is needed. Ion pumps only work on ions that are attracted by a potential difference between two electrodes, to a material that then absorbs them, effectively removing the ions from the waveguide. To elongate the track of the ions the pump is situated within a magnetic field. This causes the ions to spiral towards the electrode rather than move in a straight line, which is important because the chance of an atom entering the ion pump is random and elongating the ion path increases the chance of further ionisation of any gas atoms in the waveguide.

### Focusing coils

During acceleration the electrons have a tendency to diverge that is strongest at the gun end of the waveguide. Two factors cause this: the RF wave itself, which has a small radial component, and the electrostatic repulsion of the electrons on each other. Focusing coils surrounding the waveguide produce a magnetic field with the lines of force running lengthways along the waveguide; these stop the electrons from diverging as they are accelerated.

### Steering coils

The accelerating structure may contain minor imperfections that can affect the position of the electrons in the accelerating waveguide. The electrons will also be influenced by any external magnetic fields such as the Earth's magnetic field and, as the position of the waveguide changes in relation to these fields, the electrons may move from their optimum trajectory down the centre of the waveguide. Steering coils exert an electromagnetic force on the electrons, keeping them in the centre of the waveguide. The electromagnets are situated in pairs, two on the $x$ and two on the $z$ axis, to control for any deviation in these planes. A set of steering coils is present at either end of the accelerating waveguide.

## Treatment head

### Bending magnets

Linear accelerators with horizontally mounted accelerating structures require the direction in which the electrons are travelling to be changed before they hit the target. When the electrons leave the accelerating structure they enter the *flight tube*, which is an evacuated tube where no further acceleration takes place, transferring the electrons to the bending cavity. Bending magnets positioned either side of the cavity can be used to change the electrons' direction of travel. Three bending systems are in common use: the 90° and 270° systems, so called because of the angle the electrons are turned through, and the slalom system where the electrons take a zigzag course (Figure 8.9).

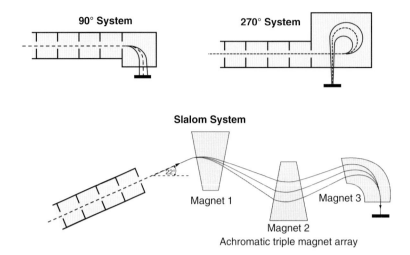

**Figure 8.9**  Bending magnets. (Slalom system diagram courtesy of Elekta Medical Systems.)

The simplest bending system, the 90° system, produces a larger focal spot on the target than the other two systems. Electrons leaving the accelerating waveguide have slightly different energies. Electrons with higher energies will be deflected less by the magnet, whereas low-energy electrons will undergo a larger angle of deflection. The other two systems bend the different electron energies to varying degrees. High-energy electrons will be bent to a greater degree than slower electrons, so allowing the electrons to be focused on a single point on the target 'achromatic'.

The 270° system has the disadvantage of needing the head to be larger to accommodate the electrons orbit. This extra height of the head raises the *isocentre* of the unit because a greater amount of space is needed to allow the head to move under the couch. An alternative to raising the isocentre height that has been utilised is a pit or sinking floor under the couch, which can open/drop when the gantry rotates under the couch. Elekta's answer to this problem was to introduce the slalom system, a variation of the 270° system that again produces the small focal spot, but without the need for a significant increase in head size.

## Target

At high energy the photons produced by the *electron target* interaction are mainly created in the forward direction. A *transmission target* allows most of the photons produced to be used and is therefore more efficient than a *reflection target*. The target is made from a metal with a high atomic number such as gold, because materials with a high atomic number are more efficient at producing X-rays. The target needs to be thick enough so that all the electrons can interact and produce X-rays, but not too thick because this will start to attenuate the beam as the X-rays have to pass through the target.

The efficiency of X-ray production at megavoltage energy is significantly better than at kilovoltage energies at approximately 30%, so less heat will be produced than in kilovoltage units. Cooling is relatively simple as less heat is produced and the target is at earth potential, so can be done by water circulating around the edge of the target structure.

## Beam-flattening filter

The spatial arrangement of X-rays produced at the target is greatest along the central axis of the beam and decreases in intensity as you move away from the central axis. This beam would be unsuitable for treatment purposes because it would be impossible to give a uniform dose at any given depth. The beam-flattening filter needs to reduce the intensity of radiation most at the central axis and then decreasingly so as you move away from the central axis. To do this the filter needs to be thicker in the middle and gradually reduce in thickness as you move away from the centre, giving a conical-shaped filter. The filter being positioned close to the point of X-ray production will have relatively small dimensions. Filters are usually made of brass or similar material. Materials with a high atomic number would make the filter smaller, but give greater changes in the beam quality across the beam. Dual energy machines will have a different flattening filter for each of the beam energies.

### Ionisation chamber

The ionisation chamber in the head of the linear accelerator is a dual, sealed, parallel plate chamber. The chamber is sealed so that it will give a constant reading at a constant dose rate regardless of the temperature and pressure. The advantage of having a dual system is that the secondary dose monitoring system can terminate the beam when the selected monitor units (MUs) are exceeded by a set limit. The ionisation chamber has a number of sectors that provide feedback to the steering coils and bending magnet, ensuring that the clinical beam is flat and has symmetry. When the change exceeds the tolerance range and automatic adjustment cannot bring it within these parameters, automatic cut-outs engage and the machine will stop.

### Optical system

As the linear accelerator does not use applicators an optical system is needed to define the *focus skin distance* (FSD) and show the beam direction. A light is positioned to one side of the head and a mirror reflects this light through 45° to run along the path the X-rays take. The mirror

is made of Mylar®, a thin strong polyester film, one surface covered with a reflective material such as aluminium that is a few micrometres thick, so as not to reduce the intensity of the radiation beam to any great extent. The geometry of this system is very important; the light beam and X-ray beam must directly superimpose on each other or the radiation beam will not correspond to the visualised field. This check that can be done with an X-ray film should be part of the routine QA programme.

## Collimators

The linear accelerator has at least two sets of collimators: the *primary collimators* and the *secondary collimators*. The primary collimator is circular and defines the maximum angle of the exiting beam. It is situated close to the target so as to reduce its size. The secondary collimators are situated after the mirror and consist of two pairs of adjustable lead blocks that restrict the radiation emerging from the head to determine square or rectangular field sizes ranging from approximately $4\,cm^2$ up to $40\,cm^2$ at 100 cm FSD, although the latter may have slightly rounded corners due to the primary collimator. The secondary collimators are calibrated so that the collimator reading will give the corresponding field size at 100 cm FSD. Due to beam divergence the field size at any other distance will be different and a calculation using similar triangles (see Chapter 1) will need to be done to determine it.

Secondary collimators can move either symmetrically around the central axis of the beam or asymmetrically. Where one of the collimators coincides with the central axis that one side of the field has no beam divergence.

Another potential issue is a *transmission penumbra* (Figure 8.10) which is caused by the beam going only through part of the collimator. To reduce this collimators do not slide straight in and out but rather move through an arc so that the edge of the collimator is always parallel to the beam edge. Transmission through the

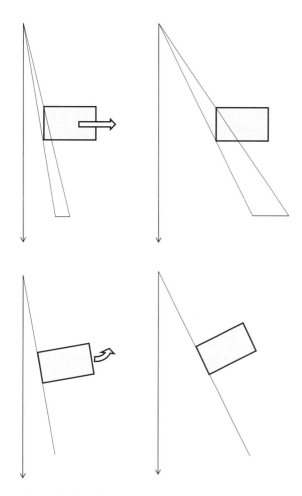

**Figure 8.10** Transmission penumbra.

collimators should be less than 2% of the primary (open) beam.

A further collimator can be positioned below the secondary collimator on one of the beam axes. This collimator consists of a number of leaves of tungsten, each of which can move independently and shape the beam. As the *multi-leaf collimators* (MLCs) are present on only one axis it is possible to have different degrees of tumour conformation depending on the collimator orientation (Figure 8.11).

For standard MLCs each leaf corresponds to a shielded width of around 1 cm at a FSD of 100 cm. This figure is reduced to values of

3–5 mm for micro- and mini-MLCs,[3] although these systems have limited field sizes. If the leaves were straight blocks of tungsten next to each other, there would be considerable leakage of radiation through the gaps. To reduce interleaf radiation leakage in the gap is kept as small as possible and the MLCs are shaped so that they have stepped or overlapping sections. The stepped and overlapping sections are not the full thickness of the blade and so cannot reduce the beam intensity by the same value as the blade. Symonds-Tayler and Webb[4] suggest a value of 14% transmission compared with 2% through the leaf. The secondary collimator is also used to reduce interleaf leakage and will be positioned just behind the leaf, the outermost leaf absorbing most of the leakage before it reaches the patient. Another issue with MLCs is the penumbra. The MLCs are not set up to move in an arc as with the secondary collimators and, to overcome the changing geometry with the beam, they are designed with rounded leaf tips. Although this shape allows some transmission of the beam through the blade tip it is independent of the position of the leaf. The greater the maximum MLC field size the greater the curvature needed.[5]

The function of all the collimators mentioned is to define the beam, which they do by attenuating the part of the beam that is not required. The collimator material needs to have a high density because the major interaction process at these energies is the Compton interaction. The most frequently used materials are lead and tungsten.

## Wedges

In older units a number of wedges, typically 15°, 30°, 45° and 60°, could physically be placed in the treatment head by the radiographer. The wedge, made from a dense material such as lead or steel attached to a backing plate that would fit into a wedge holder, was usually situated between the ionisation chamber and the mirror. The use of manual wedges has largely been superseded,

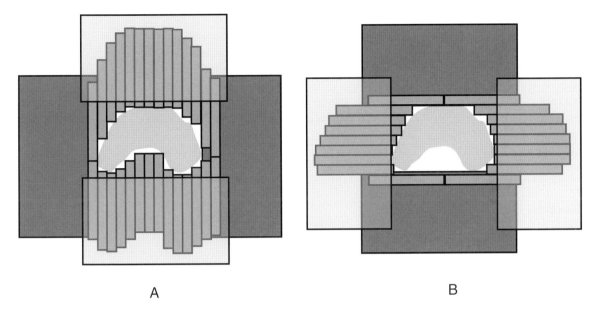

A           B

**Figure 8.11** Multi leaf collimator arrangement.

first by *motorised wedges*, which consist of a physical wedge of a large wedge angle, usually around 60°. The wedge is permanently situated in the treatment head and can be moved into the beam automatically for part of the treatment to give the desired wedge angle. Another method of obtaining a modified beam profile is through dynamic or *virtual wedges*. As the name suggests there is no physical wedge but the effect is created by moving one of the collimators across the beam at a pre-calculated speed during the treatment to give the same effect on the beam profile as a wedge. Any of the four collimator jaws could create this effect, but in practice it is limited to one set of jaws. One advantage of this system of wedging the beam is that the average beam energy remains constant across the full width of the beam. With a physical wedge there will be a degree of beam hardening that will depend on the thickness of filter traversed.

Wedges are needed to improve dose uniformity within the *planned target volume* (PTV), compensate for missing tissue and beams coming in with different *hinge angles*. The angle does not relate to the edge itself but rather the angle through which the isodose is turned, the *wedge angle* being defined as 'the complement of the angle between the central axis and a line tangent to the isodose curve at the depth of 10 cm'.[6]

## Helical tomotherapy

Tomotherapy or 'slice therapy'[7] is used to deliver *intensity-modulated radiotherapy* (IMRT). The treatment is delivered in a helical or spiral fashion. The system comprises a 6-MV linear accelerator waveguide with a megavoltage CT (MVCT) detector mounted on a rotating gantry assembly (ring gantry). For continuous rotating beam delivery slip ring technology is employed.[8]

X-rays produced by the 6-MV in-line linear accelerator are collimated into a 5-cm-wide fan beam by a primary tungsten collimator and a binary MLC. The system is dedicated to IMRT delivery and as such there is no requirement for a field flattening filter.[9] The MLC comprises 64 interleaved leaves of tongue-and-groove design.

At the isocentre each leaf width is 0.625 cm resulting in a fan-beam length of 40 cm.

The gantry aperture is 85 cm with a 40 cm CT field of view. The treatment couch translates the patient through the bore of the machine to a maximum distance of 160 cm as the gantry rotates. The integrated MVCT imaging system, mounted on the gantry opposite the beam-line, acquires images using a xenon ionisation chamber behind which is a 14-cm-thick lead beam-stop.

## Electron beams

To produce a clinical electron beam a number of changes need to be made to the linear accelerator. The most obvious is the removal of both the target and the beam-flattening filter (Figure 8.12). These structures are made of metal and being in the electron path would effectively remove all the electrons and create X-rays through bremsstrahlung interactions. Similarly the secondary collimators have to be opened because they are not used to collimate the beam and, although not in the direct path of the elec-

trons, electrons hitting the metal would produce X-rays that would contaminate the beam.

The beam-flattening filter is often positioned in a rotating carousel that also contains a number of *electron-scattering foils*. When the electron mode is selected the carousel rotates, removing the flattening filter, and the correct scattering foil for the selected energy is automatically inserted. A scattering foil is needed to spread the thin beam of electrons out over a useful area and a metal such as copper is usually used, which gives the best trade-off between scattering of the beam and bremsstrahlung X-ray production. A single foil produces a dose profile with a high central intensity of electrons, but further scattering in air and from the walls of a solid applicator produce a beam of more uniform intensity. When open-sided applicators are used the foil usually consists of two thin metal layers. The second sheet creates further scatter of the beam spreading the electrons out over a larger area because the scatter from the air alone within the applicator is not enough to produce a uniform beam. A number of different scattering foils are present

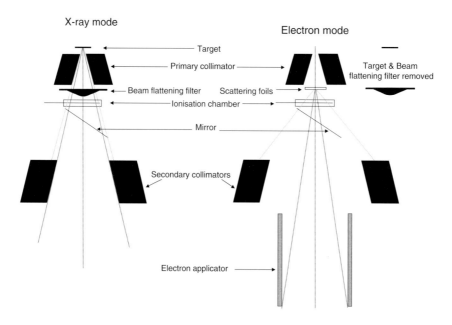

**Figure 8.12** Treatment head.

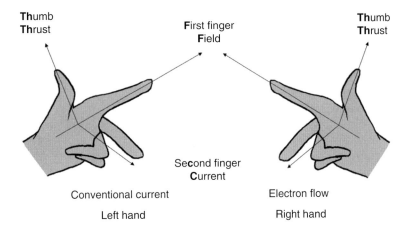

**Figure 8.13** Fleming's left-hand rule.

for the different electron energies in order to produce a suitable electron beam.

Another less frequently used method to spread out the narrow electron beam is to scan the beam over a large area using electromagnets. As there is no scattering foil in the beam this produces an electron beam with far less X-ray contamination.

Electron beams have to be collimated close to the patient's surface to reduce dose outside the treatment area from electrons that are scattered by the air. The applicators are made of a material with a relatively low atomic number, such as aluminium, to reduce the amount of bremsstrahlung X-ray production.

It is also important when changing from X-ray to electron mode that the gun current is reduced. X-ray production is inefficient and this affects the dose rate. Removal of this inefficient process would lead to a significant increase in dose rate with electron beams. For the dose rate to remain the same the gun current is reduced.

## Related principles

### The action of a magnet on an electron beam

The force causing the motion acting at right angles to both the direction of current and mag-

netic field is sometimes referred to as *Fleming's left-hand rule* (Figure 8.13) with the field (north to south) being represented by the first finger, the thumb the direction of motion and the second finger being the direction of the current flow. Although this exercise is useful for observing the three directions, it is wrong. We are looking at electron flow, which moves from negative to positive; this mnemonic was used when it was thought that current flowed from positive to negative, so in fact if you want to see the true effect you should use your right hand.

### Relativistic changes and acceleration

Equation 8.1 can be used to calculate changes in mass with velocity. Increases in mass equates to an increase in energy, but also an increase in mass will require an increase in the force applied to give the same acceleration ($F = ma$):

$$m = \frac{m_0}{\sqrt{1 - v^2/c^2}} \quad (8.1)$$

where $m$ = mass, $m_0$ = resting mass, $v$ = velocity, and $c$ = the speed of light (approximately $3 \times 10^8$ m/s).

When entering the accelerating structure the electron is travelling at approximately $0.4c$

$(1.2 \times 10^8\,\text{m/s})$ and on exiting the accelerating structure approximately $0.98c$ $(2.94 \times 10^8\,\text{m/s})$. Given the resting mass of an electron $(9.10956 \times 10^{-31}\,\text{kg})$ it is possible to calculate the mass of the electron when it exits the accelerating structure.

$$m = \frac{9.10956 \times 10^{-31}}{\sqrt{1-(2.94\times10^8)^2/(3\times10^8)^2}}$$
$$\rightarrow m = \frac{9.10956 \times 10^{-31}}{\sqrt{1-(8.64\times10^{16})/(9\times10^{16})}}$$
$$\rightarrow m = \frac{9.10956 \times 10^{-31}}{\sqrt{1-0.96}} \rightarrow m = \frac{9.10956 \times 10^{-31}}{\sqrt{0.04}}$$
$$\rightarrow m = \frac{9.10956 \times 10^{-31}}{0.20} \rightarrow m = 4.58\times10^{-30}\,\text{kg}.$$

The mass is still small, but has increased by a factor of 5 and as it gets closer to the speed of light the mass continues to increase rapidly.

## X-ray contamination of an electron beam

X-ray contamination of an electron beam typically being less than 5%, it is not usually a major issue for most treatments, but can be of concern when undertaking a total body electron (TBE) treatment. The intention is to treat the whole skin surface, but the X-ray contamination can give a significant dose to underlying tissue par-ticularly the bone marrow, which is very sensitive to radiation. The majority of the X-ray contamination is found on the central axis of the beam and this part of the beam is best avoided. Two methods can be used to overcome this. The more common method is to treat each field with two beams, one angled up 20° and one down 20°, so that the central axis of the beams passes over or under the patient. A second method that was utilised by the Hammersmith hospital was to treat the patient in the penumbra of the electron beam, which because of the scatter was quite large, but needed a modification to the dose rate in order to keep treatment times sufficiently small.

## Pressure

Pressure is measured in a number of ways; the most commonly used method, as it is used by weather forecasters, is millimetres of mercury (mmHg); 760 mm Hg is atmospheric pressure at sea level; 1 torr is equal to 1 mmHg or roughly $1.316 \times 10^{-3}$ atmospheres (atm) or approximately 133 Pa if you are more familiar with the SI units. Another measure of pressure is pound force per square inch (psi). Earlier, it was stated that the pressure of $SF_6$ in the RF waveguide was approximately 2 atm. Checking the levels of $SF_6$ should be part of the daily quality assurance procedures, the pressure being recorded in psi, 2 atm being approximately 29 psi.

## Self-test questions

1. Between which two components would a physical wedge be placed?
   (a) target and primary collimators
   (b) primary collimator and beam flattening filter
   (c) beam flattening filter and ionisation chambers
   (d) ionisation chambers and mirror
   (e) mirror and secondary collimators

2. What is the function of the encapsulated steel container in a cobalt unit?
   (a) prevent radioactive gas escaping
   (b) prevent cobalt from escaping
   (c) filter out gamma rays
   (d) filter out β particles
   (e) filter out α particles

3. Which of the following statements are true when comparing a cobalt unit with a linear accelerator?

(a) longer treatment times
(b) larger focal spot (source size)
(c) lower beam energy
(e) larger penumbra
(f) costly source changes every year

4. Which of the following components use magnets to change the direction of ions?
(a) magnetron
(b) ion pump
(c) ionisation chambers
(d) focusing coils
(e) electron gun

5. Which of the following are types of wedge?
(a) motorised
(b) manual
(c) normal
(d) virtual
(e) practical

6. Which of the following are found on a linear accelerator?
(a) beam-flattening filter
(b) reflection target
(c) quality filter
(d) stator
(e) ion pump

7. Which of the following is the most suitable target material for a linear accelerator?
(a) copper
(b) gold
(c) steel
(d) beryllium
(e) iridium

8. Cobalt has a half-life of:
(a) 5 years
(b) 5.26 years
(c) 5.5 years
(d) 5.62 years
(e) 55 years

9. What is the source of the electrons in the accelerating waveguide?
(a) scattering foils
(b) oscillator
(c) magnetron
(d) electron gun
(e) klystron

10. What is the function of the ion pump?

(a) move the beam flattening filter in and out of the beam
(b) produce a vacuum
(c) accelerate electrons
(d) maintain a vacuum
(e) circulate the $SF_6$

11. What is the function of the focusing coils?
(a) to align the electrons in the centre of the waveguide
(b) to focus the electrons onto the X-ray target
(c) to stop the electrons diverging in the waveguide
(d) to focus the X-rays
(e) to focus the RF wave into a smaller space

12. What statement is **NOT** true about a magnetron?
(a) it focuses the electrons on to the X-ray target
(b) it produces microwaves
(c) it is a high power oscillator
(d) it has a central cathode
(e) it has an outer cylindrical anode containing cavities
(f) it generates RF waves

13. In dual energy linear accelerators when the energy of the electron beam in the waveguide is increased, the magnetic field of the bending magnet required to bend the electron beam needs to:
(a) be switched off
(b) stay the same
(c) decrease
(d) increase
(e) none of the above

14. Which of the following statements are **true** about a klystron?
(a) it is predominantly used in low energy units
(b) it does not generate an RF wave
(c) it is situated in the head of the linear accelerator
(d) the structure contains $SF_6$
(e) it uses the energy of the electrons to add power to the RF wave

15. Which of the following are types of wave used to accelerate electrons?
(a) standing
(b) rotating
(c) spiralling
(d) drifting
(e) travelling

16. For a Gamma Knife unit, which of the following components make up the beam channel of the hemispherical system?
    (a) primary collimator
    (b) tungsten alloy pre-collimator
    (c) source bushing assembly
    (d) helmet
    (e) secondary collimator

17. On a unit fitted with MLCs, how many secondary collimators are there?
    (a) 2
    (b) 3
    (c) 4
    (d) 5
    (e) 6

18. Which of the following statements is **TRUE** about X-ray contamination of an electron beam?
    (a) X-ray contamination predominantly lies along the periphery of the beam
    (b) X-ray contamination, being so small, can always be ignored
    (c) X-ray contamination contributes to dose at a depth greater than the range of the electrons
    (d) X-ray contamination is usually in the order of 8%
    (e) X-ray contamination is reduced by use of scattering foils compared with beam scanning

19. Which of the following is not a component of a tomotherapy machine?
    (a) waveguide
    (b) primary collimator
    (c) binary MLC
    (d) Flattening filter
    (e) ring gantry

20. Magnets and electromagnets can be used to change the direction of charged particles. State where the following three actions occur in a linear accelerator:
    (a) force electrons through a prescribed angle of deflection
    (b) force electrons into a circular orbit
    (c) force ions into a spiral motion.

# References

1. Lindquist C, Paddick I. The Leksell gamma knife perfexion and comparisons with its predecessors. *Neurosurgery* 2007; **61**: 130–40.
2. Sulphur hexafluoride. Solvay-fluor. Available at: www.solvay-fluor.com.
3. Leal A, S'anchez-Doblado F, Arr'ans R et al. MLC leaf width impact on the clinical dose distribution: A Monte Carlo approach. *Int J Radiat Oncol Biol Physics* 2004; **59**: 1548–59.
4. Symonds-Tayler JRN, Webb S. Gap-stepped MLC leaves with filler blades can eliminate tongue-and-groove underdoses when delivering IMRT with maximum efficiency. *Physics Med Biol* 1998; **43**: 2393–5.
5. Clark BG, Teke T, Otto K. Penumbra evaluation of the Varian Millennium and BrainLAB M3 multileaf collimators. *Int J Radiat Oncol Biol Physics* 2006; **66**(4 suppl): S71–5.
6. ICRU (1976) *Determination of Absorbed Dose in a Patient Irradiated by Beams of X or Gamma Rays in Radiotherapy Procedures*. Report No 24. Oxford: ICRU Publications.
7. Mackie TR. Tomotherapy: A new concept for the delivery of dynamic conformal radiotherapy. *Med Phys* 1993; **20**: 1709–19.
8. Fenwick JD, Tome WA, Soisson ET, Mehta MP, Mackie TR. Tomotherapy and other innovative IMRT delivery systems. *Semin Radiat Oncol* 2006; 199–208.
9. Beavis AW. Is tomotherapy the future of IMRT? *Br J Radiol* 2004; **77**: 285–95.

# Chapter 9

# KILOVOLTAGE EQUIPMENT

David Flinton

## Aims and objectives

The aim of this chapter is to provide a summary of the types of kilovoltage equipment, the components of the unit and beam characteristics.

On completion of this chapter the reader should be able to:

- state the different ranges of kilovoltage energies
- describe the structure of a typical kilovoltage treatment tube
- describe the anode heel effect, and explain the need for a large target angle
- be able to explain why filters are used
- understand the importance of skin apposition at this energy.

## Background

Kilovoltage units once dominated the provision of external beam radiotherapy, until *cobalt-60 units,* and then *linear accelerators* were introduced, both of which could offer improved delivery of dose at depth and, in the case of linear accelerators, *superficial therapy* with electrons. Despite this, kilovoltage units still remain useful in the treatment of superficial conditions, especially small tumours or conditions near the eye where they have advantages over electron therapy. The current Department of Health recommendation[1] is that a superficial unit be part of the minimum compliment of treatment units present in a radiotherapy department.

## Range of kilovoltage energies

X-ray therapy of kilovoltage beams can be divided into the three areas described below[2], arranged according to their degree of beam penetration. Despite this classification of beams, treatment units will not necessarily fall into just one category because they usually offer a range of energies that may cross these boundaries (Table 9.1):

- **Very low energy:** X-rays with a half-value layer (HVL) between 0.0035 mm and 1 mm of Al. X-rays generated at an accelerating potential of <50 kV. Sometimes beams in this energy range, particularly those with a generating voltage below 30 kV are referred to as *Grenz rays*. This type of beam is not commonly used in the UK, but it is used with more frequency in both Germany and the USA. This energy is used primarily in the treatment of inflammatory skin conditions such as eczema and psoriasis, which have other safer methods of treatment available including topical use of emollients and steroid creams, non-topical treatments such as retinoids and immuno-suppressant light therapy. As a result of these 'safer' options in the UK it is recommended[3] that very low energy X-rays are used only on

**Table 9.1** Kilovoltage treatment units and their energy ranges

| Unit | Energy range (kV) | Maximum HVL | Maximum power output (kW) |
|---|---|---|---|
| Xstrahl 100 | 10–100 | 5 mm Al | 1 |
| Xstrahl 150 | 10–150 | 8 mm Al | 3 |
| Xstrahl 200 | 20–220 | 2 mm Cu | 3 |
| Xstrahl 300 | 40–300 | 3 mm Cu | 4.5 |

Medical units currently produced by Gulmay Medical.

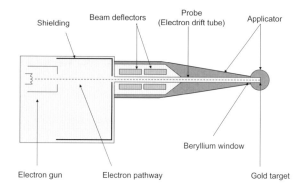

**Figure 9.1** The intrabeam intraoperative system.

inflammatory skin conditions that are either unresponsive to these other treatments or under research conditions.

- **Low energy:** X-rays with an HVL between 1 mm and 8 mm of Al. The X-rays generate a potential between 50 kV and 160 kV. Treatment is usually reserved for small superficial lesions on the skin. In the past beams using a generating voltage between 50 kV and 150 kV were referred to as *superficial*.
- **Medium energy:** X-rays with an HVL >8 mm Al, covering the X-rays generated at a potential of between 160 kV and 300 kV. Beams of these energies are primarily used in the treatment of skin tumours, but the higher-energy units can have a role to play in the palliative treatment of metastases. Beams generated using a potential of between 150 kV and 500 kV were referred to as *orthovoltage* or *deep X-ray*.

Within kilovoltage energies there are two specialised forms of treatment: contact therapy and intraoperative therapy.

Contact therapy is predominantly used in the treatment of early rectal carcinomas using a technique that is sometimes referred to as a Papillon treatment, after the doctor who developed it in the 1950s, or endocavity irradiation. The treatment utilises an X-ray unit operating at a generating voltage of 50 kV. The patient can be treated on an outpatient basis with a local anaesthetic that allows a proctoscope to be inserted and positioned over the tumour. The X-ray tube applicator then fits into the proctoscope and comes into contact with the tumour.

In 2007 Ariane Medical systems released a new contact therapy unit to replace the ageing Therapax 50 and Phillips RT-50 units which are no longer produced. The mobile unit has an in-built generator and control unit to which the X-ray tube is attached via a moveable arm. The unit utilises a transmission rod anode X-ray tube giving a dose rate of 20 Gy min$^{-1}$.

The main reason for this type of treatment is the physical property of an extremely rapid fall-off of dose in tissue rather than a radiobiological advantage. The depth dose falls from a surface dose of 100% to 15% at 2 cm depth,[4] so allowing a high local dose to the tumour while sparing normal tissue. Typical doses are of the order of 80 or 120 Gy in three or four fractions delivered every 2 or 3 weeks.[5,6]

Intraoperative therapy is similar to contact therapy and is currently undergoing trials in the treatment of small, well-defined breast cancers. The unit (Figure 9.1), developed by the Photo-electron Corporation, can be used to deliver radiation directly to the tumour bed once the tumour has been removed during the surgical procedure, or as a secondary procedure as a day-case patient if the unit is unavailable at the hospital where the surgery was performed. The unit is lightweight and small the X-ray generator body measuring $7 \times 11 \times 14\,cm$, the applicator being approximately 16 cm long. The operating voltage can vary between 10 kV and 50 kV and has an approximate HVL of 1 mm Al.

The unit utilises an electron gun to accelerate the electrons to the desired voltage. Once accelerated the electrons pass down an evacuated tube, eventually hitting a thin gold target. As they pass down the evacuated tube the electrons pass between a beam deflector that dithers the electrons across the target. The X-rays are produced isotropically and different spherical applicators maintain the tissue at a set distance from the source. The applicator's spheres range in size from 1.5 cm to 5 cm, which means that the surface dose rate will vary with applicator choice. A dose of 5 Gy is prescribed at a distance of 1 cm from the applicator, which takes between 25 and 30 minutes to deliver.[7] As with contact therapy the short treatment distance and low energy gives a rapid fall-off of dose (Figure 9.2) with distance maximising the dose to the tumour bed; at a distance of 5 mm from the applicator the dose is 8.75 Gy which equates to a *biological effective dose* (BED) of 59; a dose of 50 Gy external beam radiotherapy to the whole breast gives a BED of 60.[8] Currently the international TARGIT (*targeted intraoperative radiotherapy*) trial is trying to establish the efficacy of this single fraction treatment compared with the established pattern of fractionated external beam radiotherapy to the whole of the breast.

## Superficial and orthovoltage equipment

The main components for this type of equipment are a generator, control console, tube mounting, X-ray tube, cooling system and collimators; an optional patient information system can also be used.

### Generator

A generator serves to increase the mains voltage to the voltages required for X-ray production through the use of transformers, and then rectifies and smoothes the waveform (see Chapter 6). These actions increase the efficacy of X-ray production and increase the stability of the beam output, the electrons being accelerated by an almost constant potential difference across the tube.

At higher energies it is necessary to use two balanced generators operating together: one to supply the negative potential to the cathode, and the second the positive potential to the anode. Tubes that have this arrangement are called 'bipolar tubes'; the anode has a positive potential and the cathode a negative potential with respect to the ground potential (earth). This is a safer arrangement at higher voltages because you effectively half the maximum voltage that any one component may have. The lower-energy tubes working off one generator are termed 'unipolar', the cathode having a selectable negative potential and the anode always being at ground potential.

### Control console

Modern control consoles contain a microprocessor to monitor and manage the exposure and in

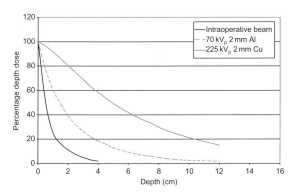

**Figure 9.2** Central axis depth–dose curves for 3 different kilovoltage energies.

some cases a dual microprocessor that allows an independent back-up timer for safety.

All operating parameters that affect or could affect dose delivery and radiation quality must be displayed on the console, which can be interlocked with numerous tube components and a select and confirm system ensures correct choice of treatment parameters, such as energy, filter and collimator. Certain units are interlocked in such a way that inserting the filter automatically defines beam energy selection.

The control panel is switched on via a key that should be kept safe when the unit is not in operation. Typical data inputted/confirmed by the operator are: dose/time set, time limit (usually 5% greater than the expected duration of treatment), filter, applicator, kV and mA. (Most modern units contain an ionisation chamber situated after the beam-flattening filter in the sub-tube assembly which allows treatment to be performed by setting dose [MU] as opposed to treatment time, which is used in the older X-ray units.) Other information available before and during treatment are: a light signifying whether X-rays are on, the dose rate and the dose administered/time treated. Pausing the treatment is possible via an interrupt key or the treatment may be terminated via the stop button. In the case of power failure an internal battery will maintain details of the treatment up to the point of power failure which can be recorded. A separate operating mode also exists that is accessible by either password or a separate key that allows physicists/engineers to calibrate the unit and configure parameters.

To prolong the tube life it is important to carry out run-up procedures. In the Gulmay Medical consoles these are automatically stored and displayed on power-up ready to be run before clinical use.

## Tube mounting

The mounting for kilovoltage units, unlike linear accelerators, is not *isocentric* (Figure 9.3). Units are usually either supported by the use of a

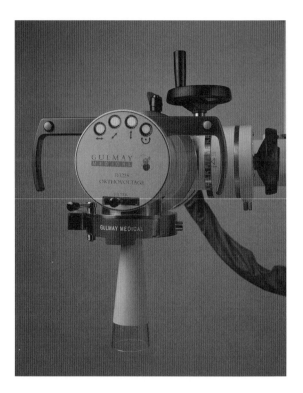

**Figure 9.3** Kilovoltage unit. (Image courtesy of Gulmay Medical Limited.)

ceiling support or have a floor-mounted stand and require manual force for any movement to occur. Movement can usually occur in three axes – longitudinal, transverse and vertical – as well as the tube being able to rotate as well as tilt. Counterweights and tensator springs help provide a consistent resistance and allow a smooth, even movement of the tube as well as allow accurate fine positioning movements. Use of electromagnetic brakes helps improve accuracy of set-up, locking the movement when desired – an advantage over the mechanical locks used on older units, which often used to give further tube movement when applied. In the case of power failure the mounting system must maintain the weight of the tube and allow the patient to be removed; this can be done by freeing all the locks except the vertical movement, so allowing the tube to be removed from the patient with no danger of the tube descending onto them.

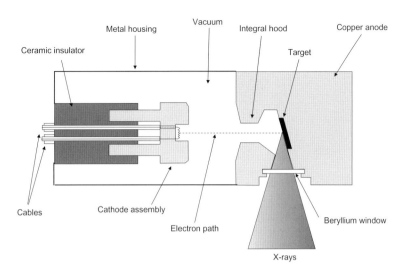

Ceramic insulator — Metal housing — Vacuum — Integral hood — Copper anode

Target

Cables — Cathode assembly — Electron path — Beryllium window

X-rays

**Figure 9.4** Unipolar tube.

## Tube design

The basic tube design is dissimilar both to the tube described in Chapter 6 and to the intraoperative tube in the previous section. The standard design used is that of a stationary anode (Figure 9.4). Recent developments in the design of kilovoltage tubes have seen the gradual replacement of the glass enveloped X-ray tube, used for over 80 years with metal-ceramic tubes. The use of metal-ceramic tubes has several advantages. Metal-ceramic are smaller and more robust than glass tubes of equivalent energy. They enable more flexibility in the electrical circuitry associated with the tube and have a higher output.

Metal ceramic tubes consist of a cathode assembly held within an evacuated tube. A ceramic insulator holds the assembly in place and electrically insulates it from the metal tube envelope. The cathode assembly consists of a single *tungsten filament* that is heated by an electrical current passing through it. When hot the filament emits electrons by *thermionic emission*. The filament is set into a *focusing cup* which has a static negative charge on it. The static charge stops the electrons from spreading out, forcing them together, and ensuring that the electron

beam moving to the anode has a small cross-sectional area. Research is currently being conducted on *carbon nanotube* (CNT) cathodes, which require no heating; they are also referred to as 'cold cathodes'. CNT cathodes have several advantages over heated cathodes. They switch on faster than the heated filaments, the electrons being emitted the instant a potential difference is applied across the tube, they consume less power, and have the ability to last longer.

The anode structure is either welded directly to the metal tube envelope or isolated from the envelope by *ceramic insulators*. The target is recessed within a copper anode, which provides a hood for the anode. Situated on one side of the hood is a *beryllium* ($Z = 4$, $A = 9$) *window*. The window allows the desired X-rays exit while the hood removes the unwanted low-energy X-rays produced by electrons hitting the anode outside the target area (extrafocal radiation).

The *target angle* is usually in the order of 30° in kilovoltage treatment tubes. This is a lot higher than the 17° used in the simulator tube or 5–17° found in the various diagnostic X-ray tubes. Having a target angle of this magnitude affects the photon beam in two ways. First the apparent *focal spot* is larger, which could have

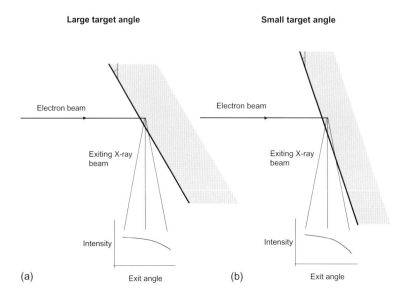

**Figure 9.5** Anode–heel effect.

the effect of increasing the geometric penumbra; however, this is negated by collimating at, or close to, the patient's surface. The second effect is to reduce the 'anode heel effect', which is caused by self-attenuation of the beam in the target. As the amount of material travelled through depends on the exit direction, we get a variation in intensity across the anode–cathode axis of the beam (Figure 9.5). This effect cannot be removed completely but is reduced in tubes with large target angles. In tubes operating over a range of energies the anode–heel effect is energy dependent: the greater the generating voltage the deeper the electron interaction in the target and the greater the degree of attenuation within the target.

All tubes have *inherent filtration* which, together with the added filtration, will give the total filtration of the beam. The inherent filtration consists of the beryllium window of the hood and the tube window.

## Cooling system

In stationary X-ray tubes most of the heat is removed from the target via conduction. *Thermal conduction* is dependent on four factors: material, cross-sectional area, temperature difference and length, the last being an inverse relationship. Copper is used because it is an extremely good thermal conductor, and it must be ensured that there is a good thermal link between the tungsten target and copper anode to allow heat to be easily transferred into the copper. The copper block in which the target is set is relatively large, allowing easy passage of the heat energy to the cooling system and also acting as a heat sink. The cooling system maintains a high temperature difference so ensuring rapid removal of heat away from the target.

At lower energies, because the X-ray tube is unipolar in design (the anode is at earth potential), water can be used to cool the anode. Either the heated water is then replaced with new cool water (lost water system) or the water can be re-circulated, having being cooled by a refrigeration unit or fan. For the higher-energy bipolar tubes, because the anode is not at earth potential, water can no longer be used as a cooling agent as it is a conductor of electricity, so oil is used instead, oil being an electrical insulator. The heated oil is then cooled using either air or water.

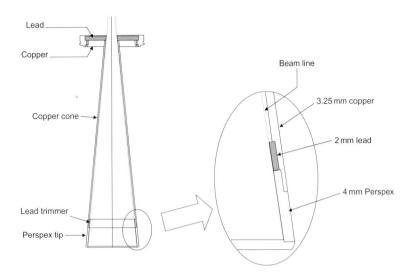

**Figure 9.6** Typical kilovoltage applicator. (Adapted from an image provided by Gulmay Medical Limited.)

## Collimation

The common method of beam collimation for kilovoltage energies is removable applicators. *Applicators* allow the operator to easily see if the beam direction is perpendicular to the skin's surface (skin apposition) and ensures that stand-off, if present, is even and minimal. This is important because stand-off and stand-in can have major consequences to the dose received (see Inverse square law). Another function of the applicator is to define the treatment distance. Applicators can be found in a range of different FSDs, ranging from about 15 cm to 50 cm, the larger FSDs generally offering larger field sizes.

The applicator assembly (Figure 9.6) consists of a rigid base plate, which is used to attach the applicator to the unit. Within the base plate is a layer of lead of sufficient thickness to collimate the beam to less than 1% of the incident intensity. Within the lead is an aperture that collimates the beam to the desired field size. A second layer of lead may be present where the wall of the applicator joins with the plastic end cap. This second lead insert acts to trim the penumbra of the beam, effectively collimating the beam near the skin's surface. A photograph of a low energy

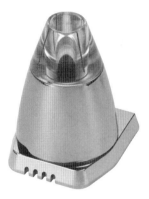

**Figure 9.7** Applicator. (Image courtesy of Gulmay Medical Limited.)

open-ended applicator is seen in Figure 9.7. Note the small indentations on the base plate that form part of the interlock system identifying the applicator when in use.

The walls of the applicator are made from either steel or copper. The walls of the applicator do not receive any primary radiation and their primary function is to attenuate any scattered radiation, which will be of low energy. The plastic end of the applicator can be of either an open or a closed design. With closed-end applicators it possible to add a little compression when treating, which can allow the smoothing out of uneven surfaces, so reducing stand-off. Compression should be avoided with open-ended tube designs because this can lead to stand-in of tissue, the soft tissue 'bulging' into the applicator, leading to a higher dose being received. The plastic end cap also has lines etched onto the plastic of visual reference marks that can aid with the correct placement of the applicator.

Applicators are available in only set sizes and shapes, and further beam shaping might be needed to limit the radiation field to the desired treatment area. This can be achieved by the use of cut-outs, sheets of lead or a low melting point alloy (LMPA). Cut-outs are shaped to the body contour and sit on the patient, covering the area needing to be shielded with a hole cut-out of the lead in the desired shape of the field. The applicator is then positioned over the cut-out. The thickness of the material used for the cut-out is dependent on the beam energy, but should reduce the dose to at least 5% of the incident beam. The cut-out effectively reduces the area of the beam, reducing the amount of scatter produced and so affecting the dose rate. As a result of this change in dose rate when a cut-out is used, a cut-out factor needs to be applied.

## Beam quality

The penetrating power of a beam varies with beam energy and it is usual with megavoltage to describe quality by stating the generating potential used. For kilovoltage beams this is not sufficient because filters are used that can significantly affect the emerging beam's quality. As a result of this it is more usual at these energies to use both the generating voltage and the HVL of the beam to describe beam quality.

## Filtration

The quality of the beam exiting the tube can be improved by the addition of filters into the beam. A filter holder is positioned after the primary collimator and is interlocked so that the machine cannot be switched on without a filter present. Quality filters are usually made of one the following three materials: aluminium, copper and tin. *Composite filters* can also be used that are made from two or more of the materials. Composite filters consist of layers of material that are always arranged in order of decreasing atomic number as you move away from the target. Each of the materials has a *k* absorption edge associated with it: the higher the atomic number of the material, the higher the energy that the absorption edge has. The absorption edge for tin occurs at 29.2 keV, copper at 9 keV and aluminium at 1.6 keV. A quality filter made of tin, copper and aluminium is sometimes referred to as a *Thoraeus filter*.

As the unit cannot work without a filter present units are provided with warm-up filters. Warm-up filters are usually made of lead, to absorb most of the primary beam, but some low-energy warm-up filters can be made from brass.

## Kilovoltage beam characteristics

At kilovoltage energy the interaction effect is a mixture of photoelectric effect and Compton scattering. Both of these interactions give rise to electrons that will be absorbed close to their site of production. Compton also gives rise to scattered photons which may travel a significant distance in tissue before depositing their energy. A significant amount of scatter is sideways and backwards (*back scatter*). The sideways scatter explains one of the characteristics of isodose curves for kilovoltage beams (see Chapter 10). The sharp edge to the beam is caused by the collimation at or near the skin's surface. Beyond this sharp edge are small amounts of radiation caused by scattered radiation moving outside the exposed area.

Back scatter depends on the field size, tissue and beam quality (Figure 9.8) used as well as the thickness of underlying tissue, but is independent of the treatment distance. The *backscatter factor*

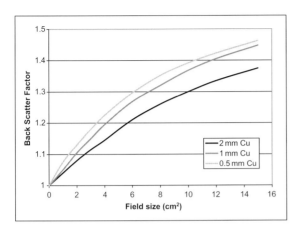

**Figure 9.8** Effect of field size and energy on backscatter.

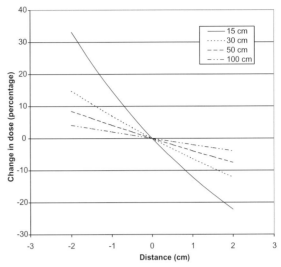

**Figure 9.9** Effect of changes in treatment distance on the dose received.

(BSF) can be calculated using equation 9.1,[9],where $K_{air,s}$ is the air kerma rate at the surface of a water phantom, $K_{air,f}$ is the air kerma rate at the same point with the phantom removed, $(\mu_{en}/\rho)_{w,air}$ is the ratio of the mass energy absorption coefficients for water and air in the presence of the scattering medium or free space. According to Klevenhagen and Thwaites[10] only small differences in beam quality occur on going from free space to surface irradiation, so although not strictly true we can assume that the $(\mu_{en}/\rho)$ terms cancel each other out and BSF can be calculated from the simpler equation – equation 9.2.

$$ BSF = \frac{K_{air,s}\left([\mu_{en}/\rho]_{w,air}\right)_s}{K_{air,f}\left([\mu_{en}/\rho]_{w,air}\right)_f} \quad (9.1) $$

$$ BSF = \frac{K_{air,s}}{K_{air,f}} \quad (9.2) $$

Backscatter can also have a major effect on dose received when lead is used as shielding behind the target volume. The interactions that occur in the lead shielding can cause a significant increase in dose on the beam side of the lead due to the high backscatter component at these energies. This can effectively be removed by coating the lead shielding with a tissue-equivalent material such as wax that will absorb the scatter before it reaches the patient.

## Inverse square law

Application of the inverse square law is especially important at kilovoltage energy due to the short treatment distances used when compared with linear accelerators. Small changes in treatment distance can lead to significant changes in dose. The importance of this variation in treatment distance, 'stand-off and stand-in' is therefore especially important at kilovoltage energy. Figure 9.9 shows how treatment distance can affect the dose received at some commonly used kilovoltage treatment distances compared with a treatment distance of 100 cm FSD.

Where stand-off and stand-in occurs a factor can be calculated that can be used to modify the dose per MU at the surface of the patient (equation 9.3):

$$ \text{Stand off} = \frac{FSD^2}{FSD + \text{Stand off}^2} $$

$$\text{Stand in} = \frac{\text{FSD}^2}{\text{FSD} - \text{Stand in}^2} \qquad (9.3)$$

These factors can then be used with the dose rate to calculate the modified dose rate due to the inverse square law. To calculate the dose at the surface, the reference surface dose rate needs to have the following factors applied: applicator factor, backscatter factor and stand-off/in factor and cut-out factor if used.

## Quality assurance tests

Monthly and annual quality assurance tests are usually carried out by physicists or radiographers. Functional checks of the treatment unit should include: tube movement in all dimensions and that the locks work; filter interlocks; beam status indicators; beam off at key off, emergency off and interrupt buttons both function correctly; the kV and mA are both correctly displayed; and correct operation of back-up timer and a check of the output using an ionisation chamber or other suitable detector at the chosen energy and filter combinations. Other checks that should also be carried out before treatment are: ensure that the patient monitoring devices work; door interlocks terminate treatment; and the couch movement and brakes all work correctly.

### Self-test questions

1. The amount of backscatter is dependent on which of the following factors?
   Applicator size
   Thickness of underlying tissue
   Beam quality
   Treatment distance
   Use of a lead cut-out

2. Which of the following should be included in the monitor unit calculation?
   Applicator factor
   Field size factor
   Backscatter factor
   Stand-off factor
   Cut-out factor

3. What is the function of the hood in the X-ray tube?
   Absorb X-rays produced outside of the focal spot
   Keep the target warm
   Decrease the tube current needed
   Increase the rate of X-ray production
   Reflect electrons onto the target

4. What property of the material dictates the order of the material in a compound quality filter?
   Work function
   Malleability
   Atomic number
   Mass number
   Melting point

5. A stand-off of 1 cm will have most effect on the dose received at which of the following treatment distances?
   20 cm
   30 cm
   40 cm
   50 cm
   100 cm

6. Which order should the materials in a compound filter be (tube side first)?
   Copper, tin, aluminium
   Tin, copper, aluminium
   Copper, aluminium, tin
   Tin, copper, aluminium
   Tin, aluminium, copper

7. What is the function of the lead situated just above the plastic endplate in an applicator?
   Attenuate the primary beam
   Join the plastic to the copper applicator
   Trim the penumbra
   Increase scatter present to flatten the beam
   Enhance electron contribution

8. Heat is primarily removed from the target through:
   conduction
   convection

radiation

insulation

adduction

9. The rate at which heat is transferred away from the target can be increased by which of the following?
Increasing the length of the material
Decreasing the cross sectional area of the material
Decreasing the temperature gradient
Choosing a material with a high thermal conductivity
Using a non-metal as the anode material

10. What is the typical target angle used in a therapy kilovoltage tube?
5°
15°
20°
25°
30°

11. Which of the following beams are synonymous with each other?
Superficial
Very low energy
Low energy
Medium energy
Supervoltage

12. To obtain a high proportion of X-rays from the target the target is made out of a material with a:
high density
low work function
high atomic number
low atomic number
poor thermal conductivity

13. The purpose of the removable filters is to:
remove characteristic X-rays
reduce the depth dose of the beam
remove high-energy X-rays
reduce the dose rate
remove low-energy X-rays

14. Which of the following is NOT a feature of a tube mounting?
Isocentric
Floor mounted
Tensator springs
Counterweights
Ceiling support

15. Which of the following is NOT present in a kilovoltage tube?
Hood
Target
Anode
Stator
Electron gun

16. The anode heel effect is affected by the:
target angle
dose rate
quality filter
generating voltage
penumbra

17. Which one of the following is best used to describe the beam quality of a kilovoltage beam?
HVL
Generating voltage
Generating voltage and the HVL
Generating voltage and the quality filter used
Generating voltage and the inherent filtration

18. Which of the following checks need to be performed on a daily basis before clinical use of the unit?
Door interlock
Treatment unit movements
The HVL of the beam
Emergency off button
Machine output

19. Why is skin apposition important in the treatment of skin tumours?

20. Why is beryllium used as the material for the window?

## Acknowledgements

My thanks go to the following people: Kirsti Gordon and Gulmay Medical for help in the early stages of the chapter and providing technical support during its writing; Mark Hulse of University Campus, Suffolk for proofreading the later drafts.

## References

1. Department of Health. *Manual for Cancer Services*. London: Department of Health, 2004.
2. Klevenhagen SC, Aukett RJ, Harrison RM, Moretti C, Nahum AE, Rosser KE. The IPMEB code of practice for the determination of absorbed dose for x-rays below 300 kV generating potential (0.035 mm Al-4 mm Cu HVL; 10-300 kV generating potential.) *Physics Med Biol* 1996; **41**: 2605–25.
3. National Institute for Health and Clinical Excellence. Grenz rays therapy for inflammatory skin conditions. *Interventional Procedure Guidance 236*. London: NICE, 2007.
4. Dale RG. The radiobiology of Papillon-type treatments. *Clin Oncol* 2007; **19**: 649–54.
5. Myrint AS, Grieve RJ, McDonald AC et al. (2007) Combined modality treatment of early rectal cancer – the UK perspective. *Clin Oncol* **19**: 674–81.
6. Sischy B. The use of endocavity irradiation for selected carcinomas of the rectum: Ten years experience. *Radiother Oncol* 1985; **4**: 97–101.
7. Vaidya JS. Intra-operative radiotherapy for breast cancer. *Recent Adv Surg* 2003; **26**: 165–81.
8. Vaidya JS, Baum M, Tobias JS et al. Targeted intra-operative radiotherapy (Targit): An innovative method of treatment for early breast cancer. *Ann Oncol* 2001; **12**: 1075–80.
9. Hassan MA, Gaber MH, Esmat E, Farag HI, Eissa HM. Standard water phantom backscatter factors for medium energy x-rays. *Romanian J Biophysics* 2004; **14**(1–4): 69–79.
10. Klevenhagen SC, Thwaites DI. Kilovoltage x-rays. In: Williams, JR, Thwaites DI (eds), *Radiotherapy Physics in Practice*. Oxford: Oxford Medical Publications, 1993.

## Chapter 10

# TREATMENT PLANNING AND COMPUTER SYSTEMS

## John Conway and Christopher M Bragg

### Aims and objectives

The aim of this chapter is to describe the fundamental physics principles behind radiotherapy treatment planning. This requires an understanding of how absorbed dose is mapped in the body when a high-energy photon beam is incident upon the surface. The basics of isodose curves, methods of beam modification and fundamental beam parameters are described.

On completion of this chapter the reader should be able to:

- understand the methods by which computer software can model the energy absorption of multiple beams traversing through a body
- understand complex planning techniques such as intensity-modulated radiotherapy (IMRT) and four-dimensional (4D) planning
- describe practical features of treatment planning systems for photon, electron, brachytherapy and stereotactic treatments.

## Introduction

This chapter describes the basic principles behind the process of radiotherapy treatment planning, with particular regard to methods employed by modern computers accurately to model the radiation beam. No attempt is made to describe the process of producing plans for a particular tumour site, and the reader is referred elsewhere

for this.[1,2] Also, the principles of radiation dosimetry are explained in Chapter 3 and a detailed description of various systems of dosimetry calculation can be found elsewhere.[3–5]

After a summary of basic dosimetry definitions, isodose data commonly employed for megavoltage therapy planning are discussed together with the corrections required when applied to the irregular structure of the human body. The first section describes the basic principles behind treatment planning followed by the fundamentals of dose modelling in the second. Here the complex computer manipulation of input data, measured from the treatment machine, enables fast and accurate predictions of absorbed dose distribution within the body. The use of advanced computer algorithms that enable more accurate modelling of the complex scatter conditions in the body is discussed.

The data input from both radiation field measurements and patient measurements is fundamental to the computer mapping of dose in tissue. A description of beam and patient data formats, methods of measurement and the quality assurance that is necessary to ensure the accuracy of the output data are discussed in the third section.

The fourth section gives a practical guide to the features found in three-dimensional treatment planning systems, and describes some of the modern planning tools that are provided by most systems to enable the production of optimum treatment plans through beam manipulation, dose assessment and plan visualisation.

Treatment planning systems are not just used for megavoltage photon calculations but are able to model particle and sealed source therapies. Brachytherapy and electron therapy planning systems are only briefly described as the number of plans produced by these are only a fraction of those produced for external beam treatments. Planning of stereotactic radiosurgery treatments has become more widespread over the last 5 years and therefore a short description of these planning methods is included. The planning of new external beam modes of treatment is also introduced in the section.

## Basic principles of treatment planning

Treatment planning has evolved from the early use of radiation for therapy, where the distribution of radioactive sources was decided by applying a set of rules, to present-day planning techniques that rely on complex computer modelling of the dose distribution from patient data and external radiation beam parameters. The overall aim of the planning process remains the translation of the therapeutic requirements of the oncologist into a set of treatment instructions that will enable the patient to be treated accurately. The treatment plan not only provides a set of instructions for the radiographer but also provides information about the distribution of dose that enables the oncologist to assess the adequacy of the beam arrangements.

The the principal steps involved in treatment planning are:

1. Localisation of the tumour and a dimensional description of the target volume by the oncologist, followed by the identification of any critical structures to be avoided during the planning process.

2. Measurement of patient data (e.g. body contours and dimensions, tissue densities) is required to enable the target volume to be defined within planar (usually transverse) contours of the body.

3. The treatment planner will determine the optimum arrangement of radiation fields to obtain a uniform dose distribution (+7 and −5% of the prescribed dose) determined by the constraints set by the clinical requirements (e.g. dose to sensitive organs). The dose distribution is calculated and displayed in single or multiple planar views to allow assessment of the plan and adjustment of field parameters to achieve optimisation.

4. The oncologist prescribes a fractionated time and dose to a reference point within the treatment volume and a set of treatment instructions is produced to allow the plan to be delivered.

The principles outlined above are described more fully below.

The International Commission on Radiation Units and Measurements (ICRU) produced a report in 1987 on the use of computers in treatment planning,[6] and subsequently produced a report on prescribing, recording and reporting procedures in external beam photon therapy[7] followed by a supplement to this 6 years later.[8] These reports are of particular importance to treatment planning in describing the parameters of volume and dose when prescribing radiotherapy treatments and the specifications from these reports are used throughout this chapter.

### Dose definitions

A first step to establishing the absorbed dose distribution in the patient is to determine the variation of dose along the central axis of the beam. The dose at depth will depend on many conditions encountered by the photon beam, such as field size, beam energy, depth in the patient, distance from the beam source and external attenuators (e.g. wedges). The dose along the centre of the field has been defined by various energy-dependent parameters, the most common of these being *percentage depth dose* (PDD) and *tissue maximum ratio* (TMR).

PDD is defined as the dose at depth in a phantom expressed as a percentage of the dose at a reference depth $d_o$ (usually the position of the peak absorbed dose, $d_o = d_{max}$) on the central axis of the beam:

$$\text{PDD}(d, d_o, A_d, s) = D_d / D_{do} \times 100.$$

The parameters shown in parentheses, as defined in Figure 10.1a, indicate the dependency of PDD on depth $d$, position of dose maximum $d_o$, area of the field $A_d$ at depth $d$ and source-to-surface distance ($s$ = SSD).

TMR is defined as the dose at depth in a phantom expressed as a ratio of the dose at the same point in relation to the radiation source but at the position of peak dose ($d_o = d_{max}$) on the central axis of the beam:

$$\text{TMR}(d, A_d) = D_d / D_{do}.$$

PDD values along the central axis of the beam may be measured using a radiation detector moved to increasing depth in a phantom with the SSD kept constant (usually 100 cm). These values can then be expressed as percentages of the peak dose on the central axis.

TMR values are measured by ensuring that the SDD remains constant with the detector always at the isocentre (usually source-to-isocentre distance, SID = SDD = 100 cm), and expressing the dose at depth as the ratio of the peak dose value.

In practice, PDD requires the phantom position to remain at a constant distance from the source while the detector moves to the point of measurement, whereas for TMR the detector remains at a constant distance from the source and the phantom (or surface) moves to provide measurement at depth. TMRs are particularly useful for isocentric treatments because the quantity is virtually independent of SSD, whereas PDD dose values require an inverse square correction for any change in SSD.

Treatment planning systems use PDD and TMR values for dose calculations and can be interconverted by inverse square and phantom scatter corrections. Another quantity used by treatment planning systems is the scatter maximum ratio (SMR), which is particularly useful for calculating scatter dose from irregular field shapes in a medium. This is defined as the

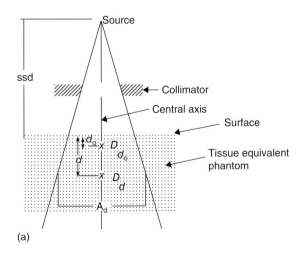
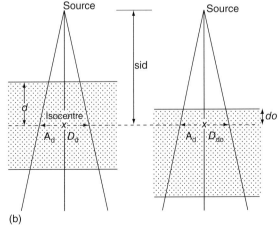

(a)                                             (b)

**Figure 10.1** (a) Percentage depth dose (PDD = $D_d / D_{do} \times 100$); (b) tissue maximum ratio (TMR = $D_d / D_{do}$).

ratio of the scattered dose at a given point ($d$) in a phantom to the effective primary dose at the same point at the position of peak dose ($d_0$; Figure 10.1b). In practice, SMR values may be obtained by subtracting the zero area field TMR, TMR($d$,0), from the finite area TMR, TMR($d$,$A_d$), and correcting for phantom scatter.

## Isodose curves and dose mapping

Isodose curves are lines joining points of equal PDD and therefore provide a means of mapping the variation in dose as a function of depth and transverse distance from the central axis of the beam. As with PDDs, the isodose distribution is affected by the beam quality (or energy), field size, SSD, attenuators and source/collimation geometry. A detailed discussion of these parameters may be found elsewhere.[3–5,9]

A single beam isodose chart typically shows a set of isodose curves that provides incremental percentage depth doses, usually ranging from the maximum value to the 10% value in steps of 10%. The chart is either normalised to the point of maximum dose on the central beam axis for a fixed SSD (100 cm), or to a reference point at depth, say 10 cm, at which the isocentre is set as an axis of rotation, i.e. source-to-axis distance (SAD) = 100 cm. The former method is the most common representation of isodose data and examples are shown in Figure 10.2 for a 6 MV open field, a 10 MV wedge field and a 6 MV asymmetrical beam. The dose distribution represents a field in a single plane with the beam at normal incidence to the surface of a water-equivalent homogeneous phantom.

Before the advent of computer planning, a set of isodose charts for open and wedged fields was required for each field size to allow the manual transcription of this data to the patient contour (usually a transverse outline of the body). Each field was traced and combined, point by point, to enable a composite isodose chart of the multiple field plan. Present computer planning systems have made these manual methods obso-lete. They require the measurement of a large amount of dose data for input into the beam model and verification of the beam model is achieved through dose analysis using computer quality analysis (QA) tools.

## Addition of isodoses

For megavoltage radiotherapy, the combination of two or more fields is usually necessary to meet the following criteria of acceptability:

- aim to achieve a uniformity of dose in the target volume within +7% and −5% of the prescribed dose at a reference point
- doses to critical structures must be maintained within specified limits
- the volume of normal tissue that is overdosed is within the tolerances specified
- the volume of the target that is under-dosed is within the tolerances specified.

In some situations a single field is employed where the tumour is superficial (e.g. spinal cord, mammary nodes). In these cases a dose distribution is not required and the treatment is prescribed to a specified depth on the central axis of the beam.

Figure 10.3a shows the simplest combination of two fields that are parallel opposed; the isodose charts are superimposed and a composite chart can be produced manually by adding the dose values from each field at points where the isodoses intersect (e.g. point A in Figure 10.3a has a composite value of 130%). Lines can be drawn that join equal values of dose; a computer system will do this automatically by adding to a matrix of dose points. The resultant dose distribution is the combined isodose data normalised to the peak dose of the individual fields (i.e. dose at $d_{max}$ = 100%).

Figure 10.3b shows a similar exercise for two fields at right angles to each other; the resultant distribution would show a dose gradient between the bottom left corner and the top right corner

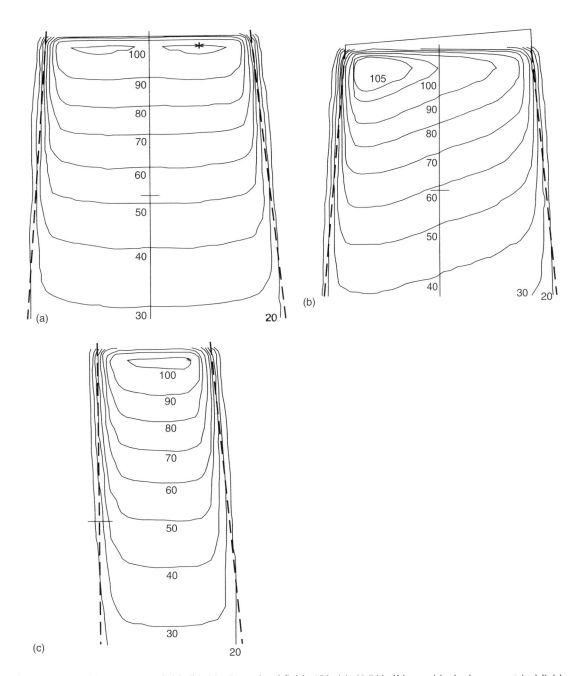

**Figure 10.2** (a) 6 MV open field; (b) 10 MV wedged field, 45°, (c) 6 MV half-beam blocked asymmetrical field.

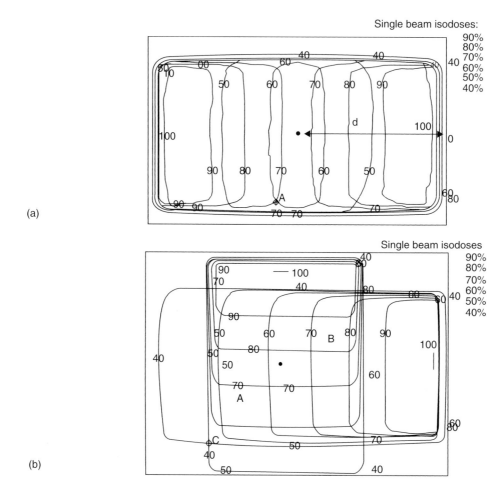

**Figure 10.3** (a) 6 MV parallel pair fields, fixed SSD; (b) 6 MV fields at right angles.

when combined ($A = 120\%$ and $B = 160\%$). A square target volume situated at the centre of each plan would indicate that the right angle field plan would not meet the above dose criteria due to this dose gradient, but the parallel pair gives a homogeneous distribution (130%) provided that adequate coverage of the target volume is maintained (i.e. large enough field size).

These field combinations are shown for the *fixed SSD method* where the axis of rotation of the machine (isocentre) is set at the surface to which the beam is incident (generally, SSD = SAD = 100 cm). Similar plans can be produced for the *isocentric method* where the iso-

centre is set approximately to the centre of the irradiated volume (the intersection point or midpoint of the fields) and the SAD = 100 cm but for each field the SSD = 100 − *d*.

## Build-up and penumbra regions

Regions of high-dose gradients in the radiation field require particular attention from the treatment planner to meet the criteria of acceptability. Tissues close to the edge of the field and near the skin surface are the areas of greatest dose uncertainty and accurate measurements are required of the spatial dose variation with an understanding of the limitations of the computer planning algorithms which model these high-dose gradient regions.

Megavoltage X-ray beams exhibit a rapid increase in dose in the first few millimetres of tissue, reaching a maximum value up to several centimetres deep depending on the incident photon energy. For a 6 MV X-ray beam, the dose increases from 20% at the surface to 85% at 5 mm deep and peaking at 15 mm depth, whereas for a 10 MV beam, the peak dose is at 25 mm depth, the dose then decreasing beyond this point. The *build-up or 'skin-sparing'* phenomena can be explained by the increase in secondary electrons, and subsequent energy deposition, beneath the surface, which reaches equilibrium at a finite depth while the photon energy fluence is continuously decreasing with depth. For treatment planning it is essential to determine whether the build-up region encroaches on the target volume, in which case some external bolus may be required.

At the edge of the radiation field the dose falls rapidly with lateral distance from the central axis; this shadow or penumbra region is caused primarily by the finite size of the radiation source and increases with the distance from the source (geometrical penumbra). However, the width of the penumbra region is also dependent on scattering from both the phantom and collimator systems. For a 6 MV X-ray beam, the distance between the 20% and 80% isodoses in the penumbra is typically 4 mm at $d_{max}$ and 6 mm at 10 cm deep. The radiation field size is defined as the lateral distance between the 50% isodoses where the field defining light on the treatment machine coincides with these points. However, in treatment planning the selection of field size may not be determined from the geometrical edge of the field but the position of, for example, the 90% isodose with respect to the target boundary. A great deal of uncertainty exists about the definition of field edges that are associated with dosimetric inaccuracies and beam positioning errors; particular caution should be taken when planning small fields (<4 cm) where these uncertainties are most significant.

## Wedges, tissue compensators and intensity modulators

### Wedges

The isodose distribution may be shaped by inserting material that reduces the radiation intensity progressively across the beam, the most widely used form of this modifying device being the *wedge filter*. A wedge-shaped metal block usually made from lead, steel or brass is physically inserted into the beam either behind or in front of the collimators at a fixed distance from the source. An example of the resulting angled isodose curve is shown in Figure 10.2b.

The *wedge angle* is defined either as the angle that a tangent drawn through a specified isodose (usually the 50%) subtends to the central axis, or as the angle through which an isodose is tilted at the central axis of the beam at a specified depth (usually 10 cm).[10] A set of wedges is usually employed on each megavoltage machine covering the angles 15, 30, 45 and 60°; these are commonly known as universal wedges because they can be used for all field sizes up to a specified maximum.

In treatment planning the wedge filter is used for two purposes:

1. Deliberately to alter the dose gradient in the patient to enable a uniform distribution of dose to be produced when beams are arranged at angles to each other. This angle is known as the hinge angle. The required wedge angle can be calculated approximately by the formula:

   Wedge angle = 90° − (hinge angle/2).

2. To compensate for surface obliquity off axis (see below), by increasing the dose (thin end of the wedge) at the region of tissue excess and reducing the dose (thick end of the wedge)

at the region of tissue deficiency, relative to the central axis. The wedge angle required for body curvature correction is approximately 50–75% of the obliquity angle (i.e. the angle subtended by a tangent line drawn at the beam entry point on the body contour, to a line normal to the central axis at the same point).

The introduction of a wedge filter into the radiation beam results in the following dosimetry effects:

- The dose output is decreased due to attenuation by the wedge and is characterised by the *wedge factor* (WF) or *wedge output factor* (WOF). WF is the ratio of dose for a given field size without and with the wedge at a specified depth on the central axis of the beam. WOF is the ratio of dose of an open $10 \times 10$ cm field to the dose of a wedged field of specified size at the depth of peak dose on the central axis of the beam measured at depth (typically 5 cm). The use of WF requires a field size variant output factor to be incorporated in the calculation of dose output, whereas WOFs are described by a table of factors for square and rectangular fields. WF and WOF, as defined here, are always greater than unity and are applied as multiplication factors to obtain correct machine settings. The wedge factor definition also assumes that the depth dose distribution is normalised to $d_{max}$ on the central axis with the wedge in the beam, as in Figure 10.2b.
- The wedge filter attenuates the lower energy X-rays in a megavoltage beam causing a 'beam-hardening' effect that alters the central axis depth dose values, particularly at large depths. This effect is more evident for steep wedges where the wedge factor is large. Most treatment planning systems take this change in beam quality into account by applying hardening factors or using measured depth dose data for wedges.

Recently, the use of physical wedges that are manually positioned in the treatment head has been superseded by the *auto-wedge* and *dynamic wedge*. The former is a steep wedge-shaped filter that is automatically introduced into the beam at a position forward of the flattening filter and is controlled by the accelerator control software. The proportion of treatment exposure with the wedge inserted relative to the open beam determines the wedge angle. The dynamic wedge feature of some linear accelerators utilises the movement of collimator jaws and control of dose rate to generate a wedge-shaped dose distribution and therefore no external beam modifier needs to be inserted into the beam. The isodose shape is the result of a summation of fields in which one independent collimation jaw is sequentially closed to create a series of decreasing field widths while simultaneously adjusting the monitor units per segment to achieve the required dose distribution.[11] The dose and jaw positions for a particular wedge are specified in segmented treatment tables (STTs).

## Tissue compensation and intensity modulators

Tissue compensation is often required when (1) the obliquity of the patient results in an unacceptable dose distribution, (2) the dose to the patient's skin must be increased, i.e. sparing is not required, or (3) the dose to a critical structure is excessive and must be reduced by shaping the dose distribution. The use of a wedge filter as a tissue compensator has already been discussed and these normally correct for obliquity in only one plane of the patient.

Tissue compensation over the full field area is simply achieved using bolus material (e.g. wax) added directly to the skin, resulting in a flat surface normal to the beam. However, such a compensator placed on the surface will result in a loss of the skin-sparing effect, which is desirable in some circumstances, although in most patients is to be avoided because of skin erythema. If the build-up effect is to be maintained, the compensating filter must be mounted on the accessory tray of the accelerator (at least 15–20 cm from the patient) and the appropriate scaling factors used.

Modern methods of dynamic collimator movement have now enabled highly sophisticated techniques for control of the dose distribution that could eventually replace the use of wedges and physical forms of tissue compensators. *Geometrical shaping* of the radiation field is made possible by the use of the multi-leaf collimator (MLC). *Dosimetric shaping* of the radiation field is made possible by intensity modulation of segments of the beam. Each field segment (or beamlet) has a specified intensity that is dependent on the required contribution at depth in the patient which itself is governed by the dose constraints to the target volumes and critical structures. The technique of IMRT is achieved by movement of the MLC leaves to specified positions while the intensity of the beam is controlled for each of these leaf positions. IMRT is applied using either 'dynamic MLC' or 'step and shoot' methods. The treatment planning methods for IMRT are described later.

### Dose corrections

The isodose data used for treatment planning is measured with the central axis of the beam perpendicular to the surface of a unit density phantom, usually a water tank as described below. A patient is neither flat nor homogeneous and therefore corrections must be made to the depth dose values. As described in the previous section, some type of compensator could be used to minimise the dose effects that the beam encounters due to these tissue variations.

### Oblique incidence

The oblique incidence of a field to the skin surface results in variation of SSD over the area of the beam and subsequently changes in attenuation due to tissue excess or deficit. Many of the manual methods of correction that can be applied

in 2D planning are briefly described but a more thorough mathematical presentation can be found elsewhere.[3–5]

- The *isodose shift method* was primarily used for manual treatment planning before the introduction of computers. This is achieved either by sliding the isodose chart forward (for missing tissue) or backwards (for more tissue) compared with its central axis position on the skin surface. Figure 10.4a illustrates a movement of the isodose curve by a distance, $x$, to

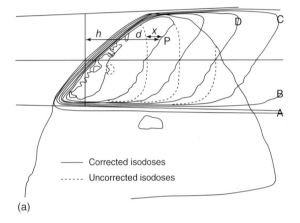

(a)

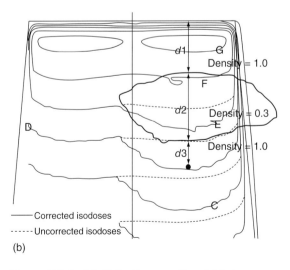

(b)

**Figure 10.4** (a) Obliquity correction; (b) heterogeneity correction.

correct for a tissue deficit of thickness, $h$; the ratio $x/h$ is almost constant (typically 0.6 for 5–15 MV photons) and can be applied to all points where dose correction for oblique incidence is necessary. This approximate method corrects for changes in beam attenuation and SSD variation. A more accurate method, and one used in computer models, is to multiply the percentage dose at the depth measured from the skin surface by the change in SSD using an inverse square correction, an *effective SSD method*.

- The *tissue-maximum ratio method* is independent of the SSD change due to tissue obliquity, and therefore the correction required to the depth dose at point P (Figure 10.4a) can be obtained from the ratio of tissue maximum ratios for depths $d$ and $d + h$. This is the most common method used for computer treatment planning and can be used for 3D calculations of depth if 3D representations of the body are available. Some systems assume that the tissue obliquity to be a tissue heterogeneity of zero density and use the corrections described below.

## Tissue heterogeneity correction

Tissue heterogeneity correction methods generally attempt to correct for changes in the primary component of the beam and ignore the complex effect on the scattered radiation in the 3D volume. However, some recently employed algorithms are able to correct for the scatter component and are described in more detail later.

The simplest method uses a depth dose correction for lung (approximately 2.5% increase in dose per centimetre for a 6 MV photon beam) and assumes no correction for small amounts of bone.

- The *effective depth method* estimates the equivalent thickness of unit density material that attenuates the beam passing through the non-uniform tissues. The effective depth at point P for a beam incident on the outline shown in Figure 10.4b is:

$$d_{\text{eff}} = d_1 + (d_2 \times 0.3) + d_3$$

The dose at this depth must now be corrected for the inverse square change due to point P being at a distance $(\text{SSD} + d_1 + d_2 + d_3)$ from the source instead of $(\text{SSD} + d_{\text{eff}})$.

- The *Batho* (or power law) *method* uses a ratio of TMRs raised to a power that is determined by the relative electron densities of the tissues. The correction factor to the depth dose at point P in Figure 10.4b is given by:

$$C_{\text{hetero}} = [\text{TMR}(d_3)]^{(\rho 1 - \rho 2)} / [\text{TMR}(d_2 + d_3)]^{(1 - \rho 2)}$$

where, $\rho_1 = 1.0$ and $\rho_2 = 0.3$ from Figure 10.4b.

- The equivalent tissue : air ratio (ETAR) method makes use of 3D arrays of CT numbers that have been converted to electron densities rather than using a regional correction of tissues with similar electron densities. This method includes the effect of scattering on the geometrical position of point P in relation to its surrounding tissues, by calculating the ratio of the tissue : air ratios (TARs obtained from TMRs) at an effective field size and effective depth against that at the true depth and field size. A weighted average of the electron densities is used to scale the field size when calculating the scatter dose at P. These corrections for heterogeneous conditions do not perform well in regions where there is lack of electron equilibrium, i.e. build-up region of the beam.

### SSD correction

SSD correction to the depth dose values is required if the actual SSD deviates from the SSD of the input data (reference data) to the treatment planning system. Often the isodose data is measured at an SSD = 100 cm and non-standard SSDs are used for isocentric treatments and extended SSDs. Changing the SSD alters the output as referenced to the dose maximum point on the central axis, $d_{max}$; if the SSD is altered to $f$ compared with the standard SSD $f_o$ (usually 100 cm), the output must be corrected by:

$$[(f + d_{max})/(f_o + d_{max})]^2$$

The percentage depth dose values change to a lesser extent with alteration in the SSD and the correction to a point at depth d is given by:

$$[(f_o + d)/(f_o + d_{max})]^2 / [(f + d_{max})/(f + d)]^2 .$$

This correction, known as the Mayneord factor, should be applied to the depth dose at the standard SSD $f_o$, using the field size measured at the SSD $f$.

## Beam weighting and normalisation

Methods of beam weighting and normalisation vary between radiotherapy centres. Two of the most common are:

1. Method 1: the beam weight for a fixed SSD treatment is a multiplying factor applied to the peak dose on the central axis of the beam, i.e. weight = 1.00, dose at $d_{max}$ = 100%; weight = 1.2, dose at $d_{max}$ = 120%.
2. Method 2: the beam weight for an isocentric treatment is the relative contribution to the dose at the isocentre, i.e. the individual dose from each beam at isocentre $d_{iso}$ = 100%. The combined dose at the isocentre may then be normalised to 100%.

However, method 1 may also be used for isocentric treatments as illustrated in Figure 10.5a where a pair of equally weighted parallel fields are each normalised (100%) to $d_{max}$. Figure 10.5b is the same plan but with the weighting of each field referred to the isocentre (method 2); hence the percentage dose at $d_{max}$ is now almost 150% for each field. The two plans are effectively identical (both have equal contributions from each field) apart for their normalisation criteria.

Figure 10.5c, d illustrates the two weighting methods with the isocentre moved from the midplane towards one of the fields; the beam weights relative to each other are now inversely proportional to the ratio of their individual depth doses at the isocentre to give equal doses at the isocentre. Again the two dose distributions are identical but are displayed differently because of the normalisation method employed.

It should be remembered at this stage that the dose distributions are relative plots of dose and that the monitor units required for each field may be easily obtained provided that the dose at the calibration reference point (usually $d_{max}$) is calculated.

## Dose prescribing and reporting

The publications ICRU50[7] and its supplement ICRU62[8] give clear recommendations about reporting of absorbed dose distributions and set out the level of complexity of dose evaluation from basic planning techniques to complex 3D dose computation.

ICRU50 gives clear and concise definitions of *gross tumour volume* (GTV), *clinical target volume* (CTV) and *planning target volume* (PTV), which are marked on the CT images of the patient before beam placement and calculation of the plan. The reports take into consideration the variations and inaccuracies of radiotherapy and the means of accounting for both the clinical uncertainties (e.g. spread of disease) and those uncertainties associated with the planning and treatment processes. The supplement publication[8] develops the concept of treatment margins that can account for geometrical changes in the CTV due to anatomical uncertainties (*internal margin*) and those added to account for uncertainties on patient position (*set-up margin*).

The ICRU publications give a general criterion for reporting dose as a point within the PTV referred to as the *ICRU reference point*; this is a point that represents the spatial variation of dose within the PTV and is generally the dose

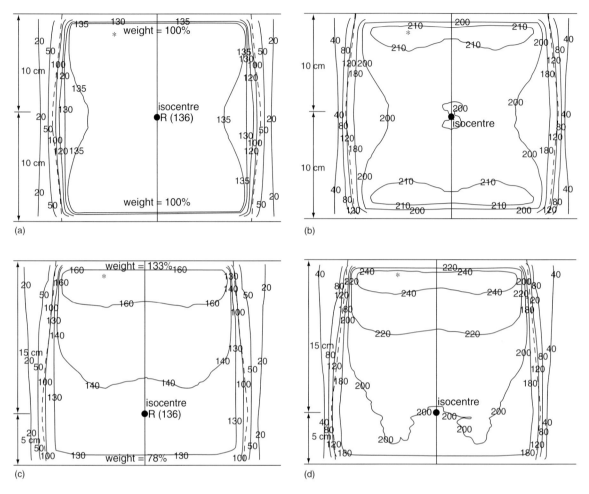

**Figure 10.5** Normalisation at (a) $d_{max}$ for each beam, equal weight at isocentre; (b) isocentre for each beam, equal weight at isocentre; (c) $d_{max}$ for each beam, equal weight at isocentre; (d) isocentre of each beam, equal weight at isocentre, a and b have their isocentre at the midplane whereas c and d have the isocentre shifted towards one field.

prescription point. This reference point is often, but not always, as with the case of half-beam blocked matched fields, at the treatment isocentre which is generally the intersection of all beams.

With the increased use of *conformal radiotherapy treatment* (CRT), which utilises geometrical shaping of beams by MLC, the concept of *conformity index* (CI) has been introduced, which is described in more detail later.

The final hard copy of the plan and associated information are important to successful imple-

mentation and must be an unambiguous set of accurate instructions. A dosimetry report sheet (Figure 10.6) will often accompany plots of the dose distribution in the required cross-sections and must contain a clear description of each field parameter, including field sizes, machine and patient angles, setting up distances and any special instructions. The sheet should also contain a step-by-step description of the monitor unit calculation for each field from the original prescribed dose distribution. All correction factors should be clearly stated (even if the value is

RT START DATE: 18/12/08
MACHINE: LA3 600C/D #737 6X
PLAN APPROVED AT: Jun 15 2008 3:19:11:000PM
Calc. grid size: 2.5 mm
Inhom. correction: Modified Batho
Isocentric norm. : None

NAME: Radiotherapy Patient
UNIT NO: XXXX-1234
CONSULTANT: ASB
1° REF POINTID: OROPHARYNX
COURSEID: 1
PLANSETUPID/NAME: OROPHARYNX. / OROPHARYNX
PLANNED USING: Eclipse version 7.1.67.4

Field Description

| FIELD No. | FIELD NAME | SSD (mm) | FIELD SIZE (mm) | SHORT AXIS | SET SIZE (mm) X | Y1 | Y2 | WEDGE | THICK END | GANTRY ANGLE | COLL ANGLE | COUCH ANGLE | Varis Wedge Code |
|---|---|---|---|---|---|---|---|---|---|---|---|---|---|
| 1 ¤ | p1_lrlat | 936 | 148×166 | VERT | 158 | 85 | 92 | EW30 Y1-IN | ANT | 270 | 90 | 0 | EDW30IN |
| 2 ¤ | p1_2saob1 | 953 | 156×169 | VERT | 164 | 92 | 85 | | | 25 | 0 | 90 | |
| 3 ¤ | p1_2saob1 | 949 | 150×168 | VERT | 158 | 92 | 85 | EW15 Y2-OUT | ANT | 90 | 90 | 0 | EDW15OUT |

TUMOUR DOSE: 30 Gy to 100% in 10 treatments

| FIELD No. | FIELD NAME | WEIGHT | Plan Normal- isation Factor | PEAK DOSE (GY) | NO. OF TRTS | PEAK DOSE /TRT. (GY) | Output Factor (MU/GY) | INV. SQUARE FACTOR | Eq Sq Eclipse (cm) | SET MU /TRT | Field Dose Contribution (GY) | Ref. Dose (GY) |
|---|---|---|---|---|---|---|---|---|---|---|---|---|
| 1 ¤ | p1_lrlat | 53% | 0.9956 | 15.83 | 10 | 1.58 | 135.9 | 0.878 | 9.3 | 189 | 0.989 | |
| 2 ¤ | p1_2saob1 | 41% | 0.9956 | 12.25 | 10 | 1.22 | 96.6 | 0.910 | 9.9 | 108 | 0.941 | |
| 3 ¤ | p1_2saob1 | 53% | 0.9956 | 15.83 | 10 | 1.58 | 114.9 | 0.903 | 9.6 | 164 | 1.070 | |

3.000

PATIENT SUPINE ¤ = Millennium 120 MLC
Set to marks on shell. Anterior distance = 96.5 cm.

Planned by: lmc                                          Checked by:

**Figure 10.6**  Radiotherapy physics planning report.

unity) to enable the calculation to be carefully checked before the start of treatment.

Electronic transfer of the patient treatment plan information to the treatment linear accelerator is highly recommended to reduce the pos-sibilities of transcription error that occurs when manual transfer is used. This electronic transfer of data is usually from the TPS to the *record and verify system* (RVS) but still requires checking to ensure correctness.

# Dose computational models for photon beams

Radiotherapy planning is almost exclusively performed using computer-based treatment planning systems, apart from some single field and parallel pair treatments for which no dose distribution is required and central axis depth doses are obtained from charts. The earliest planning systems, which became available in the 1970s, were required to calculate a 2D dose distribution for simple square or rectangular fields on a single patient contour. Advances in patient imaging and radiotherapy delivery techniques have driven the development of more sophisticated dose calculation algorithms.

The introduction of CT imaging to the radiotherapy planning process enabled more accurate localisation of the target volume, while the subsequent development of beam-shaping technology such as the MLC allowed the shape of treatment fields to be more accurately matched to that of the target. The advent of such conformal radiotherapy techniques introduced a new challenge for dose computation – the 3D calculation of dose from highly irregular fields. The other important impact of CT was the visualisation of inhomogeneities within the patient and the need to accurately account for them in the dose calculation. Subsequent developments in treatment technology, such as IMRT, have further increased the demand for more accurate dose calculation algorithms through the increased use of small fields, in which electronic equilibrium does not exist.

An understanding of the basic principles behind dose calculation models provides not only an insight into the function of the treatment planning system but also an appreciation of its inherent limitations. Different systems' calculation algorithms differ in the details of their implementation, but share many common principles. In this context, it is perhaps most useful to consider dose calculation algorithms in terms of their sophistication, from the earliest 'mass storage' models through to modern convolution-superposition algorithms.

## Storage models

The first computer-based dose calculation models, such as the Milan–Bentley storage model,[12] required the measurement of large amounts of beam data and were capable of determining the dose only from square and rectangular fields. For each square field size, open and wedged, the central axis depth dose curve and 1D dose profiles measured along the plane normal to the central axis were stored. The profiles provided off-axis ratios (i.e. the dose at a point off-axis as a ratio of the dose at the central axis in the same plane). The relative dose at an arbitrary point in a square field was calculated by interpolating between the adjacent stored off-axis ratios and multiplying the result by the central axis dose at that depth. Rectangular fields were accounted for by determining their equivalent square field size[13] and interpolating between adjacent stored square field data.

Subsequent refinements of the mass storage models went some way towards addressing their limitations, e.g. in one algorithm the measured profiles were divided into two components, a radially symmetrical envelope profile, describing the variation in off-axis ratio with distance from the central axis and depth, and a boundary profile, describing the beam penumbra as a function of depth. However, the limitation of the models' applicability only to square and rectangular fields remained.

## Correction-based algorithms

The data measured for square and rectangular fields is not easily corrected for irregular shapes produced by shielding blocks or MLC. To overcome this problem, beam sector integration was implemented in some planning systems. This method separated the absorbed dose at a point into a primary photon component and a scatter component determined empirically as a function of field size for circular fields. The sector integration method of Cunningham,[14] shown in Figure 10.7c, for determining the scatter component from an irregularly shaped beam involved subdividing the field area into 36 sectors drawn at 10° intervals. Each sector was then subdivided into lengths $d$ in centimetres, and the scatter contribution to point P calculated by summing the contribution from each segment, sectors beneath the shielding not contributing to the integration. The absorbed dose to point P is then found by adding the primary component to the scatter contribution. A more detailed account of the *primary/scatter component method* can be found elsewhere.[4]

The calculation geometry for a beam incident on a water phantom is shown in Figure 10.8.[15] The depth dose at a point $(x', y', z)$, a projection of a point on the surface $(x, y, z = 0)$ along a ray line from the radiation source to a depth $z$, is given by the product of $D_{cax}(z,A)$ – the depth

dose, at distance $z$ along the central axis for equivalent field size $A$ – and $p(r,z)$ – the profile function at the off-axis distance $r = (x'^2 + y'^2)^{1/2}$ at that depth, i.e. the dose at P is given by:

$$D(x', y', z) = D_{cax}(z, A) \times p(r, z).$$

For a realistic case in the human body and where the SSD may vary from the SSD of the measured data, then the dose at P is given by:

$$D(x', y', z) = D_{CAX}(z, A) \times p(r, z) \times C_{SSD} \times C_{OBL} \times C_{HETRO}$$

where $C_{SSD}$, $C_{obl}$ and $C_{hetro}$ are corrections for SSD change, surface obliquity and tissue heterogeneity respectively.

For the irregular field case the depth dose and off-axis values must be calculated using methods described above. The depth dose at each point on a 2D or 3D grid is calculated for each beam and finally combined into a dose matrix that enables isodose plotting.

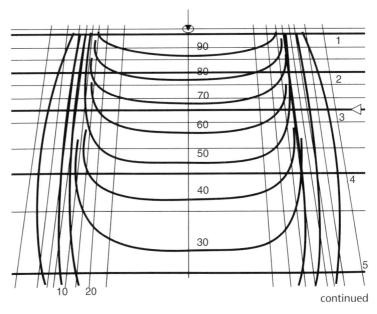

(a)

continued

**Figure 10.7** (a) Fan-line dose matrix; (b) depth dose curve and dose profile; (c) sector integration for irregular field calculation, where $d$ is the length of the sector at distance $x$ from the calculation point p.

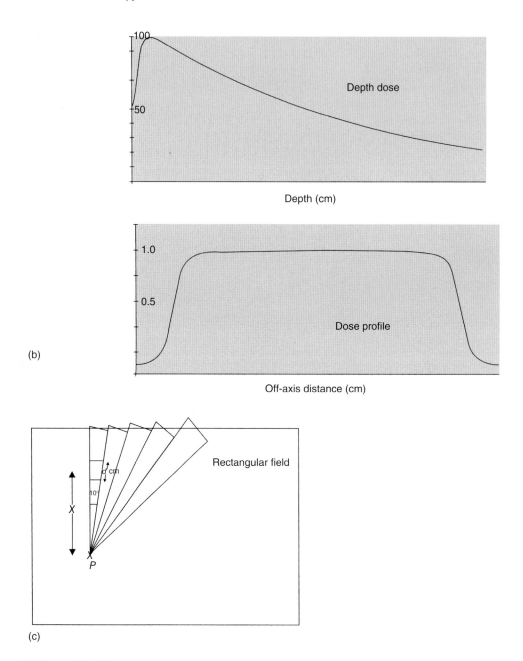

**Figure 10.7** continued

The next development in the modelling of irregular fields was the implementation of pencil beam convolution algorithms. A pencil beam kernel describes the deposition of energy around a very narrow beam, or 'pencil beam', and typi-cally represents the scatter distribution due to the primary photon fluence and secondary electron scatter. The kernels are pre-calculated during the configuration of the algorithm, either through Monte Carlo modelling techniques[15] or by

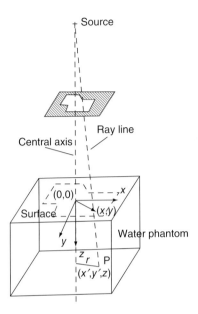

**Figure 10.8** Beam calculation geometry showing rayline projection.

processing beam data measured in a homogeneous medium.[16] Having determined the kernels, the dose distribution from a treatment field is computed by dividing the field into pencil beams and mathematically combining (convolving) their contributions over the entire field area. Making the kernels dependent upon their position within the field enables account to be taken of any beam modifiers through which the pencil beams pass, including changes in intensity and beam hardening.

Correction-based algorithms usually calculate the dose distribution with the assumption that the patient has both a flat surface and a homogeneous, water-equivalent composition. In a uniform medium with a density that is different from that of water, the water-equivalent kernels are scaled according to the relative density of the medium. More realistic patient geometries are accounted for by the subsequent application of the broad beam corrections for patient obliquity and inhomogeneity, such as those described earlier. The calculation of dose on slices away from the plane of the central axis is often achieved

by the tracing of geometric raylines from the radiation source to the calculation point, with the application of an appropriate heterogeneity correction.

## Advanced beam modelling

The beam models discussed above are capable of reasonable levels of dose calculation accuracy in a uniform medium for relatively large fields. However, the models' consideration of scatter is largely empirical and the inhomogeneity corrections used are capable of accounting for perturbations only of the photon fluence. Accurate dose calculation requires consideration of the contribution of scatter from the entire volume to the point of calculation; the impact of changes in the electron fluence is critical in this process in the absence of electronic equilibrium. The next generation of dose calculation algorithms, the *model-based* algorithms, consider electron scatter more explicitly.

Monte Carlo simulation, in which the individual interactions of millions of incident photons and the resultant photons and electrons are modelled, is currently the most accurate dose calculation model available. Despite recent advances in computational power, long calculation times prevent the widespread use of full Monte Carlo simulation in the routine clinical setting. More practical are a group of convolution-superposition (CS) models that represent the best compromise between accuracy and realistic calculation requirements.

Many different CS models are in common use; although the details of their implementations vary, most divide the dose modelling into two components. The first component describes the total energy released per unit mass, or terma. The second component, one or more kernels, describes the energy deposited around a primary photon interaction site.

The terma is the energy imparted to the medium by the interactions of the primary photons, i.e. the energy lost per unit mass from the primary photon beam. The terma at an inter-action voxel is a function of the energy fluence and is, therefore, dependent upon the depth of that voxel and the polyenergetic spectrum of the clinical beam. The terma component varies with position in a clinical beam as a result of changes in the fluence across the beam (caused by factors such as the beam hardening effect of the flatten-ing filter or a wedge). The effect of inhomogenei-ties on the terma is commonly accounted for by depth scaling, according to the relative electron densities of the tissue along the rayline.

The energy deposition kernels model the total energy imparted by the primary photons around an interaction site; this includes the energy retained by scattered photons and that trans-ferred to charged particles (electrons). The distri-bution of this energy around the interaction site defines the shape of the kernels. Commonly, sep-arate kernels are used to describe the primary energy (the primary kernel) and the scattered energy (the scatter kernel). The shape of the kernels is commonly derived for individual linear accelerators by Monte Carlo simulation, taking into account the effects of the components of different linac treatment heads. The effect of inhomogeneities is included in dose calculations by scaling the kernels – ideally anisotropically – according to the relative electron density of the tissue surrounding the interaction site.

At an individual calculation point, the total energy deposited as a result of the interactions at a particular voxel of unit mass is found by com-bining the terma at the interaction voxel with the value of the kernel specific to the location of the calculation point relative to the interaction voxel. The overall dose at the calculation point is obtained by convolving the contributions over all interaction voxels.

The more explicit consideration of electrons in model-based algorithms results in significant improvements in calculation accuracy over the correction-based models. These improvements are most clearly seen in situations where elec-tronic equilibrium does not exist:

- In low-density tissue such as lung, the simpler algorithms ignore the reduction in deposited dose caused by the increased range of scattered electrons and model only the reduction in attenuation of the primary photons, overesti-mating the dose to the low density tissue. Model-based algorithms more accurately predict the reduction in absorbed dose; this is reflected in poorer coverage of PTVs that include lung tissue.[17]
- Close to interfaces between tissues of different density (such as soft tissue and bone), correc-tion-based algorithms fail to accurately model the changes in dose, e.g. when a beam passes from soft tissue into bone, there is an increase in the dose in the soft tissue resulting from increased electron back scatter. Model-based algorithms model such effects more realisti-cally, although this is perhaps the situation in which these algorithms are least accurate.
- Fields smaller than the order of 4 cm × 4 cm exhibit lateral electronic disequilibrium due to the range of the electrons relative to the size of the field. The improved consideration of the scattered electrons by model-based algorithms enables them to more accurately predict the doses, which is of particular impor-tance in IMRT treatments, which frequently comprise large numbers of very small beam segments.

## Inverse planning calculations for IMRT

The iterative optimisation methods used by most IMRT planning systems (described later) involve the minimisation of a cost function quantifying the difference between the desired dose distribu-tion and that from the field fluences at each stage of the optimisation. This requires calculation of the dose distribution after each iteration of the optimisation.

The algorithm used in this dose calculation must be accurate and calculate the dose in a sufficiently short time that the optimisations are not unacceptably slow. This latter requirement usually necessitates compromises in the accuracy of the dose calculation, such as poor consideration of scatter and inhomogeneities and widely spaced dose calculation points.

The direction of the optimisation is dependent on the dose calculations performed after each iteration; inaccuracy in the calculations will result in fields that do not produce the desired dose distribution. (For example, if the algorithm used after each iteration tends to underestimate the PTV dose by 10% and calculates a mean PTV dose of 60 Gy, the final forward dose calculation by a more accurate algorithm would reveal that the mean PTV dose was actually over 66 Gy. The optimisation would then need to be repeated with the PTV dose constraints set approximately 10% below the dose level actually desired in order to ultimately achieve the desired dose.) This variation between the desired and actual dose resulting from inaccuracies in the algorithm used during the inverse planning is known as a 'convergence error'. Until Monte Carlo can be used routinely in inverse planning, pencil beam algorithms represent the best compromise between speed and accuracy during optimisations, ideally followed by a forward dose calculation using a more advanced algorithm.

## Data measurements for treatment planning systems

### Beam data acquisition and entry

Beam data acquisition and entry into the treatment planning system are illustrated in Figure 10.9a, which has been adapted from an original report ICRU42.[6] A large water tank fed by a reservoir is positioned in the beam using a trolley with hydraulic lift, 3D movement of a small radiation detector (<0.3 cm$^3$ ion chamber or semiconductor diode) is controlled by a PC allowing depth dose and profile data to be stored on the hard drive. Modern beam data plotting systems allow for automatic sequencing of data to enable 3D dose information to be obtained for a par-

ticular field set-up. A complete set of beam data as required by the treatment planning system together with isodose chart production may be obtained in a reasonable time period. Computer software is now provided by most manufacturers of beam data acquisition systems (BDAS) that translate the measured data into the format of a specified treatment planning system (TPS). Transfer of these files online or via digital media allows rapid input of beam data.

### Patient data acquisition and entry

Patient data acquisition and entry into the treatment planning system are shown in Fig. 10.9b, where the method employed is determined by the equipment available and the requirement for 2D or 3D data. The use of computed tomography (CT) images is the most common method of obtaining both external shape and anatomical information of the patient.

Patient contours can also be acquired using optical and ultrasonic devices that enable a 2D contour to be taken through the midplane of the target volume and other axial planes. The optical method employs laser lines projected onto the patient and imaged by two charge-coupled device (CCD) cameras. Multiple contours of the patient's skin can be reconstructed by computer manipulation of the video data.

CT provides transverse slices of the human anatomy by reconstructing the attenuation of a narrow beam of X-rays through the different tissues. The CT numbers associated with each pixel (reconstruction element) may be converted to electron density values (the parameter on which Compton attenuation is proportional) by calibrating an image produced by a phantom containing known electron densities. CT images not only provide accurate external contours of the patient but also facilitate a means of correcting for megavoltage photon attenuation in the tissues (heterogeneity correction, see above). CT information gives improved visualisation compared with non-CT planning methods, thereby

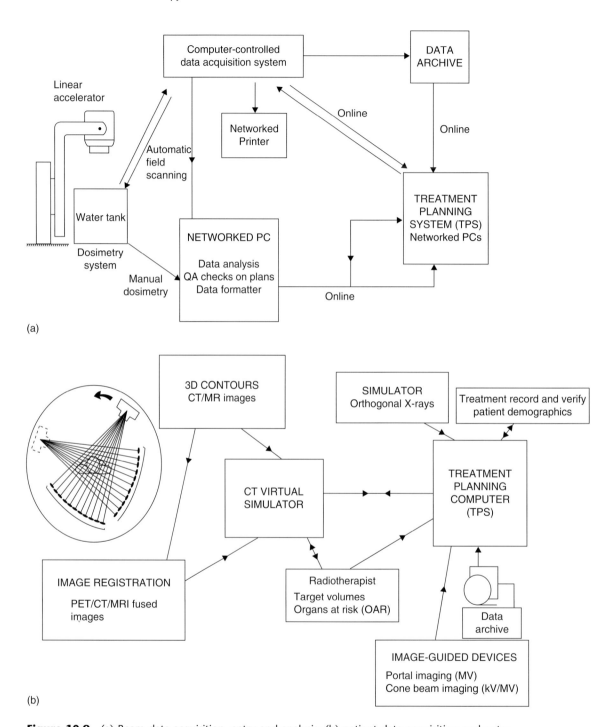

**Figure 10.9** (a) Beam data acquisition, entry and analysis; (b) patient data acquisition and entry.

enabling the clinician to delineate the target volume and surrounding structures.

The use of CT scans for treatment planning has become well established and has been shown to provide significant improvement in treatment accuracy. In recent years, the use of *magnetic resonance imaging* (MRI) for treatment planning has proved popular. Although the MRI pixel values cannot provide information for inhomogeneities, the improved soft-tissue resolution of MRI enables solid tumour visualisation and additional information for delineation of anatomical structures. Combining the target volume information obtained from MRI and transferring this to the CT images is a complex process and involves a process of fusing (or registering) the images by matching reference points common to the two types of images.

Functional imaging such as *positron emission tomography* (PET) can give additional information about the spread of the malignant disease. Some PET scanners incorporate a CT scanner (PET-CT) that provides CT images taken at the time of the PET acquisition and have inherent registration of the two imaging modalities. The use of PET-CT images for radiotherapy treatment planning requires careful consideration with regard to the fusion with the planning CT study because the patient is not in the treatment position unless provision for this has been made. Image fusion software, similar to that used for CT-MRI registration, enables any target contours (e.g. GTV) that are marked on the PET study to be automatically overlaid on the planning CT study. The increased use of images that contain additional information about the disease (e.g. post-surgery images) and can be precisely matched to the planning CT enable more accurate definition of the GTV and clinical target volume (CTV) by the clinician.

The images produced for treatment planning may be transferred directly by computer network or via a portable digital storage media (e.g. disk). The format used for this transfer is known as the *digital imaging and communications in medicine format for radiotherapy* (DICOM-RT). This format enables a common framework for data generation and exchange between radiotherapy systems although transfer between different TPSs can sometimes be problematic.

External contouring and delineation of the volumes of interest are achieved using the contouring tools provided by all planning systems. It should be remembered that accurate planning is dependent on the patient being scanned in an identical position to the treatment position. The following conditions are necessary for accurate imaging in treatment planning:

- flat-top couch insert
- large-diameter CT to accommodate the patient in treatment position
- immobilisation devices as used for treatment
- marking of reference points on the patients skin using radio-opaque catheters
- scan field size sufficient to encompass all the external contour
- minimal distortion of the image.

The treatment simulator plays an important role in target volume localisation and the verification of treatment plans (see Chapter 13). It has all the gantry and couch movements of a linear accelerator but allows radiographic or fluoroscopic visualisation of the treatment field relative to the internal organs of the body (usually bone landmarks). Some simulators have an attachment that allows the acquisition of CT data and these systems are often referred to as SIM-CT or cone beam imaging systems; limitations of this method are the inferior reconstructed image quality to diagnostic CT and the long scan times.

In the past 10 years most CT scanners have been adapted specifically to the requirements for treatment planning and the associated software is able to perform like a conventional simulator. This system, known as a CT-SIM or virtual simulation, has computer software and laser positioning equipment to provide accurate radiographic portal views using digital reconstruction from the CT data (digitally reconstructed radiographs, DRRs), and a means of marking field portal reference points on the patient. These systems also provide advanced visualisation and contouring tools that allow the rapid marking of the treatment volumes and display of field position with any associated shielding. Comparison of kV and MV portal images produced at various stages of the radiotherapy process, i.e. simulation, planning and treatment, has the potential to become a major tool that ensures quality radiotherapy treatment.

## Quality assurance

Quality assurance (QA) of planning data is essential to ensure and maintain the accuracy of the system. This subject is wide ranging and beyond the scope of this book; however, many radiotherapy publications provide a guide to commissioning and quality control for TPSs.[18,19] Quality control primarily covers software performance but must also deal with the accuracy of data transfer via digital networks. Checking the consistency of data transferred between two systems involves sending a standard data set (e.g. a test plan) and determining the accuracy of the data at the receiving system by comparing against the original sent information. All aspects of the plan parameter transfer must be checked to ensure that data has not been lost or misinterpreted during the transfer. Standard data transfer protocols, such as DICOM-RT, have been adopted to ensure that all system in radiotherapy use a common image and parameter format.

Software assurance involves testing system data integrity and the computer beam model. Beam measurements should be compared with calculations from the TPS, both at the commissioning stage and after any major upgrade of planning software. Regular quality control can be performed by comparing the output of a set of reference plans against the same distributions obtained during commissioning. These checks ensure consistency through the patient data input path and tests the basic dose calculation performance.[19]

The quality control of the system is insufficient to ensure the accuracy of treatment plans and therefore each plan must be subjected to the following (minimum) checks by a person not involved in the production of the plan:

- All measurements and contouring involving radiographic films, the CT planning scan and immobilisation device must be checked, particularly any calculations involving magnification factors.
- The accuracy of any transfer of patient outline, target definition and position of critical structures to the planning system must be confirmed and any errors investigated.
- The accuracy of transfer of the patients' treatment prescription, as specified by the clinical oncologist, must be confirmed.
- A check of the consistency of all field parameters throughout the planning reports.
- A manual calculation (or independent computer calculation) of the dose at the intersection of the field axes should be compared against the plan value.
- All calculations from the prescribed dose to the final monitor unit (MU) values for each field must be checked with particular regard to the correction factors applied. It is advisable that an independent calculation of the MUs is performed either by manual calculation using standard data or by a separate computer calculation program.
- The completion of each check should be recorded and signed; any discrepancies should be investigated.

Further checks are necessary when the planning data is transferred to the record- and-verify system (RVS), before each beam exposure and throughout the patient's treatment.

## Practical features of a treatment planning system

The rapid improvements in the speed and graphics capabilities of computers since the 1980s have enabled the development of powerful TPSs capable of performing 3D treatment planning in clinically practical timescales and at affordable prices. Although some planning continues to be done in 2D, most commonly for breast and chest wall treatments, it represents an ever decreasing proportion of the planning workload. All modern commercial TPSs are essentially 3D systems that enable 2D planning by restricting the dose calculation to the single slice on which the planning is performed. Therefore, this section will focus on the most common features of TPSs for CT-based 3D external beam planning.

### Contouring tools and features

The accurate delineation of target volumes and organs at risk is an essential element of radiotherapy planning. Planning systems' displays are commonly divided into 'windows', enabling the display of three orthogonal views. The inclusion of a 3D reconstruction of the delineated contours, with the option to hide or display individual structures, provides a helpful means of checking the continuity of structures.

Treatment planning systems offer a range of tools to assist in the contouring process, from simple, manual drawing tools to more complex algorithms for automatically defining the body outline and the positions of organs. Imaging modalities such as PET and MRI can provide additional information of use in contouring, in terms of either better target localisation or improved soft-tissue imaging. By registering the images acquired using these modalities to the planning CT scan, contouring performed on one scan can be automatically transferred to the CT slices.

The simplest tools enable the freehand contouring of structures on each CT slice. The ability to interpolate between contours delineated on non-consecutive slices or to copy contours between slices can shorten the process for relatively regular structures. The automatic addition of user-specified margins to contoured GTVs or CTVs is essential for the accurate creation of the PTV, in accordance with the recommendations of ICRU50.[7]

Automatic segmentation tools designed to reduce the time taken to contour organs at risk are increasingly becoming a feature of planning systems. Predefined settings for the typical CT numbers of organs such as the brain, spinal cord and bladder, sometimes together with knowledge of the organs' typical size and shape, enable the system to delineate the structures with minimal user input.

Tools for the manipulation and editing of contours can improve the quality of the contouring. In addition to the simple adjustment of contours on a slice-by-slice basis, the use of Boolean operators enables the combination or subtraction of structures (e.g. for removing contoured PTV outside the external contour). The addition of a specified depth of bolus to the body outline is an essential feature. Algorithms for filling cavities, removing extraneous contours and smoothing structures are particularly useful for tidying up the results of automatic segmentations.

### Beam planning

As when contouring, the beam planning display of a 3D planning system generally comprises three orthogonal views, often with a 3D view (Figure 10.10). In addition, there should be a clear indication of the most important beam parameters, including field size and location, collimator, gantry and couch angles, wedge angle and orientation, SSD and weighting. The adjustment of the field arrangement is usually done either by moving the fields on screen or by numerical entry of new values. The field size can be manually adjusted in the same way, although it is more common to automatically fit the secondary collimators to the target volume, with a user-specified margin. Non-coplanar beams, achieved through the use of collimator and couch twists, offer additional possibilities for conforming dose to the target volume.

A particularly useful display is the 'beam's eye view' (BEV) of the field. The BEV is a display of

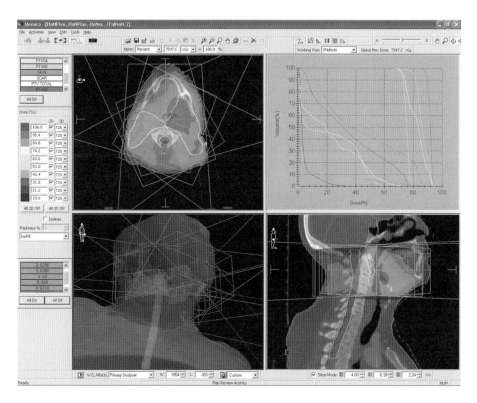

**Figure 10.10** Typical interactive screen display of a TPS (CMS Monaco) showing orthogonal CT and DVH views. (Courtesy of CMS-Elekta.)

the internal patient contours in a plane perpendicular to the beam central axis, with the observer placed at the radiation source. The field outline is shown against a perspective view of the target and any critical structure contours. Moving the fields while observing the BEV is a convenient means of identifying suitable gantry angles for avoiding critical structures. Although MLC can usually be automatically fitted to the shape of the target volume, it is often necessary to make adjustments to the positions of some leaves in order to shield critical structures. The BEV enables both this and the drawing of shielding blocks to be done easily. (Some systems can generate DRRs from the CT data which can be displayed behind the structures in a BEV, providing an efficient method for verifying the accuracy of the plan.)

The calculation options usually allow selection of the spacing between the calculation points (generally in the range 2–5 mm), the potential to choose the method of heterogeneity correction and, in systems with more than one algorithm, which calculation model is to be used. The size of the calculation dose matrix is often selectable; reducing the size of the matrix lessens the time taken for calculations until the planner is happy with the plan, at which point the calculation can be performed over the entire patient image set.

It is essential that the user be required to recalculate the dose after any changes to plan parameters that would affect the dose distribution are made (with the exception of field weights, which simply scale the contribution of each field). Within the calculated distribution, the positions of maximum dose within the plan and reference point should be available according to the definitions in ICRU50.[7] It is increasingly common for a range of plan normalisation options to be available, enabling normalisation such that either the ICRU reference point lies on the 100% isodose, or the mean target dose is equal to the 100% isodose value.

A range of options for the display of the calculated dose distribution is generally available. In addition to the basic isodoses, ideally with the option to define which isodoses are displayed, it may be possible to display the dose in three dimensions, superimposed upon the 3D view of the structures. Combined with opacity control of the 3D surfaces, this enables realistic visualisation of the dose distribution within the body.

### Plan evaluation tools

Plan evaluation tools allow the fast appraisal and optimisation of dose distributions in order to determine whether the tolerances for the target volume and critical structures have been achieved. Through their use, alternative plans for a patient's treatment can be compared and 'fine-tuning' can be performed to produce an optimal plan.

The simplest means of determining whether a plan meets the required criteria is visual assessment of the dose distribution in terms of the coverage of the target volume by the desired isodoses and the sparing of critical structures. In addition to the standard isodose display, planning systems offer a number of features to assist the visual evaluation of dose distributions. The use of a colourwash display, in which the dose levels are represented by a continuous colour gradient, may afford greater control over the display, particularly when the upper and lower displayed doses are definable. A visual indication of the location of the dose maximum within a slice or the entire calculation volume provides a convenient means of determining whether a plan's hottest point is located within the target volume. Point dose tools, indicating the dose at an arbitrary point, or line profiles, indicating the variation in dose along an arbitrary line, enable

more precise investigation of the planned dose distribution.

An alternative method of summarising the 3D dose distribution common to all modern treatment planning systems is the dose–volume histogram (DVH). The most widely used form of DVH is the cumulative DVH, a plot of the percentage volume of tissue, $V(D)$, that receives a dose greater than or equal to $D$. The DVH for a target volume can be used to easily determine the percentage of that volume receiving a dose above and below the required tolerances. Higher values of $V(D)$ for doses below the prescription dose and a sharper fall-off of the DVH thereafter indicate an improved dose distribution in the target volume. Conversely, more desirable dose distributions for critical structures are represented by lower values of $V(D)$.

Implemented in a TPS, DVHs should be customisable such that the scales can be in relative or absolute units. The DVH display is often accompanied by numerical summaries of the dose, such as the maximum and mean doses within a structure, which provide a clear indication of whether critical structure doses are within tolerance. A limitation of DVHs is that they provide no positional information, e.g. a target DVH may show a certain volume of tissue receiving a dose below the lower tolerance, but it does not indicate where that tissue is situated within the target.

The use of DVHs together with distributions enables an efficient evaluation of the quality of a treatment plan. The comparison of two alternative plans for a patient is facilitated by the ability to view the plans side by side on the screen or overlay their DVHs. The addition of the doses from several treatment plans enables evaluation of the total dose from, for example, a phased treatment. A useful variation on this plan-summing function is the ability to subtract one competing plan from another, the result being the volumetric dose difference between the two plans. Comparison of the plans' biological effectiveness (in terms of the resultant tumour control probability and normal tissue complication probability) is a capability becoming more commonplace in commercial planning systems.

Another useful means of comparing treatment plans is the conformity index, which quantifies how well the high-dose region coincides with the PTV. ICRU62[8] defines the CI as the ratio of the treated volume to that of the PTV. This parameter is not widely implemented as an evaluation tool in planning systems, partly because in the form defined by ICRU62 it is a little too simplistic for comparing plans and also because the report did not specify the isodose to be used in the definition of the treated volume. More informative indices of plan quality that are being introduced into systems quantify not only the goodness of the conformity to the PTV but also the sparing of specified OARs and the limiting of dose to all other normal tissue.

### Data export

The principal output from a planning system is a printed copy of the final plan. This hardcopy commonly displays a patient contour (with or without CT information) and target outline, the field positions and the isodose distribution in the required plane and a list of field parameters. The hardcopy must be clear and unambiguously provide all the information required to fulfil the plan objectives. In addition, a dose report containing the key plan and set-up details and a summary of the monitor unit calculations are produced (see Figure 10.6). Information is often obtained from the hardcopy long after the treatment has been completed, therefore the planning document must be a complete account of the treatment process.

Treatment planning systems tend to use a server–client architecture, i.e. the patient data and CT images are stored on a central database and pulled onto a local workstation, on which the planning is performed, before the resultant plan is pushed back to the database. The database may or may not be shared with the record and verify system; if not, a facility for exporting

the plan information to treatment units is essential. The final treatment plan may also be required to be transferred electronically to other systems such as independent monitor unit checking or virtual simulation software. Accurate transfer of the plan information between systems is essential and of particular importance when the plan contains elements that cannot be included in a hardcopy, such as MLC leaf positions. Use of the DICOM-RT protocol helps to ensure compatibility between different manufacturers' systems.

### Utilities

Utilities are provided for the configuration of machine data, the configuration of peripheral devices (such as digitisers, scanners and printers) and the administration of patient data.

As calculation algorithms have become more sophisticated, so the processing of the beam data measured on the linear accelerator into a form suitable for use by the algorithms has increased in complexity. In addition to the software for processing the data, a facility for analysing the processed data and determining how accurately it reproduces the measured data is commonly provided.

Peripheral devices used for the input or export of data during planning may require configuration within the planning system. In addition to simple items such as the printers used for producing the plan hardcopies, a calibration file for each CT scanner used must be set up to ensure accuracy of data transfer and configuration of DICOM-RT import and export processes is required.

Facilities for long-term storage of the planning data, with suitable data security measures, should be provided. Back-ups of patient data and the machine data used in calculations must be made on a regular basis and there should ideally be redundancy (such as RAID) within the system in case of disk drive failure. Other utilities allow 'house-keeping' of the disk storage systems to conserve space and remove or archive unwanted files – an increasingly important concern as the amount of data associated with each patient increases.

## Other planning modalities and advanced features

The previous section covered the most common features available in a TPS for external beam planning and many of these are available for other planning modes. The selection of beams for IMRT, electron, stereotactic radiosurgery or brachytherapy planning will often invoke special calculation models and programme modules that provide the features required for this type of planning. In some systems, particularly stereotactic treatments and brachytherapy, computer planning programs have been designed for specific therapy equipment and techniques.

### IMRT planning

IMRT represents arguably the most significant advance in radiotherapy planning since the introduction of conformal radiotherapy. The various methods of IMRT delivery are capable of producing dose distributions in which the high dose region is more closely conformed to the target volume while enabling greater sparing of normal tissue. A particular advantage over conventional treatments is the ability to produce concave distributions, enabling the sparing of organs at risk around which the target is wrapped. However, the production of IMRT plans is generally more labour intensive than conventional treatment planning. IMRT planning methods can be divided broadly into two categories: forward planning and inverse planning.

Forward planning of IMRT treatments is performed largely by the addition of additional, smaller fields within the conventional fields in order to improve the dose distribution above that achievable with conventional MLC fields and wedges alone. The degree of intensity modulation is limited by the number of fields used and

restricts the method's ability to achieve highly conformal dose distributions. However, forward planning has the benefit of requiring no more than a conventional TPS and so is not considered further here.

Inverse planning, as the name suggests, approaches the treatment planning process from a different angle from forward planning. Rather than positioning treatment fields as required and calculating the resultant dose distribution, the planner specifies the desired dose distribution and the TPS determines how best to deliver it. The inverse planning process is often known as 'optimisation' and the methods used vary between planning systems and according to the delivery technique (see Webb[20] for further information) but invariably requires the splitting of each beam into a large number of beamlets. A typical optimisation procedure is as follows:

- The desired dose distribution is specified in terms of a number of dose–volume constraints. For the target volume, there will generally be a minimum and a maximum constraint, defining the range of doses within which all the target tissue should lie. For organs at risk, a maximum dose constraint designed to limit the highest dose received by the organ and intermediate constraints to limit the dose received by a specific volume of the organ may be set.
- The TPS makes an initial guess of the required beamlet intensities (often simply uniform beams) and the resultant dose distribution within the volumes of interest is calculated. An optimisation (or cost) function quantifies the magnitude of the difference between the calculated distribution and the desired distribution – the greater the value of the function, the further the distribution is from meeting the constraints.
- The intensities of the beamlets within each field are adjusted and the dose to the volumes of interest is calculated once more. The value of the optimisation function is again recalculated; if it is lower than the previous

value, the new intensities are accepted; if not they are rejected.

- The iterative adjustment of intensities continues until the constraints are met, the user stops the process or no further reductions in the value of the optimisation function (shown in Figure 10.11) occur. It may be possible for the user to interactively adjust the constraints during the inverse planning process to assist in achieving a better outcome.

- Each field's final beamlet intensities together represent the fluence required to deliver the

final distribution. The inverse planning software then determines how to deliver the final fluences, in terms of the MLC patterns or dynamic MLC leaf motions.

- Finally, a forward dose calculation is performed, generally using the TPS's conventional algorithm to determine the dose distribution that will be delivered.

IMRT places additional demands on planning systems at several stages of the planning process. The dose calculation after each iteration of the

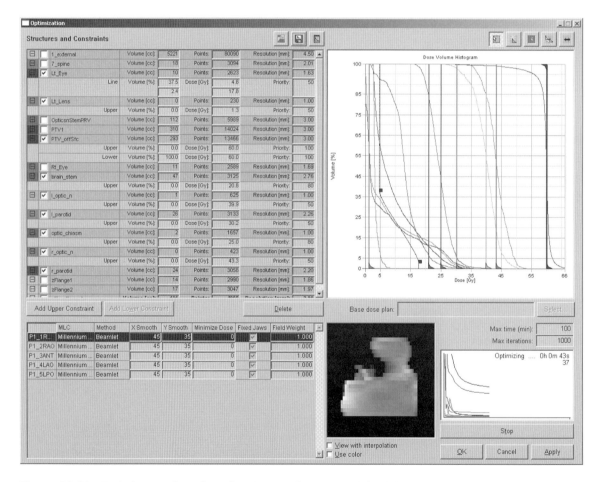

**Figure 10.11** Typical screen from the Eclipse inverse planning module of the Varian Eclipse TPS. Constraints and optimisation parameters are displayed and altered on the LHS of the screen. The RHS displays the DVHs of the volumes of interest (with constraints marked) at the present iteration, the current fluence for a selected field and a plot of the optimisation function against time. (Courtesy of Varian Medical Systems.)

inverse planning must be performed extremely rapidly – and much more rapidly than conventional algorithms are capable of, as previously described. The delivery of IMRT fields often requires more monitor units than conventional fields for the same prescription dose; the TPS must be capable of producing high-quality distributions without excessively lengthening the treatment delivery time or producing a high integral dose through high numbers of monitor units. Perhaps the greatest challenge is the frequent use of very small field segments, which requires the dose calculation algorithm to accurately model the penumbra and the effects of the lack of electronic equilibrium found in such a situation.

The complexity of IMRT treatments requires additional QA measurements to ensure that the calculated dose distribution accurately reflects the delivered dose. Planning systems increasingly have facilities to assist the process. In addition to the ability to calculate the dose from the treatment fields on a user-specified phantom, enabling comparison with film, detector array or ionisation chamber measurements, the prediction of the dose across the field as measured by an electronic portal imager allows efficient verification of the delivery.

## Electron beam planning

This usually involves the computation of dose distribution for a single field where the use of central axis depth dose data and standard isodose charts is insufficient. Situations where the irradiated tissue region is non-uniform and contains bone, lung or air cavities provide complex dosimetric problems that require evaluation using a beam model that will estimate the dose perturbations. The planning of electron beam treatments requires the choice of energy to achieve the required dose coverage (usually by the 90% isodose) at the maximum depth of the target volume within the dose restrictions to any critical structures. The field size selected is based on examination of the isodoses at the edge of the target volume and is particularly important for small fields where tapering of the peripheral isodoses requires the use of larger fields than normally chosen if photon fields were used. Field shaping by lead or lead alloy cut-outs is a common practice in electron therapy and must be included in the dosimetric calculations. The physics of electron beam therapy is covered in great detail elsewhere.[3,10]

The use of Monte Carlo-based dose calculation models for electrons is gradually becoming a more common feature of commercial planning systems. However, most TPSs use a pencil beam model based on multiple-scattering theory,[21] where the dose at a point is the sum of the contributions from all the pencil beams that make up the beam. Usually a single beam profile for each applicator at each energy is required at the depth of dose maximum to correct for the off-axis scattering that occurs within the applicator. If the applicator is not parallel to the skin surface, then correction must be made for tissue obliquity. This is achieved by an inverse square correction along the ray line from the point of calculation to the virtual source position. At angles of obliquity >45° significant changes in lateral scatter must be allowed for in the calculation. Tissue inhomogeneity is a primary cause of electron dose non-uniformity within the body and requires careful assessment to avoid underdosing the target volume or over-dosing critical structures. Correction for a slab of tissue with high (bone) or low (lung or air) electron densities can be made using an effective depth method similar to photon beams (see above). Small inhomogeneities produce hot and cold areas caused by scattering behind the edge of the structure and can be predicted only to an accuracy of about 10% with present electron beam models. Planning of electron fields is particularly useful for complex situations where fields are adjacent to each other, internal or external shielding is required or bolus material must be added to achieve an acceptable dose distribution. The planning tools used for viewing and evaluation are the same as for photon beam planning.

## 4D-CT planning

Four-dimensional CT (4D-CT) enables variations in the position of the target due to respiration to be accounted for.

The CT scan is acquired over a longer time than conventional CT, while simultaneously monitoring the patient's breathing either by tracking the motion of an external marker on the patient or by spirometry. The breathing is recorded as a waveform with which the individual CT slices are correlated (Figure 10.12).

On importing a 4D-CT dataset into the TPS, the images are separated into 'bins' according to the phase or amplitude of the respiratory waveform at the moment that each image was acquired. The result is a series of reconstructed CT scans, each representing the anatomy at a given stage of the respiratory cycle. Subsequent use of the scans is dependent upon the method of accounting for respiration to be used on treatment.

The movement of the target may be restricted during the times that the beam is on, either

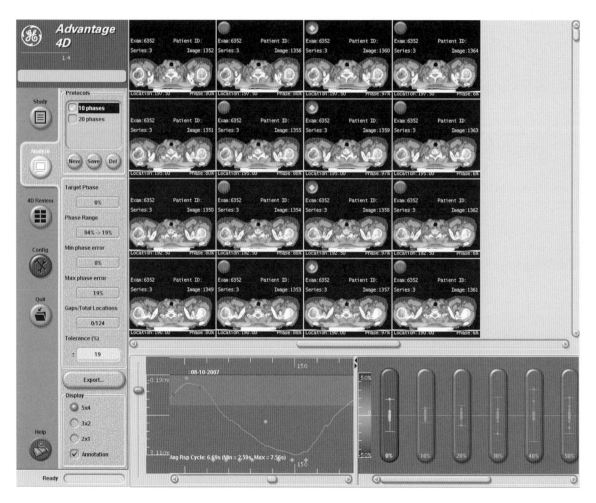

**Figure 10.12** A 4D-CT study display from GE AdvantageSim MD. The respiratory cycle is represented by the waveform at the bottom of the screen; each column contains images acquired during the same part of the cycle. (Courtesy of GE Healthcare.)

through gating the delivery according to the respiratory cycle or by a forced breath-hold method. In this situation, the planning is generally performed on a single reconstructed CT scan, corresponding to the stage of the respiratory cycle in which the dose is to be delivered. Structure delineation and planning are performed only on that scan, effectively treating it as a standard 3D planning situation.

The alternative treatment technique is to adapt the treatment fields according to the position of the target throughout the respiratory cycle. To achieve this, structures must be contoured on all of the reconstructed CT scans. This process can be made significantly faster by registering the scans to each other and copying structures between them, although careful verification of the results is required to ensure that changes in location as a result of breathing are correctly accounted for and it is wise to contour the target on each scan individually. Treatment planning becomes more involved, requiring fitting of the fields to the target and evaluation of the resultant dose distribution on each reconstructed scan. Dynamic adjustment of the MLC shape throughout the respiratory cycle is generally the most straightforward means of achieving this adaptation.

One of the most important implications of 4D techniques for planning systems is the massive increase in data involved. Typically at least 10 CT scans are reconstructed, resulting in a tenfold increase in the storage required for the CT images alone. As the technique becomes more widely implemented, it is possible that refinements to the 4D imaging process may reduce the quantities of data involved; a significant increase in required storage capacity over 3D planning will always remain.

## Stereotactic radiosurgery planning

This is required for treatment of deep-seated lesions in the brain where dedicated stereotactic apparatus, such as the Gamma Knife unit (Elekta Instruments AB) or an adapted linear accelerator, are used. The former system provides narrow photon beams, from multiple locations over a hemispherical area, focused at a point that can be positioned at the centre of the lesion.[22] Stereotactic radiosurgery or stereotactic multiple arc radiotherapy (SMART) produces an irradiated volume that is typically the shape of a walnut with variable diameter (4–30 mm) using different collimators. Treatment of these small lesions relies on accurate localisation and positioning of the patient, which is achieved using a stereotactic frame secured to the patient's head. The frame has an orthogonal coordinate system engraved on it, which is used for localisation, dose planning and alignment with the focal treatment point. Radiographic data is obtained from angiograms, CT or MR images to determine the 3D coordinates of the lesion; the shape of the skull is obtained from either the surface by measuring radial coordinates and surface interpolation or the contours obtained from CT data. The planning system produces isodoses relative to the dose at the point of maximum dose, allowing for attenuation changes along geometric ray lines to each source. The dose contribution from each source is summed into a dose matrix (as for conventional treatment planning) and plotted; multiple foci with appropriate weightings may be aligned adjacent to each other to conform the dose distribution to the shape of a lesion. The dose distribution is overlaid over the image data to give anatomical perspective of the treatment.

A commercial planning system, designed to support the Leksell Gamma Knife unit, is the Elekta Gammaplan (Figure 10.13). This system can use CT and MR scans as well as projected images from angiograms. Treatment planning is performed by defining the parameters of the cranial target and the collimator helmet to be used during treatment, and of the radiation shots to be delivered by the Gamma Knife. The user interface is similar to that of a conventional TPS for radiotherapy, but includes enhanced features

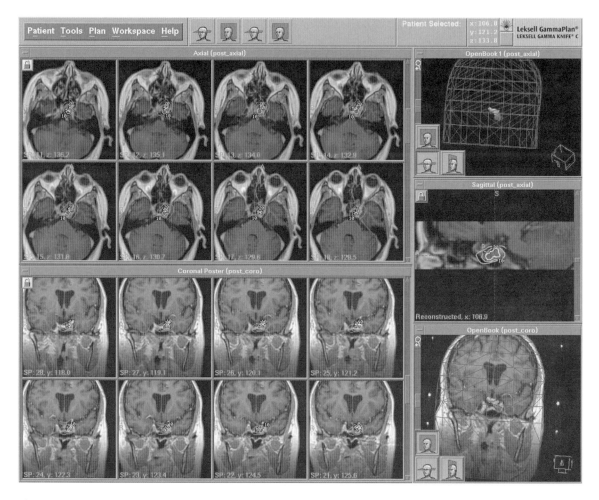

**Figure 10.13** Stereotactic radiotherapy plan (Courtesy of Elekta Gammaplan.)

to set-up and edit source patterns using collimator plugs.

## Brachytherapy planning

This is often provided as a separate TPS software package to an external beam program. The system allows calculation of individual patient treatments using various sealed sources such as iridium wire, caesium tubes or pellets, iodine seeds and gold grains. The introduction of afterloading devices for intracavitary and interstitial radiotherapy has led to computer planning packages that are tailored to the specific needs of the treatment system; Nucletron Selectron and Varian Varisource afterloading systems have a TPS that allows transfer of the treatment parameters in the required format for the machine. Pellet, seed and grain sources are usually considered as point sources, where the size of the source is small compared with the distance to the point of dose calculation, requiring inverse square, tissue absorption and scatter correction to the absorbed dose at a point. The calculation of dose distributions for line sources requires the use of integration techniques to account for the contribution of each element of the source to the dose at a point. Tables of relative dose at radial distances and angles from the centre of the source are often pre-calculated and known as Sievert integral tables.[3,4]

Computer calculation consists of summing the dose at a point for each source, the isodose curves from a cubic grid of points being plotted as for external beam models. The isodose distribution (Figure 10.14) is usually produced from the same view as the radiographs (i.e. anterior and lateral digital images). Viewing tools are similar to external beam planning and may involve the overlay of CT data. Plans may be viewed in arbitrary planes to allow visualisation

of the dose reference points defined according to the dosimetry system in use (i.e. Manchester, Paris, ICRU38[23]). A major difference between external and brachytherapy planning is that the latter has no defined target volume and therefore the minimum dose to the target tissue is ambiguous; visual assessment of the plan and dose calculation to the reference points is vital for plan evaluation.

Optimisation tools have started to appear in brachytherapy planning systems that model stepping sources such as the Selectron high-dose rate (HDR) and pulsed-dose rate (PDR) units. These allow definition of a required dose envelope and a calculation of the optimum source position and

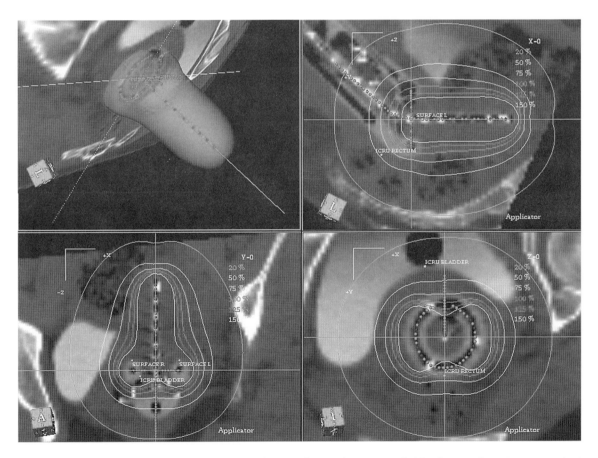

**Figure 10.14** Brachytherapy plan showing three orthogonal views and 3D dose surface for a standard Manchester insertion. (Courtesy of Nucletron.)

dwell times to accomplish this. Other planning tools that are often available are: 3D visualisation of dose surfaces; DVHs; summation of external beam dose and brachytherapy distributions; and curved plane calculations.

## Self-test questions

1. What represents a uniform dose distribution as recommended by ICRU50?
2. How does the measurement of percentage depth dose (PDD) differ from the measurement of tissue maximum ratio (TMR)?
3. Where do the regions of high-dose gradient exist in a photon beam?
4. Name three types of beam compensators that are commonly employed in radiotherapy treatment?
5. What dose corrections are employed by a TPS to accurately model photon beams in a patient?
6. What does a pencil beam kernel represent?
7. How can the sector integration be used to determine the equivalent square of an irregular field?
8. What are the main limitations of correction-based algorithms?
9. Give three uses of the beam's eye view display of a TPS.
10. What causes the convergence error in IMRT planning?

## References

1. Bental GC. *Radiation Therapy Planning*, 2nd edn. New York: McGraw-Hill, 1996.
2. Bleehan NM, Glatstein E, Haybittle JL et al. *Radiation Therapy Planning* 2nd edn. New York: McGraw-Hill, 1989.
3. Khan FM. *The Physics of Radiation Therapy*, 2nd edn. Baltimore, MD: Williams & Wilkins, 1994.
4. Williams JR, Thwaites DI. *Radiotherapy Physics in Practice*, 2nd edn. Oxford: Oxford University Press, 2000.
5. Mayles P, Nahum A, Rosenwald JC. *Handbook of Radiotherapy Physics*. London: IOP Publishing, 2007.
6. International Commission on Radiation Units and Measurements. *Use of Computers in External Beam Radiotherapy Procedures with High-Energy Photons and Electrons*. ICRU Report 42. Bethesda, MD: ICRU, 1987.
7. International Commission on Radiation Units and Measurements. *Prescribing, Recording and Reporting Photon Beam Therapy*. ICRU Report 50. Bethesda, MD: ICRU, 1993.
8. International Commission on Radiation Units and Measurements. ICRU Report 62. *Prescribing, Recording and Reporting Photon Beam Therapy* (Supplement to ICRU Report 50). Bethesda, MD: ICRU, 1999.
9. Bomford CK, Kunkler IH, Sherriff SB. *Walter and Miller's Textbook of Radiotherapy*, 5th edn. Edinburgh: Churchill Livingstone, 1993.
10. International Commission on Radiation Units and Measurements. *Determination of Absorbed Dose in a Phantom Irradiated by Beams of X or Gamma Rays in Radiotherapy Procedures*. ICRU Report 24. Bethesda, MD: ICRU, 1976.
11. Leavitt DD, Martin M, Moeller JH, Lee WL. Dynamic wedge field techniques through computer-controlled collimator motion and dose delivery. *Med Phys* 1990; **17**: 87–91.
12. Milan J, Bentley RE. The storage and manipulation of radiation dose data in a small digital computer. *Br J Radiol* 1974; **47**: 115–21.
13. Central axis depth dose data for use in radiotherapy. Appendix A. *Br J Radiol* 1996 (suppl): 25.
14. Cunningham JR. Scatter-air ratios. *Phys Med Biol* 1972; **17**: 42–51.
15. Storchi P, Woudstra E. Calculation of absorbed dose distribution due to irregular shaped photon beams using pencil beam kernels derived from basic beam data. *Phys Med Biol* 1996; **41**: 637–56.
16. Mackie TR, Bielajew AF, Rogers DWO, Battista JJ. Generation of photon energy deposition kernels using the EGS Monte Carlo code. *Phys Med Biol* 1988; **33**: 1–20.
17. Bragg CM, Conway J. Dosimetric verification of the anisotropic analytical algorithm for radiotherapy treatment planning. *Radiother Oncol* 2006; **81**: 315–23.
18. IPEM Report 68. *A Guide to Commissioning and Quality Control of Treatment Planning Systems*. York: IPEM Publications, 1996.
19. Institute of Physics and Engineering in Medicine. IPEM Report 81. Treatment planning. *Physics

*Aspects of Quality Control in Radiotherapy.* York: IPEM Publications, 1999: Chapter 4.

20. Webb S. *Intensity-Modulated Radiotherapy.* London: IOP Publishing, 2001.

21. Hogstrom KR, Mills MD, Almond PR. Electron beam dose calculation. *Phys Med Biol* 1981; **26**; 445–459.

22. Walton L, Bomford CK, Ramsden D. The Sheffield stereotactic radiosurgery unit; physical characteristics and principles of operation. *Br J Radiol* 1987; **60**: 897–906.

23. International Commission on Radiation Units and Measurements. *Dose and Volume Specification for Reporting Intracavitary Therapy in Gynecology.* ICRU 38. Bethesda, MD: ICRU, 1985.

## Chapter 11

# METHODS OF BEAM DIRECTION

Anne Jessop

## Aims and objectives

This chapter introduces the factors and methods employed to ensure accurate beam direction and delivery.

By the end of this chapter the reader will have an understanding of:
- the importance of accurate beam direction
- methods employed in the accuracy of beam direction
- advantages and disadvantages of methods used.

## Introduction

Radiation is colourless and odourless, and the recipient cannot feel it at all during exposure. This means that, for the radiographer to visualise the path of the radiation being delivered, there has to be some mechanism, visible or mechanical, by which the beam can be accurately directed. The time taken to produce complicated treatment plans would be wasted if there were no mechanism by which to replicate the required treatment parameters.

The ability to position the patient each day into the exact treatment position using various immobilisation devices and techniques leads to accurate reproducibility, beam direction and therefore treatment delivery. The beam direction methods discussed in this chapter ensure that the radiation strikes the intended target volume.

In today's radiotherapy beam direction accuracy has become even more important with the advent and development of sophisticated and complicated treatment options such as *image-guided radiotherapy* (IGRT) and *intensity-modulated radiotherapy* (IMRT) for patients with malignant disease.

## Importance of beam direction

Accurate beam direction is vitally important because this helps to ensure that a homogeneous tumour dose is delivered and received and that normal tissue is spared *normal tissue complication probability* (NTCP) versus *tumour control probability* (TCP), thus gaining the best therapeutic ratio for the patient (Figure 11.1).

There are some vital steps taken during the pre-treatment process that ensure accurate and reproducible beam direction:

- Patient positioning
- Immobilisation
- Localisation
- Field arrangement
- Dose distribution
- Verification.

196

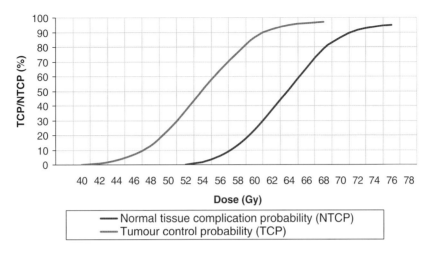

**Figure 11.1**    Radiation dose and probability of effect on normal tissue and tumour control.

## Patient positioning

This is perhaps arguably the most important factor to be taken into consideration to ensure accurate beam direction. The patient must be positioned in a stable comfortable position that minimises movement during treatment delivery and is reproducible at each subsequent visit. Simulator/CT and treatment couch tops must be compatible to allow patient positioning to be replicated at each venue. There is little value in using advanced treatment techniques and sophisticated beam delivery unless the recipient is positioned with as much care and accuracy as is taken to direct the beam of radiation that he or she is to receive.

The following are some of the more common standard positions:

- **Supine:** this is probably the most common patient position and also the most comfortable for patients.
- **Prone:** this position is best adopted when treating more posterior structures such as the spine or the rectum.

Patients should be positioned in such a way that they are stable and as comfortable as possible with the appropriate anatomy accessible and in a position that is reproducible on a daily basis. For treatment plans to remain accurate, it is important to reduce both lateral and longitudinal rotation. A high-energy beam of radiation penetrates body tissue, so the radiographer needs to be aware of the exit as well as the entry point of the radiation beam. Patients receiving direct field treatments need to be positioned in such a way that the appropriate treatment can be delivered to the specified area while avoiding critical structures that may lie within the path of the exit beam, e.g. eyes, spinal cord or bone marrow.

It may be necessary to use some positioning aids such as breast boards or T-bar to maintain the position of the patient in non-standard positions such as arms up. These positions are usually used to help maximise the therapeutic ratio. These positioning aids allow us to manipulate the movable body parts to allow a comfortable, reproducible and stable position.

### Skin marks

Radiographers need some form of skin marks on the patient to use as reference points to position and direct the radiation beams accurately. The interpretation of the marks plays a very important role in the accurate direction of the beam. By using skin marks and alignment lasers, patient orientation is reproducible at each treatment, within clinical tolerances. Skin marks and field light are symbiotic, particularly in palliative work. As well as skin marks outlining the area to be treated, orientation marks are also important on lateral aspects of the patient to facilitate accurate patient positioning and therefore accurate beam direction.

# Positioning aids/Immobilisation devices

## Breast boards

These allow comfortable arms up support for patients, moving the arms out of the path of laterally positioned beams. Breast boards position the patient so that the sternum is as horizontal as possible, thus avoiding angulation of the collimators. The disadvantage of using the breast board is that in those centres where CT planning is used the scanner needs to be of the wide-bore type to give enough clearance of the board and the patient.

## T-bar

This allows the arms to be positioned above the head when treating the chest and thorax using lateral beams.

## Beam direction shells

These are made individually, typically for patients having head and neck tumours treated. Shells can be constructed from thermoplastic or Perspex. The use of a beam direction shell enables the patient to be indexed exactly in the $x$, $y$ and $z$ coordinates of the couch on a daily basis, leading to greater accuracy in the beam delivery. Use of a bite block mounted inside the shell can increase the positioning accuracy further.

## Vacuum bags

These are bags filled with tiny polystyrene balls that can be locked into position by creating a vacuum. They can be reused after the patient has completed the course of treatment.

## Localisation

During localisation the *target volume*, critical structures and normal tissue are delineated usually with respect to the patients external body contour. Within the target volume will be included the tumour, the *gross target volume* (GTV), up to the irradiated volume. Critical structures will include organs at risk (OAR) and normal tissue with a tolerance dose close to or lower than the dose to be delivered to the target volume.

Methods of localisation may include simple clinical examination and imaging modalities such as CT or MRI.

Accurate and precise localisation techniques are paramount in order that the tumour be irradiated and the normal tissue spared. It allows for the optimum beam arrangements to be considered and can define the treatment portals.

### Clinical localisation

This is the cheapest and quickest method of tumour localisation; it can be done anywhere and needs few resources, and it could be said that clinical localisation is a mandatory aspect of the advanced imaging methods because it is necessary to know what and where to image.

# Imaging localisation

## Radiographs

This is probably the most common and cheapest imaging method available; however, radiographs can only provide two-dimensional (2D) data. Orthogonal films may be taken to enhance localisation and give three-dimensional (3D) information through a single plane.

## CT scans

CT scans provide electron density data that can be directly loaded into the treatment planning system. The data retrieved can be digitally reconstructed to produce volumetric images leading to 3D planning. There are a number of requirements of the CT scanner to ensure accuracy in the data collection. The patient must be positioned in the treatment position before the CT scan, so the scanner needs to have an identical table top to the treatment machine. As previously stated, the aperture has to be wide enough to allow immobilisation devices to pass through easily. External landmarks have to be used as registration points for future accuracy in positioning of the patient. The images have to be able to be transferred electronically to the treatment planning system.

## MR scans

Imaging using an MR scanner can be done in multiple planes; again table tops have to be identical to the radiotherapy treatment table top. MR images have a greater tissue contrast ,which is essential for more accurate tissue delineation especially in the brain and head and neck. Another advantage is that MRI involves no irradiation risk to the patient; however, there are circumstances when patients would not be suitable for MRI.

## Image fusion

As CT and MRI data is stored electronically, it is possible to manipulate the images and fuse the two together to allow better visualisation of tumour and surrounding tissue. Fusing positron emission tomography (PET) images with CT images can also enhance treatment planning options because tissue function can be considered thus allowing biological activity to be taken into consideration.

## Patient contouring

Patient contouring gives an accurate representation of the external body outline of the patient; this allows for measurements to be taken to determine depth of the tumour inside the patient and also depth of tissue that the radiation will need to traverse in order to reach the target. Depending on the amount and type of tissue that the radiation needs to traverse to the target volume, dose corrections can be applied for different tissue densities such as lung and bone.

Patients who have had CT or MRI planning will have an accurate contour taken from the images. Other methods may include the optical system for imaging and reconstruction of illuminated surfaces (OSIRIS), a manual method using a pantograph or taking a plaster of Paris cast.

## Radiation field

The treatment machine primary collimators direct the beam towards the secondary collimators, which are operated to produce the required shape and size of the radiation beam.

The geometrical shape of the radiation field delineates the beam shape and direction as it is projected from the point of origin inside the head of the machine. The physical shape of the radiation beam is defined as the area delineated by the 50% isodose curve at the isocentre.

Using multiple field arrangements it is possible to conform the dose of radiation received to closely match the shape of the target volume. This ability, however, necessitates the accuracy of patient positioning, localisation and beam direction. This conformation can be further enhanced by the use of multi-leaf collimators and IMRT planning.

## Mirror and bulb

The mirror and bulb provide evidence of the X-ray beam by producing a visible means of delineating the X-ray field. The image cast is that of the secondary beam-defining collimators. The position of the light source should be adjustable, allowing symmetrical definition about the central axis of the beam of both light and radiation and providing correct visible delineation at all distances, the bulb and X-ray target being equidistant from the mirror.

## Isocentric mounting

The three basic movable components of the treatment machine, namely the couch, gantry and floor, are positioned in such a way that all points of rotation coincide at the isocentre, usually at a distance of 100 cm from the source of radiation (Figure 11.2). This facilitates the accurate direction of the X-ray beam towards the patient.

By precise positioning of each piece of equipment to the same pre-set coordinate before the radiation exposure, the beam direction will be the same at each patient's individual delivery.

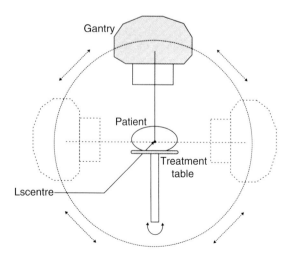

**Figure 11.2** Figure of isocentric mounting.

## Optical range finder

This determines the distance of the treatment machine from the patient. The optical range finder is not in itself a beam-direction device, although it contributes to accurate beam direction and delivery. The effects of a beam of radiation on body tissues can be influenced by the distance that the beam has travelled through air or tissue (inverse square law, half-value layer, absorbed dose, etc.), so it is important to set the correct distance at which the dose calculations have been made. A $10 \times 10$ cm field on the skin is only correct at 100 cm from the focal point of the machine, which is also the isocentre, although this may not be true for cobalt-60 units which have a different isocentre. The $10 \times 10$ cm field will then be correct at the normal isocentre for that particular machine.

## Treatment verification

With the improvement in beam shaping, dose conformation and tumour delineation methods it is essential that verification be undertaken to ensure accurate beam direction and therefore treatment delivery. Treatment verification can be done using various methods, portal films, electronic portal imaging and cone beam CT.

### Portal radiographs

Accuracy of field positioning can be checked by portal imaging using radiographic film positioned to image the beam emerging from the patient (see Chapter 13). One advantage of using film to take portal radiographs or films is that films are relatively inexpensive and easy to produce. However, at megavoltage energies, image quality can be very poor, leading to difficulties with recognition of structures and registration to the original gold standard image, so image enhancement is not an option unlike for electronic images. As a result of their size, films may present storage issues.

## Electronic portal imaging

Electronic portal imaging allows visualisation of real-time images using an electronic portal imaging device (EPID) with the option to correct patient position before treatment delivery, thus enhancing the accuracy of beam direction (see Chapter 13). As the images are acquired electronically it is possible to enhance the image to make matching and registration easier. The main disadvantage with EPIDs is the initial cost of the system and software.

## Cone beam CT

This incorporates a kV CT scanner attached to the linac. Real-time 3D images of the patient can be obtained, resulting in IGRT. The advantages of image-guided delivery is that beam positioning accuracy can be checked and verified before 'beam on', thus aiding the accuracy of beam direction.

# Beam direction devices

## Collimators

Mechanical secondary collimators provide a means of manipulating the beam to the desired shape and size. Multi-leaf collimators are used to conform the beam to the shape of the target volume, thus sparing more of the surrounding normal tissue (see Chapter 8). This is of particular importance when tumour sites are surrounded by critical structures and organs are at risk of damage from high doses of ionising radiation.

## Applicators

### Orthovoltage and superficial
These applicators are used to identify the correct source-to-skin distance (SSD) and the size and shape of the beam. The applicator is positioned in contact with the skin over the area to be treated; it also delineates beam direction. Orthovoltage applicators have a closed visible plastic end, which absorbs the secondary electron contamination, produced by X-ray interactions with the lead-lined side of the applicator. The end of the applicator defines the field size and the centre of the beam and, by observing the patient, using closed circuit television or a lead glass window, can assist in detecting patient movement during treatment.

### Electron applicators
The electron beam is delivered perpendicular to the skin surface (skin apposition) by the means of an applicator. The applicator is open ended and therefore enables the operator to see the light projection on the skin. The secondary collimators define the limits of the electron beam to a size marginally larger than the aperture in close contact with the patient. This margin is dependent on the energy of the electrons being used. The margin of definition is crucial because scattered electrons from the edge of the beam contribute to the field-edge dose, providing a uniform dose across the whole field. Applicators are a great asset to beam direction because they allow the radiographer to view the path of the radiation directly. Some applicators correctly set or identify the SSD. Electron applicators are used primarily to collimate the electrons to the necessary shape because they tend to repel each other and scatter from the path of the beam, causing the beam to bow (Bragg peak effect) just below the skin surface. This effect needs to be taken into consideration when positioning fields to avoid critical structures and also when matching photon and electron beams.

# Lasers

Typically each treatment machine will have three sets of lasers that all intersect at the isocentre, therefore giving an accurate visual representation of the treatment isocentre, either within or on the

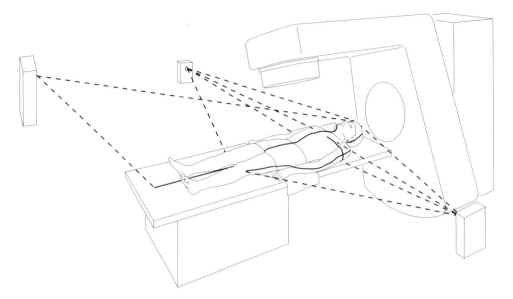

**Figure 11.3**   Laser position in treatment rooms.

patient's skin (Figure 11.3). The lasers are used for accurate patient positioning and also define the beam entry and exit points.

These aid in the accurate, reproducible positioning of the patient. Lasers are positioned at strategic points within the treatment and planning rooms. Lateral, caudocoronal and back-pointer lasers are all positioned to intersect at the machine isocentre, therefore giving an accurate visual representation of the treatment isocentre, either within or on the patient's skin. Lasers used in radiotherapy positioning are grade two lasers with less than 1 mW per beam. To aid alignment accuracy the line thickness is approximately 2 mm. The lasers are produced by a plasma tube with a particularly narrow beam profile. Lasers are projected around the room from the tube by a system of small lenses, within the laser mechanism housing, which refract the beam along the required path. Lasers can be either red or green; these have the same accuracy and usability and are little different in cost, but green lasers are more visible on darker skins.

## Methods to ensure accuracy of beam direction

### Quality assurance

Regular checks have to be made of each mechanical contributor to the accuracy of the beam direction. Lasers, field light position and machine output are checked daily to ensure that they are all within normal tolerances. The quality programme should also include treatment delivery conformance, giving the radiographer specific guidance on how a particular treatment technique should be delivered, but leaving the final determination of accurate beam direction to the radiographer.

### The treatment plan

When the patient has been imaged and a computerised treatment plan has been produced, this plan is used as a tool to ensure accurate beam direction. The plan is followed to reproduce the correct arrangement of treatment fields. The plan specifies the gantry position, diaphragm position and orientation, field sizes and SSD pertinent to an individual patient, and should be considered the primary data set. Before the course of treatment begins, the reference marks on the patient should be checked either by simulation or pre-treatment portal imaging to correct any discrepancy. By identifying the gantry position and diaphragm orientation and position, the plan gives accurate tumour skin distances which, when the patient is correctly positioned, should coincide within a specified tolerance. The plan also provides a contour of the patient's anatomy, giving a view of tumour and surrounding normal tissue. This can be invaluable when anticipating reactions to the treatment, e.g. oesophagitis in a chest patient or diarrhoea in a bladder or prostate patient.

## Conclusion

Although radiotherapy departments employ various methods of beam direction, the same fundamental rules apply: interpretation of treatment instructions, appropriate and accurate use of devices, and correct patient positioning all lead to accurate beam direction. All the factors addressed above, however, assume patient co-operation and thought should be given to the patient who, for whatever reason, cannot remain immobilised. These may be mentally ill patients who cannot comprehend the simple request to 'keep still' or children who are frightened and unable to understand the request of the radiographer. It may be necessary to resort to anaesthesia for these patients, in which case more attention should be given to patient immobilisation, if only for the patient's own safety.

### Self-test questions

1. There are various methods used for tumour localisation; consider the advantages and disadvantages for each method.
2. What is the purpose of multi-leaf collimation?
3. Consider a definition of the isocentre. How is this position determined and visualised within the treatment room?
4. What information can be found within the treatment plan that will aid accurate beam direction?
5. Why is it necessary to collimate electrons as close to the patient as possible?

## Further reading

Bomford CK, Kunkler IH. *Walter and Miller's Textbook of Radiotherapy*, 6th edn. Edinburgh: Churchill Livingstone, 2003.

Greene D, Williams PC. *Linear Accelerators for Radiation Therapy*, 2nd edn. London: The Institute of Physics, 1997.

Dobbs J, Barrett A, Ash D. *Practical Radiotherapy Planning*, 3rd edn. Oxford: Oxford University Press, 1999.

# Chapter 12

# ADVANCED TREATMENT DELIVERY

## Pete Bridge

### Aims and objectives

At the end of this chapter the reader will be able to:
- outline the less common radiation delivery systems
- understand the basic physical principles underpinning these systems
- discuss the advantages, disadvantages and future directions of alternatives to conventional radiotherapy.

## Alternatives to conventional radiotherapy

There are currently new developments in radiotherapy delivery as well as renewed interest in some modalities that have been available for many years. This chapter aims to present details of some of these less common innovative treatment delivery systems. The new tomotherapy equipment and more established but rapidly developing stereotactic and particle therapy delivery systems are discussed.

## Particle therapy

### History of particle therapy

The idea of using particles to treat cancer instead of X-rays was proposed in 1946[1] and protons were first used clinically in 1954. The most common particles, or 'hadrons' used therapeutically are protons, carbon ions and neutrons. Historically a larger range, including the pion[2] and heavy ions such as neon, has been used.

### Rationale for particle therapy

Particles are already used to treat tumours in conventional radiotherapy. Electrons created by the X-ray interactions deposit ionising energy at depth and particles produced by an accelerator interact in much the same way. The difference between the two modalities is that hadrons deposit their energy at an increased depth in the tissue. The hadrons' increased energy means that they penetrate tissue a considerable depth before delivering their maximum dose. The point at which this maximum dose occurs is known as the *Bragg peak* (Figure 12.1). The build-up region is much larger than that associated with photon beams and furthermore there is no dose delivered after the Bragg peak, because, unlike photon treatments, there is no X-ray dose-penetrating the tissue. Once the particles deposit their energy, they stop.

By carefully choosing the energy of the charged particle beam, the Bragg peak can be accurately positioned within the patient, allowing the maximum dose to encompass the whole tumour with minimal dose to the entrance and exit tracks

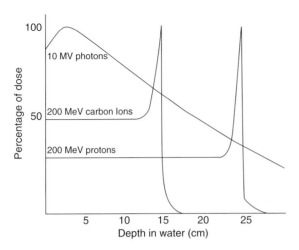

**Figure 12.1** Depth doses of particle beams.

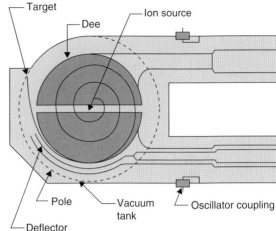

**Figure 12.2** Schematic diagram of a cyclotron. (Courtesy of SLAC.)

of the beams. Conventional photon beams deliver a relatively high dose to these volumes of normal tissue, causing side effects and potentially increasing the chance of induction of malignancy.

The resulting dosimetric benefits of hadron therapy are easily demonstrated by a range of planning studies with increased conformity and reduced integral dose over a range of tumour sites.[3,4] Simple hadron plans consistently out-perform complicated intensity-modulated radiotherapy (IMRT) plans, although intensity modulation techniques have also been successfully applied to proton planning.[5] Another potential benefit associated with hadrons is their reported increased *relative biological effectiveness* (RBE) in the Bragg peak region of between 1.1 and 2.56 even in radioresistant tissue.[6–8]

## Particle accelerators

The main difficulty associated with particle beams is in their production and the resulting costs of shielding, gantries and construction.[9] There is currently a massive initial payment associated with hadron therapy facilities due to the newness of the technology and these complicated technical specifications. A detailed explanation

of particle production, acceleration and delivery is beyond the scope of this chapter and the reader is directed to more specialist texts[10] for more details than the following overview. There are two main devices capable of accelerating protons or ions: the cyclotron and the synchrotron. Both of these accelerators work by pulling the particles in a circular manner with electromagnets. The *cyclotron* accelerates the particles between two semicircular cavities (Figure 12.2) and is relatively small in size compared with the synchrotron, which pulls the particles around a circular track. The *synchrotron* comprises a large circular waveguide with particles kept in the centre by magnets. As the particles pass around the waveguide, they are periodically accelerated by further electromagnets with each revolution until they reach their maximum speed. From the single accelerator, the particles can be guided along waveguides to several treatment delivery systems, most of which tend to be static in nature (Figure 12.3). The main technical problem with these accelerators from a therapeutic point of view is beam direction. The high energy of the beams gives them a large radius of curvature of up to 7 m, making

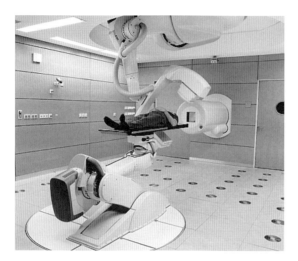

**Figure 12.3** Static proton beam line. (Courtesy of Siemens.)

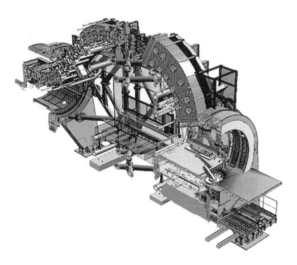

**Figure 12.4** Isocentric proton gantry. (Courtesy of Siemens.)

isocentric gantries some of the largest structures in the medical world (Figure 12.4).

Once the beam emerges from the delivery system, it has to be modulated in energy (to change the depth of the Bragg peak) and directed across the tumour. This can be achieved either by using magnets to scan the beam over the required volume[11] or by collimation and passive beam scattering with foils.[12]

## Particle therapy use

Particle therapy today remains a relatively rare modality with only around 29 accelerators worldwide producing hadrons for cancer therapy (compared with 7500 linear accelerators), according to the Particle Therapy Cooperative Group.[13] Interest in particle therapy is increasing, though, with new centres being built around the world, the recent NRAG report recommends construction of a particle beam facility in the UK.[14]

A range of tumour sites is suitable for treatment with particles, including paediatric tumours,[15] large radioresistant tumours[4] and tumours in sites close to critical structures such as head and neck.[3,16] There is a wealth of literature presenting clinical results of proton and ion therapy[17,18] and the reader is directed there for more details because a full evaluation of clinical results is beyond the scope of this book. It must be remembered that randomised trials are few and far between as centres can rarely offer both photon and particle modalities.

*Boron capture therapy* is a highly specialised form of particle therapy that uses boron to target neutron beams to tumours. An injection causes a boron compound to accumulate in the tumour, and then a beam of slow neutrons is aimed at the area of the tumour. When the boron absorbs the neutrons, it splits into short-range ions that deliver a high dose while sparing surrounding tissue.[19]

Recent years have shown increasing interest in particle therapy, causing Suit[20] to predict that protons would replace photons in 10–20 years. The key reason for this is the increased conformity that can protect normal tissue as well as allow an increase in dose and corresponding increase in survival. Reports on conventional photon IMRT concentrate mainly on the planning target volume (PTV) and organs at risk (OAR) doses, but the problem posed by increased integral dose is rarely mentioned. Avoidable secondary cancer incidence after Hodgkin's disease irradiation can be halved when protons are used instead of photons.[21] This does need to be balanced against the increased RBE of particle beams so that the inherent decreased integral dose and improved conformity reduce the chance of increased acute toxicity.

Particle therapy offers other benefits for the future such as real-time dose verification. When treating with carbon ions, fragmentation can occur, producing positron-emitting carbon-11 isotopes. This enables PET scanning to be used to pinpoint the position of the beam during treatment, enabling online verification and adaptive radiotherapy.[22] Although currently the costs and physical size of equipment associated with particle therapy are off-putting, the future should herald improved technology and reduced costs. Preliminary studies have suggested that lasers could accelerate protons instead of expensive and large cyclotrons and synchrotrons.[23] If these studies bear fruit then in the future it may be possible to make small generators using this technology to make stand-alone proton treatment machines. This would bring particle therapy away from specialist centres and into mainstream use alongside photon and electron treatments.

## Stereotactic delivery

### History of stereotactic systems

Stereotactic, meaning 'spatial movement', systems of surgery rely on highly accurate localisation methods. Although stereotactic procedures were used back in the early 1900s for animal experiments, it was not until the late 1940s that the spherical localisation system was perfected and implemented in the development of the Gamma Knife by Professor Lars Leksell.[24] This combines stereotactic immobilisation and localisation with targeted gamma ray beams to facilitate highly selective radiation damage known as 'radiosurgery'. Subsequent developments such as CT planning, robotic control and image-guidance technology have allowed stereotactic-based equipment to be used for

highly precise radiosurgery to the brain and more recently to other parts of the body.

### Rationale for stereotactic radiotherapy

The rationale for stereotactic treatment is the same as for conformal radiotherapy in that it offers the opportunity for highly targeted radiation that can be shaped to match the target volume. The difference is that stereotactic localisation equipment, combined with the small size of the radiation beams, allows for much more precision in the targeting of the treatment. As with IMRT, stereotactic treatments traditionally utilise a large number of very small beams. By training all these beams on one focus and then moving the focus around the target volume, a high dose can be delivered in a conformal manner with low intensities outside that volume.

### Stereotactic equipment

There are two main options available for stereotactic treatments: dedicated radiosurgery apparatus using multiple beams or modified linear accelerators.

#### Dedicated systems

Brain lesions can be treated using a dedicated stereotactic radiosurgery device known as the Gamma Knife. The active part of the machine is a large number of cobalt-60 gamma sources that are highly collimated to produce a fine beam of radiation. They are arranged and focused in a hemisphere surrounding the isocentre where the patient lies (Figure 12.5). The patient has a metal frame attached to the skull, allowing for highly accurate localisation of small volumes within the brain (Figure 12.6). The large number of beams and rigid immobilisation mean that the Gamma Knife produces very conformal dose distributions.[25]

Another dedicated system is the CyberKnife.[26] This comprises a 6-MV linear accelerator mounted on an industrial robotic arm (Figure

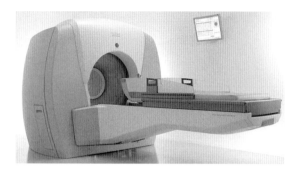

**Figure 12.5** Leksell Gamma Knife Perfexion. (Courtesy of Elekta.)

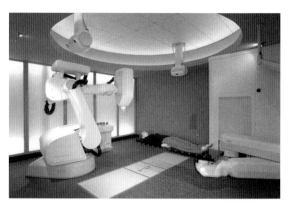

**Figure 12.7** CyberKnife Robotic Stereotactic Radiosurgery System. (Courtesy of Accuray Inc.)

treatment and thus track the tumour during respiratory motion.[29] Organ deformation complexities currently render this four-dimensional (4D) approach difficult in clinical situations, however.

The Novalis system is similar to the CyberKnife in that orthogonal kilovoltage X-rays guide localisation, although real-time tracking is performed by infrared guidance.[30] This equipment resembles a conventional linear accelerator (Figure 12.8) and is capable of fully conformal arc radiotherapy using dynamic multi-leaf collimator (MLC) technology.[31] The couch top is capable of full automatic adjustment including tipping along the longitudinal and transverse axes.

### Linear accelerator-based systems

In addition to these dedicated devices, several manufacturers and clinical centres have developed adaptations for existing linear accelerators that can facilitate delivery of stereotactic treatments. These do not generally offer the small multiple beams of dedicated systems but utilise stereotactic immobilisation devices and image-guided radiotherapy (IGRT) technology. Tomotherapy equipment has also been used to deliver stereotactic treatments using specialised immobilisation devices[32,33] and this equipment is discussed in more detail below. Recent innovations such as micro-MLCs and CT-based image guidance have dramatically improved the

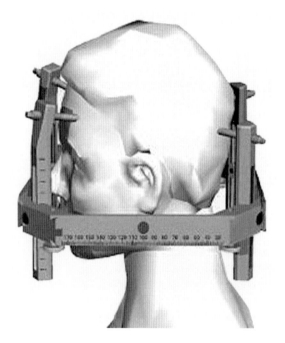

**Figure 12.6** Leksell Coordinate Frame G. (Courtesy of Elekta.)

12.7.) A series of small collimators produce a range of circular beams as small as 5 mm diameter.[27] Orthogonal kilovoltage imaging systems provide the possibility of real-time image-guided radiotherapy and the CyberKnife system has been used successfully to treat a range of tumours and metastatic deposits throughout the whole body, as opposed to just the brain.[28] The robotic arm offers the potential to move the beam during

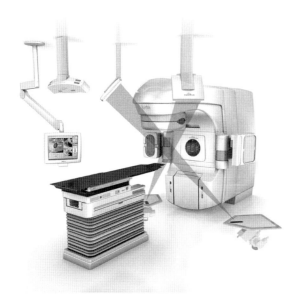

**Figure 12.8** Novalis Shaped Beam Surgery. (Courtesy of BrainLab AG.)

conformity of linear accelerator-based stereo-tactic radiosurgery.[34]

## Stereotactic use

Common indications for cranial stereotactic radiosurgery include arteriovenous malforma-tions[35] as well as malignant and benign brain tumours[36,37] and brain metastases.[38] More recently, with the increased confidence in posi-tioning afforded by IGRT, stereotactic radiosur-gery has been used to treat spinal metastases[39] (although at increased expense compared with conventional RT[28]). Lung and upper abdominal tumours have also been treated with stereotactic radiosurgery,[29,40] and in general there is increas-ing interest and use of this modality.

## Tomotherapy

### History of tomotherapy

Tomotherapy is a relatively new modality in the radiotherapy arena, although the underpinning research started in the early 1990s.[41] Tomother-apy Inc. is currently the sole supplier of dedicated tomotherapy equipment and has supplied over 200 installations since the first patient was treated clinically in 2003. More recently, adapta-tions have been designed to allow helical fan-beam treatments to be delivered using standard linear accelerators.

### Rationale for tomotherapy

The fundamental rationale for tomotherapy is that, if the components of a linear accelerator and associated megavoltage imaging system are mounted in a sealed ring gantry, they can be moved safely around the patient at high speeds. This allows for an increased number of beam angles to be used for treatment and for rapid megavoltage CT image acquisition. Thus the equipment combines the conformality of IMRT treatment with the confidence provided by inher-ent IGRT capability. The ease of imaging presents daily pre-irradiation localisation as a feasible option and in turn allows for increased confi-dence in target coverage with associated reduc-tion in margins,[42] as well as the possibility of adaptive radiotherapy[43] and potential for dose escalation.

### Tomotherapy equipment

Dedicated tomotherapy equipment basically con-sists of a ring gantry containing a megavoltage accelerator, binary MLC and image detector (Figure 12.9). The couch passes through the ring aperture as the beam is delivered, creating a con-tinuous spiral pattern of dose delivery. The accel-erator produces X-rays of 6 MeV for treatment and 3.5 MeV for imaging, and the binary MLC collimates this into a fan beam with a maximum isocentre width of 40 cm. By constantly changing the MLC size as the accelerator rotates and the couch moves longitudinally, fully continuous IMRT can be achieved. The treatment couch can extend a considerable distance into the aperture,

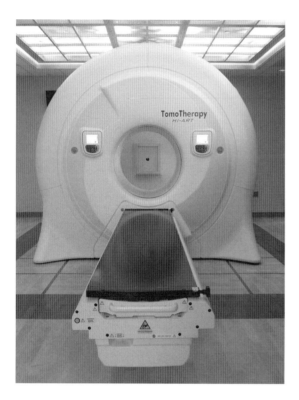

**Figure 12.9** Hi-ART tomotherapy system. (Courtesy of Tomotherapy Inc.)

## Tomotherapy use

Although tomotherapy is suitable for treating the whole range of tumour types and sites, most centres have chosen to use their units to treat sites traditionally selected for IMRT or those requiring IGRT. Studies have demonstrated tomotherapy's ability to deliver conformal distributions to the prostate,[45,46] rectum,[42,47] and head and neck[48] (including nasopharynx,[49] and parotid,[50]) breast,[51] spine,[32] meninges[52] and lung.[53] Results from these studies indicate improved sparing of critical structures as with conventional IMRT. Tomotherapy has also been used successfully for palliation,[54,55] suggesting that it has a potential role to play in everyday workloads. There are some implications associated with this modality, with one study suggesting that tomotherapy treatment times averaged 25 min[56] due to a combination of daily imaging and IMRT being used for all patients. Some studies have attempted to compare tomotherapy with conventional IMRT[57] and stereotactic radiosurgery,[58] and seem to suggest that certain sites are better suited for particular modalities than others, although a full evaluation of these comparisons is beyond the scope of this text. Future directions for this modality as with conventional radiotherapy indicate the potential for 4D treatment of lungs[59,60] and adaptive radiotherapy.[43,61]

ensuring that large volumes can be made available for treatment. The manufacturers claim that a cylindrical volume of 40 cm diameter and 160 cm length can be treated. NomosSTAT is a serial tomotherapy adaptation that comprises an add-on binary collimator and associated software. This allows helical fan-beam IMRT to be delivered, but the lack of a ring gantry means that the accelerator cannot spin around the patient as fast as with dedicated hardware.

Research is currently being undertaken into the possibility of developing a magnetic resonance (MR)-based tomotherapy system.[44] This would use MR to image the patient before and potentially during treatment. The high magnetic fields involved would render accelerators useless, so it is proposed to use cobalt-60 gamma rays as the sources of radiation.

### Self-test questions

1. What is the difference between proton (hadron) and X-ray interactions in tissue at depth?
2. How does the build-up region vary for protons compared with that for photon beams?
3. What does the term 'stereotactic' mean?
4. Describe the basic technology incorporated in a tomotherapy unit.
5. What is the advantage of using this integrated technology?

# References

1. Wilson RR. Radiological use of fast protons. *Radiology* 1946; **47**: 487–91

2. Raju MR. Particle radiotherapy: Historical developments and current status. *Radiat Res* 1996; **145**: 391–407.

3. Cozzi L, Fogliata A, Lomax A, Bolsi A. A treatment planning comparison of 3D conformal therapy, intensity modulated photon therapy and proton therapy for treatment of advanced head and neck tumours. *Radiat Oncol* 2001; **61**: 287–97.

4. Zurlo A, Lomax A, Hoess A et al. The role of proton therapy in the treatment of large irradiation volumes: A comparative planning study of pancreatic and biliary tumors. *Int J Radiat Oncol Biol Phys* 2000; **48**: 277–88.

5. Oelfke U, Bortfeld T. Optimization of physical dose distributions with hadron beams: comparing photon IMRT with IMPT. *Technol Cancer Res Treat* 2003; **2**: 401–12.

6. Kraft G. Tumor therapy with ion beams. *Nuclear Instruments and Methods in Physics Research Section A: Accelerators, Spectrometers, Detectors and Associated Equipment* 2000; **454**: 1–10.

7. Paganetti H, Niemierko A, Ancukiewicz M et al. Relative biological effectiveness (RBE) values for proton beam therapy. *Int J Radiat Oncol Biol Phys* 2002; **53**: 407–21.

8. Kagawa K, Murakami M, Hishikawa Y et al. Preclinical biological assessment of proton and carbon ion beams at Hyogo Ion Beam Medical Center. *Int J Radiat Oncol Biol Phys* 2002; **54**: 928–38.

9. Suit H. The Gray Lecture 2001: Coming Technical Advances in Radiation Oncology. *Int J Radiat Oncol Biol Phys* 2002; **53**: 798–809

10. Delaney TF, Kooy HM. *Proton and Charged Particle Radiotherapy*. Philadelphia, PA: Lippincott Williams & Wilkins, 2007

11. Park, BS, Cho YS, Hong IS. Development of a MeV proton beam irradiation system. The review of scientific instruments. *Medical Physics* 2008; **79**(2 Pt 2): 02C718.

12. Lu HM, Brett R, Engelsman M, Slopsema R, Kooy H, Flanz, J. Sensitivities in the production of spread-out Bragg peak dose distributions by passive scattering with beam current modulation. *Med Phys* 2007; **34**: 3844–53.

13. Particle Therapy Co-operative Group (PTCOG). http://ptcog.web.psi.ch (last accessed 27 June 2008).

14. Price P, Errington RD, Jones B. Report on the UK meeting September 2001 to discuss the clinical and scientific case for a high-energy proton therapy facility in the UK. *Clin Oncol* 2002; **15**: S1–9.

15. Hardy P, Bridge P. What are the potential benefits and limitations of particle therapy in the treatment of paediatric malignancies? *J Radiother Pract* 2008; **7**: 9–18.

16. Schulz-Ertner D, Haberer T, Scholz M et al. Acute radiation-induced toxicity of heavy ion radiotherapy delivered with intensity modulated pencil beam scanning in patients with base of skull tumors. *Radiother Oncol* 2002; **64**: 189–95.

17. Grob KD, Pavlovic M, eds. *Proposal for a Dedicated Ion Beam Facility for Cancer Therapy*. Darmstadt: GSI, 1998.

18. Orecchia R, Zurlo A, Loasses A et al. Particle beam therapy (hadrontherapy): basis for interest and clinical experience. *Eur J Cancer* 1998; **34**: 459–68.

19. Coderre JA, Turcotte JC, Riley KJ, Binns PJ, Harling OK, Kiger WS. Boron neutron capture therapy: cellular targeting of high linear energy transfer radiation. *Technol Cancer Res Treat* 2003; **2**: 355–75.

20. Suit HD. Protons to replace photons in external beam radiation therapy? *Clin Oncol* 2003; **15**: S29–31.

21. Schneider U, Lomax A, Lombriser N. Comparative risk assessment of secondary cancer incidence after treatment of Hodgkin's disease with photon and proton radiation. *Radiat Res* 2000; **154**: 382–8.

22. Enghardt W, Debus J, Haberer T. The application of PET to quality assurance of heavy-ion tumor therapy. *Strahlenther Onkol* 1999; **175**(suppl 2): 33–6.

23. McKenna P, Ledingham KWD, Spencer I et al. Characterization of multiterawatt laser-solid interactions for proton acceleration. *Rev Sci Instrum* 2002; **73**: 4176–84.

24. Kelly PJ. *Tumor Stereotaxis*. Philadelphia, PA: WB Saunders Co., 1991.

25. Nakamura J, Verhey LJ, Smith V et al. Dose conformity of gamma knife radiosurgery and risk factors for complications. *Int J Radiat Oncol Biol Phys* 2001; **51**: 1313–19.

26. Quinn AM. Cyberknife: A robotic radiosurgery system. *Clin J Oncol Nurs* 2002; **6**: 149–56.

27. Kuo JS, Yu C, Petrovich Z, Apuzzo ML. The Cyberknife stereotactic radiosurgery system: Description, installation and an evaluation of use and functionality. *Neurosurgery* 2003; **53**: 1235–9.

28. Sahgal A, Larson DA, Chang EL. Stereotactic body radiosurgery for spinal metastases: A critical review. *Int J Radiat Oncol Biol Phys* 2008; **71**: 652–65.

29. Lu XQ, Shanmugham LN, Mahadevan A et al. Organ deformation and dose coverage in robotic respiratory-tracking radiotherapy. *Int J Radiat Oncol Biol Phys* 2008; **71**: 281–9.

30. Verellen D, Soete G, Linthout N et al. Quality assurance of a system for improved target localization and patient set-up that combines real-time infrared tracking and stereoscopic X-ray imaging. *Radiother Oncol* 2003; **67**: 129–41.

31. Jin JY, Chen Q, Jin R. Technical and clinical experience with spine radiosurgery: A new technology for management of localized spine metastases. *Technol Cancer Res Treat* 2007; **6**: 127–33.

32. Kim B, Soisson ET, Duma C et al. Image-guided helical tomotherapy for treatment of spine tumours. *Clin Neurol Neurosurg* 2008; **110**: 357–62.

33. Holmes TW, Hudes R, Dziuba S, Kazi A, Hall M, Dawson D. Stereotactic image-guided intensity modulated radiotherapy using the HI-ART II helical tomotherapy system. *Med Dosim* 2008; **33**: 135–48.

34. Hazard LJ, Wang B, Skidmore TB et al Conformity of linear accelerator-based stereotactic radiosurgery using dynamic conformal arcs or intensity modulation and micro-multileaf collimator. *Int J Radiat Oncol Biol Phys* 2008; in press.

35. Starke RM, Komotar RJ, Hwang BY et al. A comprehensive review of radiosurgery for cerebral arteriovenous malformations: outcomes, predictive factors, and grading scales. *Stereotact Funct Neurosurg* 2008; **86**: 191–9.

36. Lipani JD, Jackson PS, Soltys SG, Sato K, Adler JR. Survival following cyberknife radiosurgery and hypofractionated radiotherapy for newly diagnosed glioblastoma multiforme. *Technol Cancer Res Treat* 2008; **7**: 249–56.

37. Kobayashi T, Kida Y, Mori Y, Hasegawa T. Long-term results of gamma knife surgery for the treatment of craniopharyngioma in 98 consecutive cases. *J Neurosurg* 2005; **103**(suppl): 482–8.

38. Andrews DW, Scott CB, Sperduto PW et al. Whole brain radiation therapy with or without stereotactic radiosurgery boost for patients with one to three brain metastases: Phase III results of the RTOG 9508 randomised trial. *Lancet* 2004; **47**: 291–8.

39. Gerszten PC, Burton SA. Clinical assessment of stereotactic IGRT: Spinal radiosurgery. *Med Dosim* 2008; **33**: 107–16.

40. Schweikard A, Shiromi H, Adler J. Respiratory tracking in radiosurgery. *Med Phys* 2004; **31**: 2738–41.

41. Mackie TR, Holmes T, Swerdloff S et al. Tomo-Therapy: A new concept for the delivery of dynamic conformal radiotherapy. *Med Phys* 1993; **20**: 1709–19.

42. Tournel K, De Ridder M, Engels B et al. Assessment of intrafractional movement and internal motion in radiotherapy of rectal cancer using megavoltage computed tomography. *Int J Radiat Oncol Biol Phys* 2008; **71**: 934–9.

43. Geets X, Tomsej M, Lee JA et al. Adaptive biological image-guided IMRT with anatomic and functional imaging in pharyngo-laryngeal tumors: impact on target volume delineation and dose distribution using helical tomotherapy. *Radiother Oncol* 2007; **85**: 105–15.

44. Kron T, Eyles D, Schreiner JL, Battista J. Magnetic resonance imaging for adaptive cobalt tomotherapy: A proposal. *J Med Phys* 2006; **31**: 242–54.

45. Lee HL, Baisden JM, Skinner HD, Schneider BF. Improved rectal sparing with simultaneous integrated boost in the treatment of localized prostate cancer using helical tomotherapy. *Int J Radiat Oncol Biol Phys* 2007; **69**(suppl 1): S375–6.

46. Chen SS, Shah AP, Strauss JB et al. Tomotherapy treatment of the prostate and pelvic lymph nodes with a sequential conedown. *Int J Radiat Oncol Biol Phys* 2007; **69**(suppl 1): S692–3.

47. De Ridder M, Tournel K, Van Nieuwenhove Y et al. Phase II study of preoperative helical tomotherapy for rectal cancer. *Int J Radiat Oncol Biol Phys* 2008; **70**: 728–34.

48. Lee C, Langen KM, Lu W et al. Assessment of parotid gland dose changes during head and neck cancer radiotherapy using daily megavoltage computed tomography and deformable image registration. *Int J Radiat Oncol Biol Phys* 2008; in press.

49. Lee N, Xia P, Quivey JM et al. Intensity-modulated radiotherapy in the treatment of nasopharyngeal carcinoma: an update of the

UCSF experience. *Int J Radiat Oncol Biol Phys* 2002; **53**: 12–22.

50. Lee TK, Rosen II, Gibbons JP, Fields RS, Hogstrom KR. Helical tomotherapy for parotid gland tumors. *Int J Radiat Oncol Biol Phys* 2008; **70**: 883–91.
51. McIntosh A, Read PW, Khandelwal SR et al. Evaluation of coplanar partial left breast irradiation using tomotherapy-based topotherapy. *Int J Radiat Oncol Biol Phys* 2008; **71**: 603–10.
52. Christodouleas JP, Latronico D, Kleinberg L. Brain-sparing total meningeal radiation for a patient with widespread progressive meningiomas using helical intensity modulated radiation. *Clin Neurol Neurosurg* 2008; **110**: 310–14.
53. Sterzing F, Sroka-Perez G, Schubert K et al. Evaluating target coverage and normal tissue sparing in the adjuvant radiotherapy of malignant pleural mesothelioma: helical tomotherapy compared with step-and-shoot IMRT. *Radiother Oncol* 2008; **86**: 251–7.
54. MacPherson M, Montgomery L, Fox G et al. On-line rapid palliation using helical tomotherapy: a prospective feasibility study. *Radiother Oncol* 2008; **87**: 116–18.
55. Bauman G, Yartsev S, Rodrigues G et al. A prospective evaluation of helical tomotherapy. *Int J Radiat Oncol Biol Phys* 2007; **68**: 632–41.
56. Bijdekerke P, Verellen D, Tournel K et al. Tomo-Therapy: implications on daily workload and scheduling patients. *Radiother Oncol* 2008; **86**: 224–30.
57. Mavroidis P, Ferreira BC, Shi C, Lind BK, Papanikolaou N. Treatment plan comparison between helical tomotherapy and MLC-based IMRT using radiobiological measures. *Phys Med Biol* 2007; **52**: 3817–36.
58. Khoo VS, Oldham M, Adams EJ, Bedford JL, Webb S, Brada M. Comparison of intensity-modulated tomotherapy with stereotactically guided conformal radiotherapy for brain tumors. *Int J Radiat Oncol Biol Phys* 1999; **45**: 415–5.
59. Zhang T, Lu W, Olivera GH et al. Breathing-synchronized delivery: a potential four-dimensional tomotherapy treatment technique. *Int J Radiat Oncol Biol Phys* 2007; **68**: 1572–78.
60. Smeenk C, Gaede S, Battista JJ. Delineation of moving targets with slow MVCT scans: implications for adaptive non-gated lung tomotherapy. *Phys Med Biol* 2007; **52**: 1119–34.
61. Vonk D, Jaradat H, Mehta M, Khuntia D. Adaptive tomotherapy planning for integrated boost doses in rapidly responding lung cancers. *I Int J Radiat Oncol Biol Phys* 2007; **69**: S525.

## Further reading

Chin L, Regine W. *Principles and Practice of Stereotactic Radiosurgery*. New York: Springer-Verlag, 2008.
Van Dyk J. *Modern Technology of Radiation Oncology*, Vol. **2**. Madison, CT: Medical Physics Publishing, 2005.
Wieszczycka W, Schaf WH. *Proton Radiotherapy Accelerators*. London: World Scientific Publishing Co., 2001.

# Chapter 13
# TREATMENT VERIFICATION

## Cath Holborn

### Aims and objectives

By the end of this chapter the reader should be able to:
- provide definitions for the types of error that can occur during treatment
- outline the key factors that should be considered within a verification protocol
- discuss the different imaging modalities available for treatment verification
- describe the different methods used for verifying the dose delivered
- explain the rationale behind adaptive and predictive radiotherapy
- discuss the role of record and verify systems in ensuring an accurate treatment delivery.

## Introduction

Treatment verification is an integral part of the treatment process. Techniques aimed at maximising the therapeutic ratio such as *three-dimensional conformal radiotherapy* (3DCRT) and *intensity-modulated radiotherapy* (IMRT) are now used routinely within many radiotherapy departments, and treatment verification plays a vital role in ensuring that this ultimate aim is achieved. Both geometric and dosimetric verification can be performed, the latter being particularly significant when considering the irregular and concave isodose distributions created using IMRT.

The verification protocols implemented must be rigorous to effectively ensure that the treatment is delivered to the intended planned position. A sound knowledge of the sources and types of error that may occur is essential.

Conventional approaches to treatment verification have relied on the use of two-dimensional (2D) images acquired using portal film and more recently the use of electronic imaging devices (EPIDs), at megavoltage energies. Field placement set to skin marks is verified relative to bony anatomy used as a surrogate for the planned planning target volume (PTV) position. However, many studies have since found that for many sites internal organ motion is evident[1] and therefore direct visualisation of the target, often in 3D, may be more accurate in verifying a treatment.

As the imaging modalities available and approaches to verification have advanced, the term 'image-guided radiotherapy' (IGRT) has been more recently used to describe the process of treatment verification. More specifically it is used to describe those approaches that identify and correct for positional variations in both external patient set-up and internal anatomy. At the time of this book's publication, research and development into IGRT, the equipment available

214

and how it may be used are extensive and continually being modified and updated.

## Geometric uncertainty

As previously mentioned in Chapter 10, the ICRU 62 guidelines[2] separate the PTV into an internal margin (IM) and a set-up margin (SM), accounting for changes in organ motion and external set-up error, respectively. Errors within these margins may also be categorised as either random or systematic.

A systematic error occurs as a result of discrepancies between the planning process and the actual treatment. It results in a fixed deviation of the clinical target volume (CTV) from the intended planned position over all fractions for a particular patient.[3] Initial steps to minimise any systematic set-up error have been recommended by a number of studies[4-6] and include: setting a couch height using a vertical scale, using comparable solid or carbon fibre couch tops in all pre-treatment and treatment areas, and using the planned *digitally reconstructed radiographs* (DRRs) as the verification reference image instead of simulator check films.

As the name suggests, a random error is unpredictable and can vary between fractions (inter-fraction) or even within a fraction (intrafraction). Factors such as poor immobilisation, poor set-up, movable skin marks and internal organ motion could all contribute to the occurrence of a random error.

As systematic errors are consistent for every fraction, the dosimetric consequences of a deviation from the intended planned position are arguably more significant, although certain techniques and regimens such as the sliding window approach for IMRT and larger daily doses associated with hypo-fractionation will make the dose coverage more susceptible to random error.

Errors may also occur or 'drift' during a course of treatment and are often referred to as a *time trend errors*. These are more likely to occur in those sites where changes in a patient's anatomy, e.g. as a result of weight loss, are common and alter a patient's set-up.

The treatment site provides an indication as to what factors may contribute to geometric uncertainty. Perhaps more importantly, however, imaging modalities should be used to determine the degree and types of error within a patient population as a means of ensuring that an appropriate PTV is allocated. As stated in a 2002 report[4] by the Royal College of Radiologists (RCR), each department should measure their own set-up accuracy and compare these with published data.

## Verification protocols

Verification protocols are primarily used throughout a treatment course to ensure that field placement stays within the intended PTV. This is particularly important given the increased conformity and tighter margins used with 3DCRT, which increase the risk of a geographical miss. The steep dose gradients associated with IMRT make the occurrence of a geographical miss even more significant. When designing a verification protocol, several important factors should be considered.

First, any errors that are measured during treatment can be corrected either online or offline.

*Online correction* is where an image is acquired and any error is corrected for before the treatment is delivered for that fraction. It is often used to identify gross errors before treatment, and is particularly useful on the first fraction or for regimens using a larger daily dose, e.g. weekly fractionation. As random error varies between fractions, it can be corrected for using only online imaging.

*Offline correction* is used to reduce the systematic error and involves acquiring an image that is then reviewed retrospectively after the treatment has been delivered. Any error is corrected for in subsequent fractions.

It is important to consider the frequency of imaging. Applying a correction based on only one image provides merely a 'snapshot' of the error that day and may not be representative of the error occurring in subsequent fractions. The systematic error component can be more accurately determined by increasing the frequency of imaging in the first week. An example of this is the 'no action level' (NAL) protocol[7] which rules that a set number of initial images should be acquired for each patient and used to determine an average set-up error. Irrespective of its magnitude, one set-up correction is then applied for all subsequent fractions.

Variations on this approach may exist, e.g. some departments may choose to apply a correction only if the error measured is above a predetermined action or tolerance level. Is it important that an appropriate action level is decided upon if this is the case because this is essentially the point at which you would decide to correct for a measured error or, perhaps more importantly, the magnitude of error that you would deem acceptable. One should therefore consider the technique itself and how susceptible it is to a geographical miss, plus what the consequences of this would be, e.g. on any adjacent organs at risk. It would also be important to consider the inherent accuracy of the method used to measure the error.

Departments may also choose to repeat images on a weekly basis thereafter to ensure that the accuracy is maintained throughout treatment. Although it is argued that a more rigorous approach to detect such time trend errors may be needed, using daily imaging with a 4-day rolling average measurement, to detect errors >5 mm.[5]

Daily online imaging may be more advantageous when the random error is greater than the systematic error, but raises more questions around additional dose and increased workload. When evaluating this for a given patient population, knowing the source of this random error is an important consideration, e.g. if it was mostly attributable to internal organ motion, one would have to question the overall benefit of daily online imaging if this was based only on visualisation of bony anatomy and not the target itself.

The following section provides further detail on the imaging modalities available. There is now a wide variety of imaging modalities available for treatment verification with many departments moving towards those that offer the opportunity for visualisation of both bony and soft tissue anatomy (image-guided radiotherapy or IGRT).

## Megavoltage portal imaging

Megavoltage (MV) portal imaging has been the main modality used for treatment verification for many years. Only bony anatomy is visible, however, and as such stable bony landmarks are relied upon for the verification of field placement. As previously mentioned this means that only external set-up error can be corrected for. Image quality is poor relative to radiographs acquired at kilovoltage (kV) energies due to the differences in the predominant attenuation processes occurring. This results in lower differential tissue attenuation and poor contrast resolution. However, there have been a number of developments in portal imaging technology that have improved their use as a verification tool.

Initially, only radiographic film and cassette technology was available for treatment verification, and the image quality achievable with the most recent systems, e.g. the Kodak EC-L, demonstrates superior contrast resolution. In fact it is deemed superior to the older EPID systems and is comparable to that achieved with the most recent amorphous silicon (a-Si) detectors. However, the image is not available immediately and must be processed before the image analysis can be performed. There are also issues associated with the storage and, where required, the subsequent retrieval of the hard copies.

The digital nature of EPI overcomes these immediate problems but also offers a number of additional advantages. Instant image availability enables the option for online verification before treatment delivery and the incorporated software allows manipulation for image enhancement. Simple measuring tools such as digital rulers can be used to determine the distances between field edges and/or the isocentre and relevant bony landmarks. These are useful for quickly assessing the set-up and detecting gross errors, but more sophisticated tools for quantitative image analysis are now available with many systems offering automated matching algorithms for image alignment. These advantages reduce the level of subjectivity associated with portal film analysis. It has been determined that simple visual inspection of images can detect errors only >5 mm[8] and that treatment portal errors can be quantified more accurately using EPID systems.[9] As images are obtained in real time, EPIDs can also acquire what is known as a movie or cine loop, whereby multiple images are acquired during a single fraction. These are useful for monitoring intrafraction motion, e.g. due to breathing. Most departments using EPI will now be equipped with a-Si detectors, but brief descriptions of older EPID systems are provided below as well.

Initial devices were based on a system that uses a video camera, 45° mirror and a phosphor-coated metal plate, which acts as an X-ray to light converter. The light diffuses through the phosphor screen and is reflected by the mirror through a lens to the video camera. The video signal is digitised and processed for viewing. The structure of these devices tends to make them bulky and can restrict machine manoeuvrability. Detector efficiency is limited in that only a very small amount of the emitted light photons reaches the camera system. Electronic noise (an unwanted signal) in the camera system is also a problem.

Matrix ion chamber devices consist of a $256 \times 256$ matrix of straight wire electrodes. An organic liquid iso-octane (hydrocarbon) fills the gap between the electrodes. The electrodes along one axis are connected to a high voltage (300 V) supply, which is applied to each of the electrodes lines in turn. The electrodes along the other axis are connected to electrometers and measure the resulting ionisation currents. As only one electrode line is activated at any one time, a large fraction of the radiation beam that interacts with the device is not used to generate a signal, again limiting detector efficiency. Background noise level is in the region of 0.25%.

The most recent a-Si devices produce a much higher image quality. Similar to the camera-based systems they contain a phosphor screen which converts X-rays into light. In contrast, however, this is then detected by an array of hydrogenated a-Si photodiodes, which have a high resistance to radiation damage and thus can be placed in contact with the screen. This results in a compact imaging device that is more efficient in detecting the light emitted. Within each pixel, a photodiode is accompanied by a *thin film transistor* (TFT). Once light has accumulated within the photodiodes, electronic readings from the a-Si array are taken one row at a time, by applying a voltage that causes the TFTs to become conducting. This acts like a switch allowing current to flow between neighbouring photodiodes (Figure 13.1). Commercial systems currently available include the Varian PortalVision and Elekta iView GT.

*Computed radiography* (CR) is a digital alternative to film and may be used instead of or as a back-up for EPI. The image contrast is comparable to Kodak EC-L film and a-Si detectors and they are DICOM compatible, allowing the transfer of images and use of the software tools for image analysis. However, real-time imaging is not possible because the images must still be processed.

## Use of fiducial markers

Markers may be used to improve the accuracy of treatment delivery in a number of ways. They act as a localisation aid and surrogate for target position and may be placed externally or implanted internally.

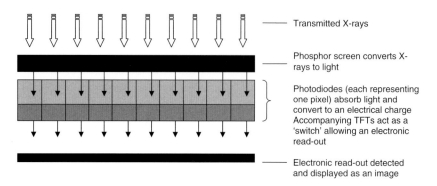

Transmitted X-rays

Phosphor screen converts X-rays to light

Photodiodes (each representing one pixel) absorb light and convert to an electrical charge Accompanying TFTs act as a 'switch' allowing an electronic read-out

Electronic read-out detected and displayed as an image

**Figure 13.1** Diagram to illustrate the main components of the amorphous silicon detector and the process of image production.

Research has focused particularly on the use of implanted markers in the prostate. The seeds are implanted using transrectal ultrasound guidance and it therefore involves an invasive procedure for the patient, although the main area of concern reported is that of marker migration. Any marker movement measured should indicate prostate motion only for it to be a reliable method for treatment verification. To date, the evidence presented has indicated that marker migration is minimal (a few millimetres at most).

The markers can be easily detected using an existing MV EPID or more recent on-board kV devices. The 'centre of mass' (COM) of the markers may be used as a reference point, although intermarker distances and individual seed measurements can also be used. Three or more markers are more often used to act as a coordinate system for image registration. Markers cannot highlight the target contour, although assessment of marker distances over time may 'indicate' a possible change such as prostate deformation, which could be investigated further with CT if needed.

Markers placed either externally or again internally can also be used to monitor and correct for intrafraction motion, during treatment delivery. This is known as *real-time tumour tracking* and is used together with a 'gating' system that tracks the position of markers during treatment delivery and will switch the beam on only when the markers are within the intended planned position. The beam will switch off whenever this is not the case. The Varian RPM (real-time patient management) system uses externally placed reflective markers and an infrared tracking camera to monitor the patient's breathing cycle and correlate tumour position with this.

**Ultrasound verification**

Much research has been undertaken investigating the use of ultrasonography as a verification tool, primarily for 3DCRT and IMRT to the prostate. The outline of the prostate and the interface between the prostate and bladder, and to a lesser degree the prostate and rectum, can be visualised in order to determine the daily prostate position. This is then matched to that on the original CT plan and the accompanying software calculates the couch shifts necessary to correct for any positional changes. For further detail on how an ultrasound image is produced see Chapter 5.

Several systems are available and examples of these include the BAT (B-mode acquisition and targeting) system (NOMOS Corp., USA), the Son Array (Varian) and Restitu (Resonant Medical, Canada). The mechanisms for registering anatomical position do differ, but essentially the location and orientation of the US probe must be tracked in relation to the isocentre.[10] The BAT system uses an infrared tracking system and a 2D probe that captures images in both sagittal and transverse directions. The Son Array uses a free-hand, optically guided, 2D probe to capture and correlate a series of images into a 3D reconstructed data set. Restitu uses a 3D probe with infrared tracking and is the only system that compares the verification ultrasound image to another ultrasound image, acquired at the planning stage.

Ultrasonography has the advantage of being non-invasive, relatively quick and easy to use, with no discomfort experienced by the patient.[11] There is no associated radiation dose, which would be particularly significant if daily online imaging were applied.

However, image quality may not always be acceptable enough to allow accurate patient positioning. A full bladder volume is needed and other characteristics, such as a smaller distance from the abdominal surface to the prostate isocentre, less thickness of tissue anterior to the bladder and a greater amount of prostate gland superior to the pubic symphysis in the anteroposterior direction, have all been associated with good image quality.[12] A certain degree of probe pressure is needed to achieve a good quality image but this itself could actually move the prostate and mean that the image acquired may not be a true representation of the prostate position.[12–14]

## Computed tomography

The theoretical benefits of using CT as a verification tool are that the images are matched 'like for like' with the planned CT volumes and, in contrast to ultrasonography, the prostate contour is arguably more easily identified, allowing for changes in the position, size and shape to be determined. However, the prostate still has regions of very low contrast on CT images[15] and

the image quality does vary between the different CT modalities available.[16]

One option is to design a treatment room so that it incorporates a linear accelerator and a diagnostic CT scanner. The planning and verification CT volumes are both of diagnostic image quality. The patient does not need to move between procedures and remains on the same treatment couch as the two different machines move on rails into the required positions. The Primatom (Siemens) is an example of one such commercially available 'CT on rails' system.

Another option is to integrate the imaging equipment within the linear accelerator itself. *Cone beam CT* (CBCT) is used in this instance. CBCT images can be acquired using both MV and kV energies. In contrast to the thin collimated beam used to take multiple slices throughout the volume in conventional CT, the X-ray source used in CBCT covers the complete volume all at once, throughout either a 180° or 360° gantry rotation (Figure 13.2). Multiple 2D images are acquired and then reconstructed into a 3D volume, although they are not of diagnostic quality. Intrafraction motion can also cause reconstruction artefacts and the larger field of view (FOV) used with CBCT can cause image artefacts and streaking due to the increased amount of scattered radiation. It also means that

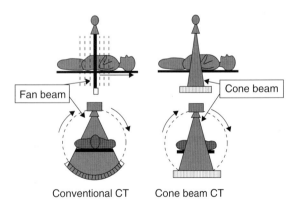

**Figure 13.2** Diagram to illustrate the differences between conventional CT and cone beam CT. (Courtesy of Dr Jonathon Sykes, St James' Hospital, Leeds.)

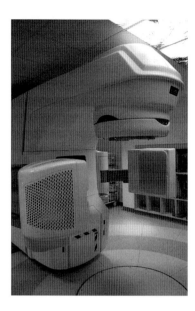

**Figure 13.3** Varian On-Board Imager (OBI) incorporating an additional kV-X-ray source and detector. (Courtesy of Western Park Hospital, Sheffield.)

the CT numbers (used for dose planning and calculation) are less reliable than diagnostic CT.

Kilovolt CBCT uses an additional kV X-ray source attached to the gantry, perpendicular to the MV EPID detector (Figure 13.3). The kV tube can also be run in plain radiographic or fluoroscopic modes, the latter being used during the CBCT gantry rotation. Examples of commercially available systems are the Elekta Synergy and the Varian OBI.

Megavolt CBCT adapts the existing treatment machine and EPID detector, making it a relatively inexpensive option. The increased penetration with MV energies means that more of the incident dose reaches the detector, which may be of benefit particularly for larger patients. However, detector efficiency is low and as a result a proportion of the X-rays is not stopped and passes straight through. The high linac dose rate must also be lowered, otherwise the dose delivered in a 1- to 2-min acquisition time would be much higher than a conventional MV portal. This also means that much less radiation will reach the detector. In addition to this, the image quality

with MV CBCT has a lower contrast resolution compared with kV due to the attenuation process that dominates at MV energies. This can be a benefit, however, for those patients with a hip replacement because they can be imaged without causing major streak artefacts.

*Tomotherapy* is a relatively new development within radiotherapy and involves the use of an entirely 'new' treatment machine combining treatment planning, image-guided CT verification and treatment delivery into one integrated system. The treatment is effectively delivered in slices that arc around the patient, in much the same way as a CT scan is obtained (see Chapter 12). With this in mind, both serial and helical tomotherapy units are available, the latter resembling the appearance of a CT scanner rather than a linear accelerator. Commercial systems available are the NomosSTAT (serial) and Tomotherapy Inc. HiART (helical).

## Comparison of different methods

The preceding section has provided an overview of the key modalities available for treatment verification. For those treatment sites where organ motion or even tumour shrinkage is evident, the need to visualise soft tissue is clearly an advantage. In this respect, portal imaging based on bony anatomy alone may be insufficient. There are a number of different IGRT methods available but each has their own individual benefits and limitations.

Image quality is one factor that may impact on the accuracy of the technique. Research into the use of ultrasonography has demonstrated this to be a problem when contouring and aligning the images[17,18] and measured differences between operators (interobserver variability) and the same operator (intraobserver variability) have been observed.[12,19]

Although most research has focused on prostate cancer, there is significant interest in the use of implanted markers as a surrogate for target position. In contrast to CT and ultrasonography, minimal training in marker identification is required, and thus the level of subjectivity and associated observer variability is much less. Several studies[20-22] have demonstrated the benefit of using implanted markers for image registration, instead of contour- or anatomy-based techniques. Markers could still be used together with CT verification, as this provides the advantage of highlighting other changes such as weight loss or organ deformation, if these were likely to be an issue.

Ongoing research is essential in order to determine which is the most effective modality and indeed which verification protocol is the most appropriate, for each treatment site, in order to ensure the most accurate treatment delivery. An ideal outcome would be where a further reduction in error could be achieved, allowing a reduction in the PTV margin. This would hopefully reduce normal tissue toxicity and/or facilitate an escalation in the dose delivered, where appropriate.

## Adaptive and predictive radiotherapy

Variations in external set-up and internal anatomical position are both site and patient specific. As previously mentioned, imaging protocols should be used locally to develop knowledge of the random and systematic error associated with differing treatment sites. The benefits of this are twofold: first, it ensures that the PTV margin allocated is appropriate and, second, it helps to ensure that the most appropriate verification protocol is selected, given the type of error that predominates.

*Adaptive radiotherapy* takes this a step further and adapts the plan based on patient-specific variations measured during their treatment, e.g. an initial PTV margin of 1 cm may be allocated based on previously researched population data. For an individual patient, imaging in the first week may then allow a reduction of the systematic error such that the PTV margin could be reduced and the treatment re-planned accordingly.

Image guided techniques arguably offer the biggest potential for adaptive radiotherapy because error due to both external set-up error and organ motion can be corrected for. Yan et al.[23] used diagnostic CT scans in the first week of treatment to determine a patient-specific PTV in the second week for 3DCRT to the prostate. Interestingly, it was noted that 2 weeks of daily CT measurements would be needed to have the same effect when delivering IMRT. CT verification techniques offer a further advantage in allowing visualisation of the target contour and therefore changes in the size and shape as well as position can be detected. Again, if this was to occur, the plan could be adapted accordingly based on the new CTV contour.

It is also possible to use previously determined patterns of change to 'predict' the shape and location of the target at the point of radiation (*predictive radiotherapy*), e.g. Hoogeman et al.[24] determined that the initial rectal volume on the planning CT could be used to predict average prostate and rectal wall rotations. Using this pretreatment information, it was found that the average systematic rotation could be reduced by 28%.

Adaptation of the 'standard' plan, based on individual data gathered either in the first weeks of treatment or before this at the planning stage, can be achieved in a number of ways. One option would be to have a pre-selection of probable estimated plans based on prior predictive knowledge gathered. However, if predictions or patterns were not possible and the change in the plan were entirely patient specific, then individual re-plans would be needed. In this case, depending on the change, this may require a repeat planning CT. Integrated CT options in the treatment room, i.e. CBCT and tomotherapy, could arguably streamline this process. Even though the CT numbers are less reliable than those produced with diagnostic CT, CBCT images can be used to produce a plan,[25] although research in this area is ongoing. As previously mentioned, tomotherapy units include a fully integrated planning system, easily facilitating a 'scan, plan and treat' approach. For both these modalities, however, it would also be important to consider the image quality and the ability to accurately re-contour the CTV and organs at risk.

It is important to note that, if any adaptations are made, ongoing verification checks and effective immobilisation (internal and/or external) would be needed to ensure that this level of accuracy were maintained.

## An issue of additional dose

When using an MV EPID it may be possible to subtract the monitor units used to acquire the images from those intended for that treatment field. Orthogonal reference images are most often acquired, however, so this may not be possible if the treatment fields are at oblique angles. Additional dose outside the planned treatment volume will also be incurred if a double exposure is used, as a means of identifying relevant anatomy needed for the match.

Volumetric (tomography) imaging is associated with higher concomitant doses than plain radiographic portal imaging. For both types of imaging, kV energies will deliver a lower concomitant dose than MV. Obviously with ultrasonography, there is no ionising radiation dose at all.

It has been highlighted earlier that an increased frequency of imaging is needed to effectively reduce the systematic error associated with a set-up and that daily online imaging would be needed to fully eliminate the random error. With particular reference to the latter, the choice of imaging modality and the benefits associated with this must be balanced against the additional dose delivered.

With any imaging protocol, the additional dose delivered must be justified under the regulations set out by IR(ME)R 2000.[26]

## Dosimetric verification

Dosimetric verification is just as crucial as verifying field placement (geometric verification), particularly considering the increased need for accuracy with conformal treatments and specifically the complex dose distributions associated with IMRT. In fact, verifying the dose delivered is the most obvious way of assessing the ultimate accuracy of a patient's treatment.

In 2008, the publication, *Towards Safer* Radiotherapy,[27] stated that in vivo dosimetry can detect some significant errors and recommended that all radiotherapy centres should have protocols in place for in vivo dosimetry. It was recommended that this should be in routine use at the start of treatment for most patients.

There are several methods available for verifying the dose delivered to the patient, also known as in vivo dosimetry. They include the use of *thermoluminescent dosimeters* (TLDs), *semiconductor diodes* and radiographic film or more recently EPIDs. There are more recently developed systems such as *MOSFETs* (metal oxide-silicon field effect transistors), but this section focuses on the former systems.

TLDs contain impurities that effectively alter the properties of the crystal such that they 'trap' electrons produced as a result of irradiation within intermediate energy levels. To return to their normal energy level, they require energy. This is applied in the form of heat and as the electrons are released they emit light. This light is detected by a photomultiplier with the total light output being proportional to the total number of trapped electrons, and therefore the absorbed dose within the crystal. Different crystalline materials may be used, the most common being lithium fluoride. One of the main disadvantages is that an immediate read-out is not possible. TLDs are most commonly used for measuring the dose to organs at risk such as the lens of the eye.

Semi-conductor diodes have a high sensitivity and are more frequently used to measure central axis and off-axis entrance and exit dose measurements. Most clinical semi-conductor detectors comprise p-type silicon (silicon doped with boron) bonded to a very thin wafer of n-type silicon (silicon doped with phosphorus). A 'depletion region' exists either side of this p–n junction containing no mobile charge with a potential difference of around 0.7 V across it. During irradiation of the diode ionisation occurs within the detector and ion pairs are swept across the depletion region, thus creating a current. The current is proportional to the ion pairs produced and thus the absorbed dose within the diode. The current can be measured by connecting the detector to an electrometer. A number of multi-channel electrometers are available. The major advantage of semi-conductor systems is that they allow real-time assessment of dose. In practice this means that, where the ratio of measured dose to expected dose exceeds a specified tolerance (typically ±5%), set-up can be investigated while the patient remains on the couch.

Thorough commissioning combined with the careful application of locally determined correction factors and regular calibration can result in the implementation of accurate and precise dose verification using diodes. Appleyard et al.[28,29] provide comprehensive reports on the implementation of diodes for entrance dosimetry and the determination of appropriate tolerance levels.

TLDs and semi-conductor diodes are, however, point dosimeters and therefore somewhat limited for verifying the accuracy of dose fluence during delivery of IMRT. Diode arrays may be used to assess this but EPIDs offer greater flexibility in that they offer the potential to simultaneously verify both field placement and dose fluence. The transmitted dose at any point within a portal image can be determined through evaluation of the pixel signals or grey-scale values. These are related to the portion of radiation transmitted through the patient and hence also the dose absorbed. These 'measured' portal dose images (PDIs) can be compared with 'predicted' PDIs calculated using algorithms and the CT data.

Dosimetric verification is a necessity for the verification of IMRT, specifically the intended beam fluence. As a minimum, this is verified through the acquisition of pre-treatment PDIs using the EPID (pre-treatment quality assurance or QA) and with the use of a phantom. As proposed by McDermott et al.,[30] verification could equally involve the use of EPID in vivo dosimetry once a patient started treatment. For prostate IMRT, they recommended combining dosimetric information taken from three fractions as a means of determining clinical relevant systematic errors.

## Record-and-verify systems and computer-controlled delivery

The focus of this section is on the role of record-and-verify systems. However, in today's increasingly complex and technical environment, this system is in fact one small part of a much larger patient information and management system. Each patient will have their own electronic medical record (EMR), which will include the records associated with other aspects of their patient journey, e.g. the verification images acquired and a record of any corrections made, clinic reviews and test results.

In addition to the sources of error already outlined, error in the delivery of treatment can also occur, albeit rarely, due to the incorrect selection of planned treatment parameters. This was a particular risk when 'manual' delivery methods were used and parameters were input into the console on a daily basis. 'Random' transcription errors from the treatment plan were possible.

Some aspects of machine operation were verified, e.g. interlocks, electronic beam flatness monitors, dose rate monitors. Such monitoring circuits helped to ensure that the machine was operating effectively. However, the installation and use of computerised record-and-verify systems began in the mid to late 1970s. Such systems have been shown to dramatically reduce this random error, even with increasing plan complexity.[31]

All geometrical and physical data required for the irradiation of a specific patient with a selected field is entered into the system at the planning stage. Such parameters should include the following:

- Patient identification (name and number)
- Mode of treatment (photons or electrons)
- Technique (static or dynamic)
- Treatment field
- Field size (including offset jaw positions)
- Fraction number
- Beam energy
- Monitor units (open and wedged fields)
- Daily tumour dose (a series of reference doses are optional)
- Cumulative doses
- Wedge angle and orientation
- Gantry angle (plus stop angle and increment angle for arc therapy)
- Collimator angle
- Couch position (reliant on positioning devices being fixed at set points on the table)
- Electron applicators and field sizes.

This planned 'prescription' can then be retrieved for each treatment session. Any deviations in the daily set-up from the planned parameters will be highlighted by the system and prevent the operator from initiating an exposure, unless an override is requested. Some departments choose to limit this responsibility to senior staff.

Small, accepted, patient variations can occur on a day-to-day basis. A record-and-verify system must be able to accept minor deviations from values specified on the database. This is achieved by specifying maximum possible deviations or tolerances from prescribed values in the form of tolerance tables. It is essential to undertake an appraisal of the treatment techniques employed before its clinical use. Such a process determines those parameters that remain fixed, those that may vary and others where monitoring is impractical. Tolerances that are too tight will result in the excessive need to override, and those that are too large will risk an inaccurate set-up. A balance between the two is needed.

A limitation of the initial record and verify systems was that they still relied on the accurate entry of treatment parameters to start with and this was still done manually. Any error introduced at this planning stage would then remain throughout the treatment unless detected, resulting in a 'systematic' transcription error. Nowadays, however, the treatment parameters can be directly downloaded from the computer planning system to the record-and-verify system via the DICOM network, removing the chance of transcription errors.

Once integrated into the planning and delivery system, the record-and-verify system arguably 'controls' the parameters, rather than simply verifying them. It is part of a much larger computer-controlled delivery system.[32]

Computer-controlled delivery is driving treatment delivery more and more. It would be very difficult to deliver IMRT and its associated multiple multi-leaf collimator (MLC) segments, in particular those that are delivered dynamically, without this. The imaging options used for treatment verification are also guided by computer-assisted hardware and software packages and several systems will even use remote couch control to make the necessary positional changes.

Although computer-assisted systems are important in improving the accuracy of treatment delivery, they must not replace the diligence of the radiographer and QA procedures must be in place to monitor their inherent accuracy and reliability.

The presence of any record-and-verify system should never replace the level of diligence displayed by the radiographer.[33] It is particularly important to be aware that the system cannot verify everything. In a study by Huang et al.,[34] missing information or the incorrect positioning of beam modification devices such as bolus increased the risk of error.

## Conclusion

As technology advances, the potential to deliver a more accurate treatment delivery increases. Developments in the field of treatment verification contribute significantly to this and the most effective protocols should ideally combine the use of both geometric and dosimetric verification strategies.

The exact verification protocol adopted will depend on treatment site, the sources of error and the types of error that predominate. Although sites that are affected by organ motion and/or tumour shrinkage will benefit from the use of IGRT, in which direct identification of the target is possible, other sites may equally benefit from a rigorous protocol using conventional portal imaging based on bony anatomy only. One must also consider the type of correction strategy employed. If random error predominates, daily

online imaging may be required. Any imaging strategy must work within the IR(ME)R 2000[26] regulations and any additional dose incurred should be justified.

In contrast to geometric verification, dosimetric verification is not widely implemented at present, although it is anticipated that this will soon change given the recent recommendations from the *Towards Safer Radiotherapy* document.[27]

The integration of increasingly complex technology into all aspects of the treatment delivery process has necessitated the need for computer control of the systems that we use. With this in mind, all computer-controlled systems should be subject to routine QA checks that monitor their inherent accuracy. We must also still be aware that these systems cannot control everything and thus we must not become reliant on them. We must still be able to detect and question any unusual parameters and be aware of those components of a technique that cannot be automatically verified or controlled.

### Self-test questions

1. Differentiate between a systematic error and a random error.

2. List the factors that may contribute to random error.

3. Random error can only be corrected for using online imaging. TRUE or FALSE.

4. Describe what is meant by offline correction.

5. Imaging on day 1 only is an effective means of reducing the systematic error. TRUE or FALSE.

6. With reference to amorphous silicon detectors, once the transmitted X-rays are converted to light, describe how this is then converted into an electronic readout.

7. For treatment sites where organ motion contributes to the associated error, explain why IGRT is preferable to conventional portal imaging.

8. State ONE advantage of using the following IGRT options:

Ultrasonography
EPID using implanted markers
CBCT.

9. State ONE possible disadvantage of using the following IGRT options:
Ultrasonography
EPID using implanted markers
CBCT.

10. List the options available for dosimetric verification.

11. Why are TLDs and semi-conductor diodes unsuitable for the dosimetric verification of IMRT?

12. Explain the rationale behind adaptive radiotherapy.

13. Explain how modern record and verify systems can help to significantly reduce the error associated with the incorrect selection of treatment parameters.

14. What are the potential limitations of computer-controlled treatment delivery systems?

# References

1. Langen KM, Jones DTL. Organ motion and its management. *Int J Radiat Oncol Biol Phys* 2001; **50**: 265–78.
2. International Commission on Radiation Units and Measurements. *Prescribing, Recording, and Reporting Photon Beam Therapy* (Supplement to ICRU Report 50). ICRU Report 62. Bethesda, MD: ICRU Publications, 1999.
3. Hurkmans CW, Remeijer P, Lebesque JV, Mijnheer BJ. Set-up verification using portal imaging; review of current clinical practice. *Radiother Oncol* 2001; **58**: 105–20.
4. Royal College of Radiologists. *Development and Implementation of Conformal Radiotherapy in the United Kingdom BFCO(02)2*. London: The Royal College of Radiologists, 2002.
5. Langmack K, Routsis D. Towards an evidence based treatment technique in prostate radiotherapy. *J Radiother Pract* 2000; **2**: 91–100.
6. Griffiths SE, Stanley S, Sydes M, RT01 Radiographers Group on behalf of all the RT01 Collaborators. () Recommendations on best practice for radiographer set-up of conformal radiotherapy treatment for patients with prostate cancer: experience developed during the MRC RT01 trial (ISRTCN 47772397). *J Radiother Pract* 2004; **4**: 107–17.
7. de Boer HC, Heijmen BJ. A protocol for the reduction of systematic patient setup errors with minimal portal imaging workload. *Int J Radiat Oncol Biol Phys* 2001; **50**: 1350–65.
8. Perera T, Moseley J, Munro P. (1999) Subjectivity in interpretation of portal images. *Int J Radiat Oncol Biol Phys* **45**: 529–534.
9. Kruse JJ, Herman MG, Hagness CR et al. Electronic and film portal images: a comparison of landmark visibility and review accuracy. *Int J Radiat Oncol Biol Phys* 2002; **54**: 584–91.
10. Fung A, Enke C, Ayyangar K et al. Prostate motion and isocenter adjustment from ultrasound-based localization during delivery of radiation therapy. *Int J Radiat Oncol Biol Phys* 2005; **61**: 984–92.
11. Kuban DA, Dong L, Cheung R, Strom E, De Crevoisier R. Ultrasound-based localization. *Semin Radiat Oncol* 2005; **15**: 180–91.
12. Serago CF, Chungbin SJ, Buskirk SJ, Ezzell GA, Collie AC, Vora SA. Initial experience with ultrasound localization for positioning prostate cancer patients for external beam radiotherapy. *Int J Radiat Oncol Biol Phys* 2002; **53**: 1130–8.
13. McGahan J, Ryu J, Fogata M. Ultrasound probe pressure as a source of error in prostate localization for external beam radiotherapy. *Int J Radiat Oncol Biol Phys* 2004; **60**: 788–93.
14. Artignan X, Smitsmans M, Lebesque J, Jaffray D, van Herk M, Bartelink H. Online ultrasound image guidance for radiotherapy of prostate cancer: impact of image acquisition on prostate displacement. *Int J Radiat Oncol Biol Phys* 2004; **59**: 595–601.
15. Court L, Dong L, Taylor N et al. Evaluation of a contour-alignment technique for CT-guided prostate radiotherapy: an intra- and interobserver study. *Int J Radiat Oncol Biol Phys* 2004; **59**: 412–18.
16. Ling C, Yorke E, Fuks Z. From IMRT to IGRT: Frontierland or neverland? *Radiother Oncol. Radiother Oncol* 2006; **78**: 119–22.
17. Chandra A, Dong L, Huang E et al. Experience of ultrasound-based daily prostate localization. *Int J Radiat Oncol Biol Phys* 2003; **56**: 436–47.
18. Little D, Dong L, Levy L, Chandra A, Kuban D. Use of portal images and BAT ultrasonography to measure setup error and organ motion for prostate IMRT: implications for treatment margins. *Int J Radiat Oncol Biol Phys* 2003; **56**: 1218–24.
19. Langen K, Pouliot J, Anezinos C et al. Evaluation of ultrasound-based prostate localization for image-guided radiotherapy. *Int J Radiat Oncol Biol Phys* 2003; **57**: 635–44.
20. Létourneau D, Martinez A, Lockman D et al. Assessment of residual error for online cone-beam CT-guided treatment of prostate cancer patients. *Int J Radiat Oncol Biol Phys* 2005; **62**: 1239–46.
21. Langen K, Zhang Y, Andrews R et al. Initial experience with megavoltage (MV) CT guidance for daily prostate alignments. *Int J Radiat Oncol Biol Phys* 2005; **62**: 1517–24.
22. McNair H, Mangar S, Coffey J et al. A comparison of CT- and ultrasound-based imaging to localize the prostate for external beam radiotherapy. *Int J Radiat Oncol Biol Phys* 2006; **65**: 678–87.
23. Yan D, Lockman D, Brabbins D, Tyburski L, Martinez A. An off-line strategy for constructing a patient-specific planning target volume in adaptive treatment process for prostate cancer. *Int J Radiat Oncol Biol Phys* 2000; **48**: 289–302.
24. Hoogeman M, van Herk M, de Bois J, Lebesque J. Strategies to reduce the systematic error due to

tumor and rectum motion in radiotherapy of prostate cancer. *Radiother Oncol* 2005; **74**: 177–85.

25. Ding G, Duggan D, Coffey C et al. A study on adaptive IMRT treatment planning using kV cone-beam CT. *Radiother Oncol* 2007; **85**: 116–25.

26. *Ionising Radiation (Medical Exposure) Regulations*. Statutory instrument 2000 No. 1059, 2000.

27. Royal College of Radiologists, Society and College of Radiographers, Institute of Physics and Engineering in Medicine, National Patient Safety Agency, British Institute of Radiology. *Towards Safer Radiotherapy*. London: The Royal College of Radiologists, 2008.

28. Appleyard R, Ball K, Hughes FE et al. Systematic in vivo dosimetry for quality assurance using diodes 1. Experiences and results of the implementation of entrance dose measurements. *J Radiother Pract* 2004; **3**: 185–96.

29. Appleyard R, Ball K, Hughes FE et al. Systematic in vivo dosimetry for quality assurance using diodes 2. Experiences and results of the implementation of entrance dose measurements. *J Radiother Pract* 2005; **4**: 143–54.

30. McDermott LN, Wendling M, Sonke J, Van Herk M, Mijnheer BJ. Replacing pretreatment verification with in vivo EPID dosimetry for prostate IMRT. *Int J Radiat Oncol Biol Phys* 2007; **67**: 1568–77.

31. Fraass BA, Lash KL, Matrone GM et al. The impact of treatment complexity and computer-control delivery technology on treatment delivery errors. *Int J Radiat Oncol Biol Phys* 1998; **42**: 651–9.

32. Fraass BA. QA Issues for computer-controlled treatment delivery: This is not your old R/V system any more! *Int J Radiat Oncol Biol Phys* 2008; **71**: S98–102.

33. Patton GA, Gaffney DK, Moeller JH. Facilitation of radiotherapeutic error by computerized record and verify systems. *Int J Radiat Oncol Biol Phys* 2003; **56**: 50–7.

34. Huang G, Medlam G, Lee J et al. Error in the delivery of radiation therapy: results of a quality assurance review. *Int J Radiat Oncol Biol Phys* 2005; **61**: 1590–5.

## Further reading

Herman MG. Clinical use of electronic portal imaging *Semin Radiat Oncol* 2005; **15**: 157–67.

Langmack KA. Portal imaging. *Br J Radiol* 2001; **74**: 789–804.

# Chapter 14

# INTRODUCTION TO RADIATION PROTECTION

Pete Bridge

### Aims and objectives

- To provide an overview of the relevant ionising radiations legislation
- To outline the basic principles underpinning radiation protection
- To explain the application of radiation protection principles and legislation to practice.

At the end of this chapter the reader will be able to:
- understand the importance of radiation protection
- be conversant with the legislation governing the use of ionising radiations
- understand radiation protection in practice.

## Dangers of ionising radiations

The purpose of *ionising radiation regulations* is to enable the safe use of radiation and it is important to understand the dangers that radiation presents in order to appreciate the importance of the regulations. Much of our knowledge concerning the hazardous nature of ionising radiation has been gained at the expense of early radiation workers and victims of nuclear accidents and weaponry. Common practices in the early days of radiography seem foolhardy today, but stemmed from a lack of understanding of the hazards associated with these new unseen rays.[1]

Early radiotherapy was conducted by patients holding radioactive isotopes to their tumours, while common practice among X-ray workers was to check functioning of fluoroscopy screens by watching to see if an image of their watch was visible when placed on the opposite side of their head to the source of X-rays. Radiodermatitis of the hands was common in these early workers, often leading to necrosis and amputation. Over-treatment of patients in the early days, as well as use of radiation for treatment of benign conditions such as ringworm[2] led to many cases of overdosing and development of side effects drastically worse than the original symptoms. It was not just medical use that caused problems; it was common practice for painters of radium dials on watches to lick the ends of their brushes to produce neat dots on the watch face. Ingestion of the radium paint led to increased bone cancer incidence.[3] Long-term follow-up studies of the survivors of the Nagasaki bomb showed an increased leukaemia incidence of 1.5 extra cases per million people per centigray per year.[4]

## Rationale for radiation protection

It should be appreciated, then, that not only does radiation injure all the cells of the body, causing acute and long-term damage to tissues, but it can also increase the chance of secondary malignancies and genetic mutations in offspring of exposed people. We categorise these effects as 'stochastic', meaning 'random in nature' or 'deterministic'. Stochastic effects can occur with even a small radiation dose, with the incidence of the effect increasing with higher doses. Deterministic effects occur only after a 'threshold' dose has been given and there is an increase in severity with increasing dose. It is the aim of radiation protection legislation to minimise the chance of a stochastic effect occurring. It is important for therapy radiographers to understand the dangers of radiation in order to reassure patients and also ensure that respect for the radiation leads to safe working practices.

## Radiation protection organisations

The International Commission on Radiological Units and Measurements (ICRU) is an international body established in 1925 to ensure consistency in radiation measurement and reporting. The International Commission on Radiological Protection (ICRP) is an international advisory body founded in 1928 to advise on radiation protection issues and form recommendations. In the UK, the Health Protection Agency (HPA) is responsible for developing these into regulations and ensuring compliance. The HPA enforces the two sets of regulations: the Ionising Radiation Regulations (IRR 1999)[5] and the Ionising Radiation (Medical Exposure) Regulations (IR(ME)R 2000).[6] The IRR 1999 superseded the previous IRR 1985 and covers any situation involving ionising radiation, be it medical, industrial or military. The IR(ME)R 2000 superseded the previous Protection of Persons Undergoing Medical Examination or Treatment (POPUMET 1988)[7] and is specifically concerned with the medical uses of ionising radiation. Clearly the IRR 1999 has relevance for all radiation use, such as the nuclear power industry, so this chapter is concerned only with those elements that are directly relevant to radiotherapy. All of the IR(ME)R

2000, on the other hand, is directly relevant and is discussed in detail. The reader is urged to read the regulations in conjunction with this chapter.

## Radiation protection legislation

### IR(ME)R 2000

Overview

The IR(ME)R 2000 is primarily aimed at ensuring that people working with radiation in the medical field are aware of their responsibilities and that it is easy to identify who has what responsibility. There is also an emphasis on justification of doses and keeping them as low as possible to minimise the chance of stochastic effects. Throughout the regulations, there is reference to 'practical aspects'. This term refers to exposing someone to radiation or any supporting task that is contributing to the delivery of that exposure. It encompasses such diverse tasks as handling of the equipment, identification of the patient and development of films.

Role definitions

As the IR(ME)R 2000 forms a legal document, some of the language used can be hard to understand and it is imperative that the reader be able to translate the terms (Table 14.1).

In most of the above definitions, there is reference to 'the employer's procedures'. These procedures are written by the employer and Schedule 1 of IR(ME)R outlines a list of essential procedures, which are the key to determining where responsibility lies and who is playing a particular role in the department. The essential employers' procedures include:

- Patient identification
- Identification of referrers, practitioners and operators
- Check for female patients' pregnancy status
- Quality assurance programmes
- Assessment of patient doses

**Table 14.1** IR(ME)R 2000 role definitions

| Role | Definition | Translation |
|------|-----------|-------------|
| Employer | 'Any natural or legal person who, in the course of a trade, business or other undertaking, carries out (other than as an employee), or engages others to carry out, medical exposures or practical aspects, at a given radiological installation.' | Someone who employs people to perform medical exposures (or practical aspects) or is self-employed) |
| Operator | 'Any person who is entitled, in accordance with the employer's procedures, to carry out practical aspects including those to whom practical aspects have been allocated pursuant to regulation 5(3), medical physics experts as referred to in regulation 9 and, except where they do so under the direct supervision of a person who is adequately trained, persons participating in practical aspects as part of practical training in practical aspects as part of practical training as referred to in regulation 11(3)' | Someone who an employer entitles to do practical aspects A specialist that the employer entitles to do practical aspects Medical physics experts Unsupervised students |
| Practitioner | 'Registered medical practitioner, dental practitioner or other health professional who is entitled in accordance with the employer's procedures to take responsibility for an individual exposure.' | Health professional entitled by the employer's procedures to take responsibility for exposures |
| Referrer | 'Registered medical practitioner, dental practitioner or other health professional who is entitled in accordance with the employer's procedures to refer individuals for medical exposures to a practitioner.' | Health professional entitled by the employer's procedures to refer patients to a practitioner |

- Provision of patient information and written instructions
- Dose evaluation
- Reduction of chance of accidental exposure.

### Duties and responsibilities

A major part of the IR(ME)R 2000 is the clear delineation of duties and responsibilities for each of the roles. The employer, as has already been determined, has to write the procedures listed above and ensure compliance with them. The employer also has to write protocols (or work instructions) and recommendations for quality assurance (QA) checks and dose levels. Other responsibilities include staff training and investigation of incidents, with associated notification of authorities.

The practitioner, operator and referrer must all comply with the employers; procedures, highlighting their importance within the IR(ME)R 2000. The practitioner must be able to justify all exposures, while the operator is responsible for practical aspects and, depending on the employers' procedures, can authorise exposures under certain conditions. The referrer has the responsibility to provide all relevant medical data in order to prevent repeat exposures being undertaken.

### Justification

IR(ME)R 2000 Regulation 6 outlines when an exposure can be justified. It is the responsibility of the practitioner to determine if there is sufficient net benefit to the exposure and this is the main source of justification. Authorisation is also dependent on women having been asked if they are pregnant or breast-feeding and on the referrer's medical data having been used.

Regulation 7 highlights the importance of keeping doses low. Clearly radiotherapy doses cannot be low in order to ensure tumour kill, but doses must be planned in order to ensure that normal tissue doses are low. Non-radiotherapy doses such as simulation procedures must be minimised with equipment and methods chosen to assist with this. All doses must be recorded and evaluated, even in the pre-treatment area. Another key element of dose minimisation is provision for clinical audit and the IR(ME)R 2000 state that this should be an integral part of practice.

## Advice

Regulation 9 ensures that medical physics experts are available in all departments and are closely involved with all radiotherapy practice. They must be involved to optimise treatments, help with dosimetry and QA, and advise on radiation protection for medical exposures.

## Training

Regulation 11 clarifies that neither practitioners nor operators can carry out medical exposures or practical aspects without adequate training and certification. Provision is made for students to train so long as an adequately trained person supervises them. Employers must keep records of staff training and, when agency staff are employed, the agencies must give their employee records to employers. Schedule 2 of the IR(ME)R 2000 outlines the key knowledge and understanding that should be included in training programmes.

## IRR 1999

### Overview

IRR 1999 comprises a more extensive set of legislation than IR(ME)R 2000 because it covers all uses of ionising radiation. They contain sections concerned with arrangements for control of radioactive items and details of how radioactive quantities of different substances are. Clearly these sections are essential reading for those departments that routinely use sealed or unsealed sources. There are also details of organisational arrangements and procedures, dose limits and personal monitoring, and duties of employers, which need to be applied to all radiotherapy departments.

### Local rules

Regulation 17 of the IRR 1999 stipulates that the employer has to write local rules using the advice of the radiation protection adviser (see Personnel below). The purpose of these rules is to inform employees of the correct practices that must be used to minimise exposure. In radiotherapy, the dose to staff is negligible so the purpose of radiotherapy department local rules is to prevent accidental irradiation. Local rules list the relevant radiation protection personnel, detail where radiation protection hazards and protective features are, as well as outline systems of work. There are general rules to be followed everywhere and area-specific rules. General rules ensure that warnings are heeded, dosimeters are worn and that the patient is alone in the room when radiation is present. Furthermore, the operator must not be distracted, faults must be listed and the machine must remain supervised when switched on. Area-specific rules describe safety devices and procedures, e.g. the 'closing-up' procedure for ensuring that the patient is alone when the beam is on.

### Personnel

IR(ME)R 2000 insisted that medical physics experts be available to give advice on radiation protection for medical exposures. In addition, IRR 1999 Regulation 13 stipulates that every employer has to consult a specialist physicist nominated the 'radiation protection adviser'. The radiation protection adviser provides advice on how to follow the regulations, designation of areas (see later) and monitoring of installations. They also need to be involved with plans for new installations and purchasing of new equipment. The IRR 1999 ensure that 'radiation protection supervisors' are appointed within the department to assist with compliance with regulations. They have a range of duties:

- Ensure that local rules are understood and followed
- Regulate entry into areas
- Ensure that personal dose meters are worn and checked
- Check protective equipment
- Liaise between staff regarding changes that might affect protection
- Remain aware of good practice and help train staff
- Ensure that low doses are used
- Ensure that records are kept.

### Dose limits

Radiation dose limits represent the absolute maximum dose a person or organ can receive in a year. Dose limits are much lower than the threshold doses required for deterministic effects, so the aim of dose limits is to limit the risk of stochastic effects taking place. The unit of measurement for dose limits is the sievert (Sv), which is the unit of *dose equivalent*. This ensures that dose limits are valid for a range of different modalities of radiation. It takes into account the biological effect of the radiation so that 1 Sv delivered with neutrons does the same amount of damage as 1 Sv of X-rays. When determining dose limits, the aim is to ensure that the risk of working with radiation is acceptable by making the same level as other acceptable risks. We compare the risk with the annual accidental death rate in other industries, which is 0.8 in 100 000.[8] Radiation dose limits are set to maintain stochastic effect risk at a comparative level. For therapy radiographers, however, who are not 'classified workers', the annual dose limit is the same as for the general public (assuming frequent exposure), which is 1 mSv.[5]

### Area designation

According to the IRR(1999), employers are responsible for designating areas of their department by radiation risk. 'Controlled areas' are those in which people working there are likely to receive an effective dose greater than 6 mSv a year. In the radiotherapy department, this includes treatment rooms, mazes and pre-treatment rooms containing simulators or CT scanners. People entering these areas need to follow special procedures in order to restrict their exposure. An example of this is the 'closing up procedure' to ensure that no one is in the room when there is radiation present. Controlled areas must be described in the local rules, be obviously demarcated and highlighted with suitable and sufficient warning signs. (Figure 14.1). The only people who can enter a controlled area are *classified people* (those receiving >6 mSv per year), patients receiving an exposure, Health and Safety Inspectors and people following a written system of work (e.g. local rules). Therapy radiographers are not classified people because they receive minimal dose and are able to enter controlled areas via the latter provision. Entry to a 'supervised area', on the other hand, is less strict, although these need to be constantly under review to check whether they should be controlled or not. People working there are likely to receive an effective dose >1 mSv a year. Examples of these in radiotherapy departments are the control desks and any waiting rooms immediately adjacent to treatment rooms.

## Radiation protection in practice

### Risks and benefits

The risks associated with radiation and ways in which they can be minimised have been discussed. Despite the risks, there are clearly benefits associated with medical radiation. The IR(ME)R 2000 requires all medical exposures to be justified, meaning that there is an overall benefit compared with the level of risk. Potential benefits of ionising radiation include cure of disease or improvement in quality of life, accurate diagnosis, early disease detection or accurate placement of catheters, stents, etc. If the potential benefit is seen as less than the risks associated

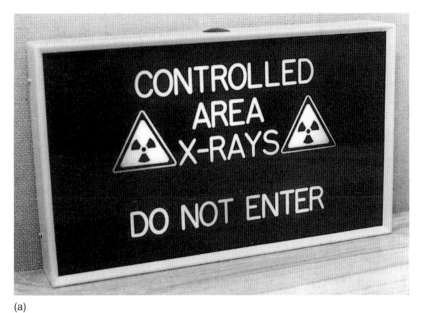

(a)

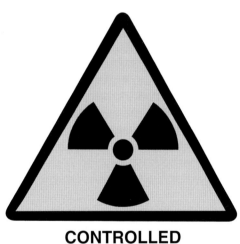

CONTROLLED
AREA
GAMMA RAYS

(b)

**Figure 14.1** Warning signs.

with the radiation, we should not use it. IR(ME)R 2000 Regulation 6(2) lists the factors to be considered when *justifying exposures*. These include patient characteristics, benefits and risks of the exposure, and consideration of alternatives to radiation.

## ALARA

The concept of *ALARA/ALARP* (as low as reasonably achievable/practicable) is that people working with radiation should try to keep their exposure and that of others to a minimum. It is important to ensure that the aims of the exposure are achieved to avoid it having to be repeated. This is achieved by following established protocols using good equipment and effective procedures. The three basic principles of radiation protection are time, distance and shielding. For most radiotherapy working practices, time is not a radiation protection issue because the radiation can be switched off. The ALARA principle is embedded in IR(ME)R 2000 Regulation 7. For non-radiotherapeutic procedures, the dose must be kept low, so settings must be carefully chosen to ensure that images do not need repeating and equipment such as image intensifiers, auto-exposure controls and image-capture software must be used. Furthermore, the employer has a responsibility to ensure that each exposure is evaluated and recorded. Fluoroscopy times and image exposures need to be noted and monitored to ensure that best practice is being followed. For radiotherapeutic procedures, target dose must be maximised, but Regulation 7 stipulates that exposures must be planned in order that non-target tissue doses are as low as reasonably practicable. This necessitates the use of shielding blocks, multi-leaf collimators, conformal planning, and appropriate immobilisation equipment and methods. This dose reduction must not be at the expense of tumour dose, which must be maintained at a radiotherapeutic level. The IR(ME)R (2000) again states that the employer must ensure outcomes of exposures are recorded. The verification and recording software usually performs this task.

## Personal monitoring

All staff members working in the radiotherapy department participate in *personal dose monitoring*. Monitoring is performed whenever people could receive 10% of the annual dose limit. Therapy radiographers usually receive slightly more than background dose (2.6 mSv/year)[9] so the main aim of personal dosimetry in most areas within the radiotherapy department is to check

for problems with radiation shielding and local rules or staff compliance/understanding with the local rules. The exception to this is, of course, brachytherapy, where the nature of the radiation is such that dose to staff is more likely. Radiation protection issues relating to this area are covered in more detail in Chapter 16. Records are kept for 50 years. Personal dosimeters should be portable, tough, sensitive, reliable and relatively cheap. For more details on personal dosimeters, see Chapter 3.

## Radiation protection by design

The three main principles of radiation protection are speed (which is not relevant to electrically produced radiation), distance and shielding. The latter elements are combined when treatment and simulation bunkers are designed and the final section of this chapter focuses on this issue.

### Equipment design

The primary factor affecting room design has to be the equipment that is to be located in it. Radiation generators are categorised according to their radiation protection needs (Table 14.2). Category 1 and 2 equipment produces low-energy radiation that operates in the photoelectric absorption dominant range of energies. With the exception of simulator and CT equipment, kilovoltage equipment is non-isocentrically mounted, so the main beam can be directed at any wall. This presents a different challenge for

**Table 14.2** External beam equipment

| | |
|---|---|
| Category 1 | X-ray tubes producing 10–150 kV photons |
| Category 2 | X-ray tubes producing 150–400 kV photons |
| Category 3 | Gamma ray beam units |
| Category 4 | Accelerators producing 1–50 MV photons |

radiation protection than category 3 and 4 equipment. There are three main sources of radiation associated with X-ray-producing equipment: the primary beam, scattered radiation produced by interactions of the primary beam and leakage radiation from the radiation generator itself. Manufacturers have a responsibility to maintain radiation leakage levels as low as possible. It is down to the room design to minimise the impact of the primary and scattered radiation.

## Barrier design

For isocentrically mounted radiation generators, it can be seen that the primary beam is only capable of irradiating a rigidly defined section of the room (Figure 14.2). This band of walls, floor and ceiling is known as the *primary barrier*. The remaining boundaries of the room that receive only secondary (leakage) radiation from the machine and scattered radiation from the patient and other materials are known as *secondary barriers*. It is important to distinguish between these barriers because only the primary barrier needs to be thick enough to attenuate the primary beam and choosing a thinner secondary barrier can save money. A variety of building materials can be used for barrier construction as seen in Table 14.3 and the density of the chosen material will clearly affect how thick the barrier needs to be.

Major factors affecting barrier thickness include the daily workload and energy of the machine. This will determine the dose rate at the isocentre and it is the aim of the barrier to reduce the dose rate outside the room to no more than the safe limit (for public areas this should be around 0.3 mSv/year).[10] Typical thickness requirements are 6 or 7 tenth value layers (TVLs) for a primary barrier and around 3 TLVs for a second-

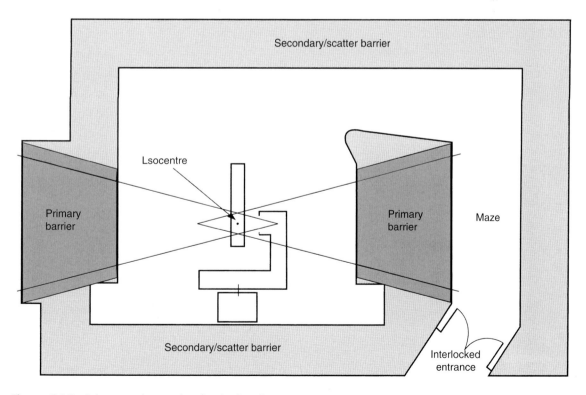

**Figure 14.2** Primary and secondary barrier location.

**Table 14.3** Barrier construction

| Material | Density (kg m$^{-3}$) |
|---|---|
| Brick (common red) | 1920 |
| Breeze block | 1200 |
| Concrete | 2370 |
| Barytes concrete | 3100 |
| Earth fill | 1520 |
| Glass | 2580 |
| Glass (lead) | 4360 |
| Steel | 7849 |
| Lead (solid) | 11 340 |

ary barrier. The size of the room will influence barrier thickness with the inverse square law reducing intensity and therefore barrier thickness for a large room. Converse to this, a larger distance to the barrier will require a wider primary barrier due to beam divergence.

The width of the primary barrier is dependent on the maximum area that can receive the primary beam. Beam divergence, collimator rotation and multiple gantry angles need to be considered when determining how much of the room needs to be a primary barrier. Penetration of barriers for cable access, for example, needs to be planned using angled access tubes and shielding to ensure that radiation cannot escape through the ducts.

For non-isocentrically mounted apparatus such as kilovoltage radiotherapy units, the primary beam direction is not so restrained and the entire room has to act as a primary barrier. As a result of the relatively low beam quality, however, the walls can be much thinner than those required for megavoltage installations.

## Treatment room entrance

The room entrance design plays a large role in radiation protection. Clearly any treatment or simulation rooms where patients are left alone need to be accessible in case of emergency, yet an entrance presents an opportunity for radiation to escape. For this reason, treatment rooms using high-energy megavoltage photons will usually use a maze entrance[11] to attenuate radiation via scatter processes (see Figure 14.2). This allows for ease of access but denies scattered photons passage out of the room. At lower kV energies, a shielded door may be sufficient, but, as the energy increases, the required door thickness presents technical difficulties such as the need for a motorised opening mechanism. At photon energies over 20 MeV, a shielded door impregnated with boron is necessary to absorb thermal neutrons that are produced. The choice of entrance will largely be dictated by availability of space while balancing the need for protection against the need for easy access to the patient. The control area must be remote to the radiation generator, with CCTV or lead glass screens allowing visualisation of the patient at MV and kV respectively.

## Treatment room location

Another important factor affecting radiation protection is the position of the room itself in relation to its surroundings. Adjoining treatment or simulation rooms can benefit from sharing of primary barriers, thus saving on shielding materials. Any other rooms need to be shielded according to their typical occupancy. Rooms that are used sporadically, such as toilets or corridors, have a lower 'occupancy factor' than offices or wards so shielding needs to reflect that. Apart from being adjacent to other radiation generators, bunkers can benefit from being single-storey buildings (thus avoiding the need for reinforced and shielded floors and ceilings). Backing into a hill is ideal because earth fill can be used as a cheap shielding material, ensuring that it is only the occasional passing earthworm or mole that receives a dose.

## Additional safety features

Any controlled areas must have warnings in place identifying prohibited access and displaying the radiation caution trefoil, as illustrated in Figure 14.2. In addition to *warning signs*, there should be *warning lights* and an *audible alarm* to alert visually impaired visitors. A range of *interlocks* should be present to ensure that the patient is the only person being irradiated and that he or she is receiving the correct dose. *Access interlocks* such as barriers, infrared beams, doors or motion sensors will terminate the exposure if broken by

an intruder. Various systems such as verification software, 'select-and-confirm' protocols and accessory interlocks ensure that the correct parameters are used in the exposure. *Performance interlocks* within the radiation generator are designed to maintain correct beam quality, intensity and dosimetric consistency. It can be seen, therefore, that there are a great number of design features that help ensure radiation protection being achieved in the radiotherapy department. These can only be effective, however, in the context of commitment to staff training and compliance with legislation, local rules and protocols.

---

### Self-test questions

1. What are the characteristics of stochastic effects?
2. What are the two main pieces of ionising radiation legislation in the UK?
3. What are 'practical aspects'?
4. Under what circumstances could a student be classed as an 'operator'?
5. Who is responsible for writing work instructions/protocols?
6. Who is responsible for justification of an exposure?
7. Who is responsible for designating areas as controlled or supervised?
8. Who is responsible for regulating entry into controlled areas?
9. What is the unit of dose equivalent?
10. What is the annual dose limit for a member of the public likely to be exposed frequently?
11. Is a radiotherapy linear accelerator maze likely to be a controlled or supervised area?
12. How can ALARA be achieved in radiotherapy?
13. How can ALARA be achieved in pre-treatment?
14. What is the aim of personal monitoring in radiotherapy?
15. What are the three sources of radiation to be found in a radiotherapy treatment room?
16. Why is the primary barrier thicker than the secondary barrier?
17. Name two factors affecting primary barrier thickness.
18. Name two factors affecting primary barrier width in a linear accelerator room.
19. What advantages does a shielded door offer over a maze entrance?
20. Why might designing a department with adjacent treatment rooms save money?

---

## References

1. Mould RF. *The Early Years of Radiotherapy with Emphasis on X-ray and Radium Apparatus.* Bristol: Institute of Physics Publishing, 1993.
2. Ron E, Modan B, Boice JD. Mortality after radiotherapy for ringworm of the scalp. *Am J Epidemiology* 1988; **127**: 713–25.
3. Polednak AP, Stehney AF, Rowland RE. Mortality among women first employed before 1930 in the US radium dial-painting industry. A group ascertained from employment lists. *Am J Epidemiology* 1978; **107**: 179–95.
4. Finch SC. Radiation-induced leukaemia: lessons from history. *Best Pract Res Clin Haematol* 2007; **20**: 109–18.
5. Statutory instrument 3232. *The Ionising Radiation Regulations 1999.* London: HMSO, 1999.
6. Statutory instrument 1059. *The Ionising Radiation (medical exposure) Regulations 2000.* London: HMSO, 2000.
7. Statutory instrument 778. *The Ionising Radiation (protection of persons undergoing medical exam-*

*ination or treatment) Regulations 1988*. London: HMSO, 1985.

8. Health and Safety Executive. *Statistics of Fatal Injuries 2006/07*. London: Health and Safety Executive, 2007.

9. Hughes JS. *Ionising Radiation Exposure of the UK Population: 1999 review*. London: Health Protection Agency, 1999.

10. Allisy-Roberts P, ed. *Medical and Dental Guidance Notes. A good practice guide on all aspects of radiation protection in the clinical environment*. London: Institute of Physics and Engineering in Medicine, 2002.

11. Stedeford B, Morgan HM, Mayles WPM. *The Design of Radiotherapy Treatment Room Facilities*. London: IPEM, 2002.

## Chapter 15

# USE OF RADIONUCLIDES IN IMAGING AND THERAPY

David Duncan

## Aims and objectives

On completion of this chapter you should be able to:
- describe the basic operation of a nuclear medicine generator system
- list the components of a gamma camera and explain each part's role in acquiring an image
- discuss basic principles of imaging and radionuclide therapy in nuclear medicine, especially in oncology
- list the advantages and disadvantages of the use of hybrid imaging in nuclear medicine
- describe radiation protection principles used in nuclear medicine
- state the different factors that affect patient radiation dosimetry.

## Introduction

This chapter is not intended to be a comprehensive explanation of the discipline of nuclear medicine but rather provide a taste of those areas that are particularly relevant to the patient with cancer. Radionuclides have a dual role to play in the management of cancer. Radionuclide imaging is used for the diagnosis, staging and monitoring of cancers. Radioactive iodine has been used in the treatment of thyroid and others cancers for many years. In recent years, methodologies have been developed specifically for tumour imaging and the targeting of nuclides to tumours for local therapy. The materials and methods for this are described. These activities bring with them problems of radiation protection because patients become radiation sources (and sometimes leaky ones) for a period of time. The regulations and procedures for dealing with this are also summarised.

By introducing substances into the body that follow specific physiological pathways while emitting radiation, it is possible to detect and map penetrating radiation from outside the body to produce images or to use non-penetrating radiation for therapy. In therapeutic applications the activities administered are much higher than for diagnosis.

Radionuclides are localised to the desired tissue by being chemically attached to, or incorporated into, some compound that is designed to follow a known biodistribution in the body. There are a number of different mechanisms by which this is achieved. The radionuclide and compound together are called the radiopharmaceutical.

## Radionuclides for therapy

For therapy the energy from the radiation needs to be deposited in the tissue to be destroyed. Depending on the volume of this tissue and hence the desired range of the particles, radionuclides emitting beta rays of varying average energies and occasionally alpha particles can be used. The range of particle emission has to be considered because, if it is too small, there may be incomplete irradiation and hence potential tumour recurrence and, if it is too large, the surrounding tissue will be irradiated with consequent damage.

If pure alpha or beta emitters are used, the radiation will not be emitted from the patient's body. This is clearly an advantage in radiation protection terms. If, however, the nuclide also emits gamma rays, it enables simultaneous imaging of the biodistribution.

## Radionuclides for imaging

For imaging, the emissions need to leave the body to be detected and only gamma rays have sufficient range. To minimise the patient dose, ideally nuclides that emit only gamma rays should be used.

The nuclide must decay slowly enough that the activity remaining will still be adequate for imaging when the radiopharmaceutical has reached its destination. It must also be short enough not to linger in the body for days or weeks after the imaging study, adding to the radiation dose to no useful effect. The element has to have a chemical affinity for the compounds to which it is to be labelled and there must be no toxicity.

Synthetic isotopes with optimum characteristics for imaging and for various therapies are continually sought and produced. For most imaging purposes, technetium-99 m ($^{99m}$Tc) is used, which is a pure gamma emitter with 140 keV characteristic energy and a half-life ($t_{1/2}$) of 6 hours. The 'm' in $^{99m}$Tc shows that this radionuclide is metastable. Metastability can be defined as an excited state of an atom with a measurable half-life or a nucleus that takes time to decay.

## Radioactive decay

Radioactive substances decay at an exponential rate. Despite decaying by different means with the emission(s) of varying particles or amounts of energy, the decay process always follows this pattern. The rate of decay cannot be altered and is not affected by such things as heat, magnetic or electrical fields. Radioactive isotopes are known as *radioisotopes*. When discussed in relation to nuclear medicine, they are commonly known as *radionuclides*. Radionuclides bound to pharmaceuticals are known as *radiopharmaceuticals*.

*Radioactive decay* is an event originating in the nucleus of the atom, hence it is sometimes described as nuclear decay. The physical half-life of a radioisotope is the time taken for the amount of radioactivity of a substance to reach half its original value. This is a distinctive time for each individual type of radioisotope. Radioactive decay is a random event, but the law of averages enables us to determine physical half-lives. This can vary from microseconds to millions of years depending on the type of radioisotope involved.

Radioactive decay can be calculated using the equation:

$$A = A_0 e^{-\lambda t}$$

where $A$ = amount of radioactivity present at a given/desired time, $A_0$ = initial amount of radioactivity present, or at time 0, and $\lambda$ = the transformation (or decay) constant.

The transformation constant is the same for all radionuclides with the same physical half-life. The SI unit for measuring radioactivity amounts is the *becquerel* (Bq): 1 becquerel equates to one radioactive disintegration per second. Doses used in diagnostic nuclear medicine are usually stated in megabecquerels (MBq), whereas those used for radionuclide therapy, where higher doses are used, can be stated in gigabecquerels (GBq). The non-SI unit used in some countries is the *Curie* (Ci): 1 mCi is equivalent to 37 MBq.

## Radionuclide generator systems

Logistically, to use radionuclides that have half-lives of less than a day, a local source is necessary.

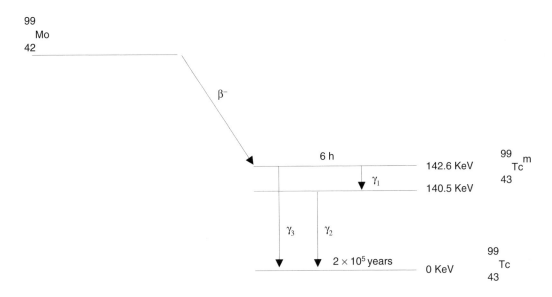

$^{99}_{42}Mo$

$\beta^-$

6 h — 142.6 KeV — $^{99m}_{43}Tc$

$\gamma_1$ — 140.5 KeV

$\gamma_3$ $\gamma_2$

$2 \times 10^5$ years — 0 KeV — $^{99}_{43}Tc$

**Figure 15.1** Simplified decay scheme for $^{99}$Mo showing production of $^{99m}$Tc and associated decays.

One way of doing this is to keep a supply of one radionuclide (the parent or mother) that decays to another, useful radionuclide (the daughter) in a form in which parent and daughter can be separated. This storage and separation system is called a generator.

Most commonly used nowadays is the molybdenum/technetium ($^{99}$Mo/$^{99m}$Tc) generator. The parent is $^{99}$Mo, which decays to $^{99m}$Tc in 86% of events. The $^{99m}$Tc decays in turn to $^{99}$Tc which has a half-life of $2.1 \times 10^5$ years and can thus be considered effectively stable (Figure 15.1). The generator system allows the technetium to be separated from the molybdenum in radiation and microbial safety (Figure 15.2). As the daughter radionuclide is to be administered to patients, it is essential that the entire internal generator system is a sterile environment.

The $^{99}$Mo, as ammonium molybdate $(NH_4)^+(MoO_4)^-$, is adsorbed onto an alumina column on which the $^{99m}$Tc is formed as $^{99m}$TcO$_4$ and which can then be removed by ion exchange. When physiological or 0.9% saline is passed through the column, a process known as elution, the chloride ions exchange with the TcO$_4$ but not the MoO$_4$ ions, because these are more tightly bound to the column, and a solution of sodium pertechnetate Na$^+$TcO$_4^-$ is produced and known as the eluate. The saline can be pushed or pulled over the column in either a positive or negative pressure system. Negative pressure is safer for radiation spill but may draw in bacteria so microbial filters are included (see Figure 15.2).

After elution there is very little $^{99m}$Tc left on the column and this needs time to build up again before the process can be repeated. The maximum individual yield from a column is obtained 23 hours after the last elution, after which time the rate of decay matches that of build-up and the level does not increase but decreases with the decay rate of the parent radionuclide. Generators can be eluted more frequently, yielding less activity each time but providing more activity in total over the course of a day. The amount of activity obtained depends on the time since the previous elution, the size of generator delivered (the original activity of the parent) and the age of the generator (how long it has been in the department). $^{99}$Mo/$^{99m}$Tc generators are replaced weekly.

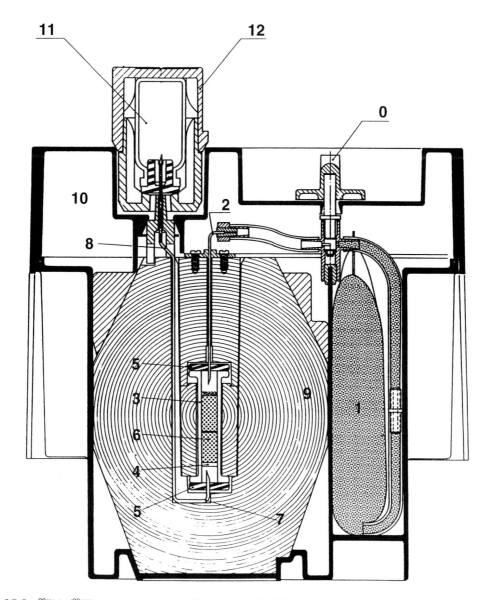

**Figure 15.2** $^{99m}$Mo/$^{99m}$Tc generator system. (Courtesy of CIS UK.)

Before patient use, the eluate undergoes several quality control checks, either on a daily or a weekly basis. These include checks for $^{99}$Mo and aluminium breakthrough into the eluate, as well as radiochemical purity and sterility.

Departments buy the minimum size generator possible for their activity needs, not just for financial reasons but also to reduce the amount of activity they are storing and the radiation dose to the operators. $^{68}$Ge–$^{68}$Ga and $^{82}$Sr–$^{82}$Rb generators may also be used in positron electron tomography (PET; discussed later).

Further, radionuclides less commonly used in nuclear medicine can be obtained from other sources. Iodine-131 ($^{131}$I), used mainly for therapy applications, can be obtained from nuclear reactors. $^{131}$I is a superfluous by-product of common fission reactions and as a result is usually inexpensive to obtain. Other radionuclides, including indium-111 ($^{111}$In) and gallium-67 ($^{67}$Ga), are cyclotron produced. Cyclotron-produced radionuclides are relatively expensive to purchase compared with other radionuclides.

## Radiopharmacy

The production of radiopharmaceuticals or *radiolabelling* is carried out in a radiopharmacy. Radiopharmaceuticals can be bought from commercial manufacturers if they are compounds of a longer-lived nuclide but most are made either in a large hospital centre that supplies smaller centres in the area or (for larger departments) on site. For the more common radiopharmaceuticals this is done by the addition of the eluate to pre-prepared, freeze-dried kits bought from manufacturers. Larger centres will also radiolabel autologous blood products and some label antibodies and cell receptors.

## Imaging equipment

### The gamma camera

After the administration of a radiopharmaceutical, the patient contains radioactivity in a distribution corresponding to a physiological process. This is mapped into an image using a gamma camera. Although there are several producers of gamma cameras internationally, the components and construction of the gamma camera by each company are essentially the same. The following is a brief description of the design of a gamma camera.

The collimator is used to select the desired rays for use in the image. Gamma rays are emitted from a patient in all directions. When they are detected in the crystal there is, therefore, no way of knowing where they came from and so the distribution cannot be mapped. It is necessary to confine the rays reaching the camera face to those

perpendicular to it, thus producing a 1:1 map of the distribution in the body. As can be seen in Figure 15.3, this is done by cutting out as many of the other rays as possible by absorbing them in lead. To do this, a collimator or lead block is interposed between the patient and crystal; this collimator contains a honeycomb of equally sized and spaced holes, the size, spacing and thickness of the block differing according to use. Collimators are interchangeable on a given camera and different ones are used for different characteristic energies, different fineness of detail or *resolution* (better resolution can be gained only at the expense of the images taking significantly longer), and sometimes to manipulate the shape of an image.

The crystal is located directly behind the collimator. It is made of sodium iodide (NaI) into which impurities of thallium have been introduced. This material will *scintillate* or give off flashes of light when a gamma photon imparts its energy into it. Crystals are fragile and the camera has to be handled with extreme care, especially when the collimator is being changed because the crystal is particularly vulnerable to mechanical damage. The crystal is also highly sensitive to moisture (hygroscopic) and light and for protection is encapsulated in a thin aluminium cover.

Once the *gamma photon* enters the crystal, its energy is transformed into a shower of light photons by a process in which electrons excited by the gamma ray are liberated from the valence band and move into a higher-energy level band and 'hole' caused by an atom of the impurity. Their excess energy will be emitted as flashes (or photons) of light or a scintillation. The number of light photons released is proportional to the energy deposited. All the energy of the gamma ray must be used up in this process to make the system work. This usually happens as a result of Compton scatter events in which kinetic energy is lost and is followed by a photoelectric interaction. These interactions occur within a very small distance so that they can be considered as happening at one point on the camera face. Light

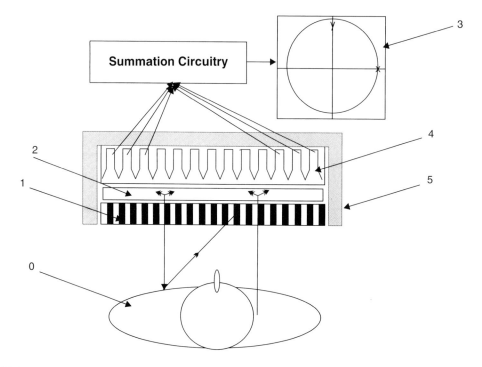

**Figure 15.3** Gamma camera.

close to the crystal edges is reflected from the sides of the aluminium casing, allowing it to be included. Some photons pass straight through the crystal and are not detected. For any given crystal substance, the efficiency (proportion of the activity detected) depends on the thickness of that crystal and the energy of the incident ray. Research into more efficient crystal materials is ongoing.

Each gamma event is processed separately but as the luminescence decay is in the order of nanoseconds, the camera is ready to process the next incoming photon so rapidly that count rates up to $10^4$ s$^{-1}$ can be handled. The time that it takes the camera to generate and process a reading from a single photon interaction is known as dead-time (the camera cannot detect any further gamma events during this time). This is usually only a problem with very high count rate studies and rarely occurs.

The light is directed to the next stage, the photomultiplier tubes, by a light guide. This is made of Plexiglas and optically couples the crystal to the front face of the *photomultiplier tubes* (PMTs) (Figure 15.4). The light flashes are detected by the PMTs adjacent to it, which ultimately turn that flash into a detectable current by converting light energy to usable electrical energy. The light guide diffuses the light around it to increase the number of PMTs involved in detecting light and improves positioning efficiency. The number of PMTs per camera head varies for different manufacturers and camera head dimensions.

Inside an evacuated glass tube the PMT contains the *photocathode*, which is made of caesium antimonide. Light energy ejects a few electrons from this material in a manner analogous to the photoelectric effect. When it receives a flash of light from the crystal, the number of electrons ejected is still proportional to the incident light and hence the energy of the photon.

Inside the tube are a number of *dynodes* or metal plates also coated with caesium antimo-

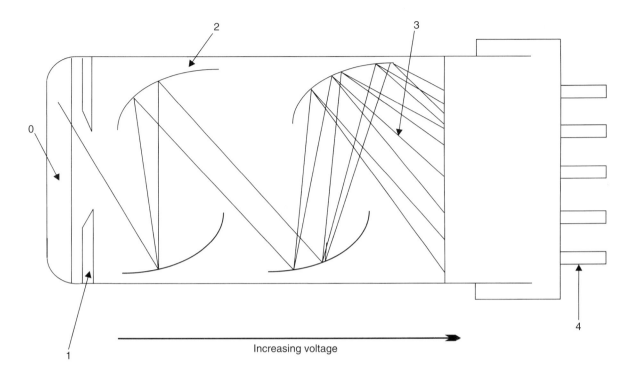

**Figure 15.4** Photomultiplier tube.

nide and positively charged, because there is an applied voltage between cathode and each successive dynode of about 200 V. This causes an electron to be accelerated towards the dynode. When it strikes the dynode, a secondary emission occurs, i.e. several electrons are ejected for each one that impinges. This happens at each succeeding dynode thus multiplying the number of electrons at each stage. If there are 10 dynodes the current will be increased by $10^6$. This is a respectable current and the proportionality of this current to the characteristic energy of the photon is maintained.

These bursts of current are converted into voltage pulses and shaped in the preamplifier. They all need to be multiplied by the same factor before sorting and positioning. The amplifier converts millivolts to tens of volts.

Pulses from a gamma event arriving at the end of the amplifier part of the circuit are then examined in two ways. *Pulse height analysis* and summation circuitry are used to select and position the events into an image. Only those gamma rays that had the original characteristic energy need to be recorded in the image. Pulses corresponding to other energies are from either scattered rays or electronic noise and are not required. Before a pulse is accepted as part of the image, the total amount of current from all PMTs is summed and passed to the *pulse height analyser* (PHA).

The system is not perfect and there is a small variation in amplifications in the pulses, so a range of voltages corresponding to energies about 10% above and below the characteristic energy are likely to correspond to genuine events. Thus, only pulses corresponding to energies between these preset levels should be accepted for further processing. The PHA looks at the size of the incoming pulse and compares it with the *lower level discriminator* and rejects it if it falls below that level. It then compares it with the *upper level discriminator* and again rejects it if it is greater.

To detect the position of the original photon, the strengths of the signals from the various PMTs are compared in the summation circuitry, e.g. if the light flash happens on the right side of the field, the signals from the combined PMTs on the right will be larger than those on the left. The difference in signal size will give a measure of how far to the right of the midline the event occurred. This procedure is repeated for each event accepted for left and right (or X) coordinates and top and bottom (or Y) coordinates. This positions the flash of light onto a cathode ray tube or in a computer matrix, which then forms the final image. The forming image can usually also be seen on a persistence scope so that the position can be adjusted before the image acquisition is started.

The signals are digitised in an *analogue digital converter* and assigned to a certain *pixel* (short for picture cell) in a computer matrix. The memory in this pixel then increases by one unit so that a distribution of numbers in different cells is collected over the period of the acquisition; these numbers can be translated into intensities on a screen. This can be viewed directly and stored digitally for future display and manipulations. In the past, the images were recorded on film, but are now stored digitally on acquisition stations and on systems such as PACS (picture archiving and communications system). As the information now consists of a series of numbers in a matrix it can be manipulated and different areas numerically compared, e.g. left and right kidney uptakes. This is called *quantitation* and allows for numbers equating to physiological function to be obtained as well as images.

## SPECT

Just as computed tomography (CT) added an extra dimension to conventional planar radiography, single photon emission computed tomography (SPECT) uses analogous techniques and reconstruction algorithms to extend the usefulness of radionuclide imaging and produce cross-sectional images of the distribution of a radiopharmaceutical in the body.

There are several advantages to SPECT. Similar to all tomography it removes overlying structures from the image and also gives more information on the position of a structure. It can determine size and, more importantly, volume, which allows for quantification, and it can reduce the effects of attenuation. These advantages can be very important for relative uptake measurements.

The gamma camera gantry needs to be structured to be capable of rotating around the patient and acquiring data at varying angles over 360°. A computer for manipulating the data is essential. Specially shaped collimators can be used to allow the camera to be brought as close as possible to the patient. Increasing the number of camera heads used simultaneously increases the amount of information collected in a given time. Cameras with two and three camera heads (Figure 15.5) are common. Often these heads can be configured in various positions depending on what body area is being imaged and how much information is required.

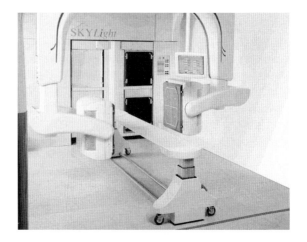

**Figure 15.5** A multi-headed gamma camera. (Image courtesy of Philips.)

## SPECT/CT

One of the more recent developments in patient imaging utilises hybrid imaging. An example of this is SPECT/CT, in which a gamma camera is physically combined with a CT machine and images from both modalities are taken sequentially. Images are acquired from both modalities and can be viewed separately and together (co-registered). This benefits the nuclear medicine image in two major ways. The use of X-rays allows the application of non-uniform attenuation correction to the nuclear medicine image, therefore helping to compensate for patient variables such as obesity and giving a more accurate representation of radionuclide distribution. Hybrid imaging also allows for co-registration of both modalities so that areas of radionuclide uptake can be more accurately localised. This can be important for, among other things, differentiating localised from extracapsular tumour spread. Hybrid imaging therefore combines functional (nuclear medicine) with structural (CT) information.

When SPECT/CT was first developed, CT machines were installed in proximity to existing nuclear medicine cameras. The CT component of such machines was generally considered non-diagnostic. Now manufacturers are manufacturing combined hybrid machines with truly diagnostic CT machines so that patients can potentially undergo their nuclear medicine study and diagnostic CT study in one appointment (Figure 15.6).

## PET imaging

PET (positron emission tomography) is based on similar principles to general nuclear medicine scanning. The two main differences are in the type of radionuclide used and the image acquisition equipment.

Positrons are emitted from a nucleus that has too many protons. A proton will decay to a

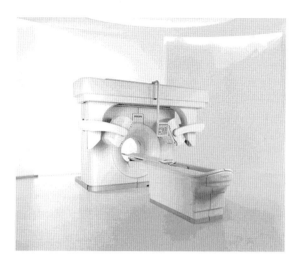

**Figure 15.6** SPECT/CT machine. Note the gamma camera component is the same as in Figure 15.5, with the addition of an in-built CT machine. (Image courtesy of Philips.)

neutron with the emission of a positron and a neutrino. The positron travels only a very short distance before combining with an electron. An annihilation event occurs at this time with the creation of two 511 keV gamma photons travelling at 180° to each other (Figure 15.7). It is these photons that are detected. As further gamma photons are detected, an image starts to appear.

As opposed to a camera head employed by nuclear medicine gamma cameras, PET machines are composed of a ring of detectors within which the patient is positioned (Figure 15.7). The gamma photons emitted travel at the speed of light. Rather than register the gamma photons as two separate events, the PET machine registers them as a paired event. It does this through the establishment of time windows. If two gamma photons are detected within the same (small) time window, the camera records them as coming from the same annihilation event. As the gamma photons travel at 180° to each other, the camera draws a line of flight between the two events and determines that the annihilation must have occurred along this line. This type of acquisition

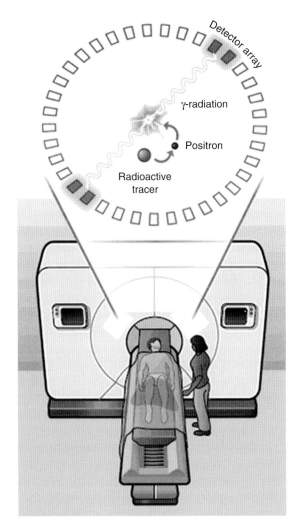

**Figure 15.7** PET camera detector array and diagram of annihilation event after positron emission (top). (Image courtesy of Jiang Long & Science Creative Quarterly.)

is not faultless and some errors do occur, especially at high count rates (when very high levels of emissions are being detected). Some errors occur that can contribute to noise and background, appearing in the image.

## PET radiopharmaceuticals

PET radionuclides are produced within a cyclotron. When incorporated into a radiopharma-

ceutical, they generally resemble substances naturally taken up by the human body and as such are considered metabolically active or biologically useful tracers. This makes them useful for accurately showing natural biodistribution within the body. They are usually short-lived radionuclides (short physical half-lives) ranging from seconds to minutes. As a result of this, departments need to be close to the supplying cyclotron, or use a suitable generator that is stored in the department.

When first developed, it was believed that PET imaging's main use would be in studying cardiology and neurology, with a small role in oncology. With the development of effective radiopharmaceuticals, this has shifted the focus towards oncology so that currently 85–90% of the disease processes studied with PET are oncology based. PET is a functional imaging modality and as such the information that it provides complements that provided from structural imaging approaches such as CT and MRI. As a result, one of its many roles is in distinguishing scarred or necrosed tissue from viable tumour in follow-up studies post-treatment.

## PET/CT

Just as SPECT/CT cameras were developed, PET/CT cameras have also evolved. This has provided similar benefits for PET studies as for SPECT studies (attenuation correction, co-registration). This development has been so significant for PET imaging and considered so useful that PET cameras are now produced only as hybrid PET/CT machines. As with SPECT/CT, the CT component has increasingly become diagnostic. This has led to a role in radiotherapy planning and is especially useful in cases where a tumour is poorly defined. This also has the potential to combine what once may have been separate appointments for PET, CT and planning into a single appointment, and therefore has great potential to speed up the process between diagnosis and treatment.

The role of PET imaging is continually increasing. Several new radiopharmaceuticals are being researched and both hardware and software are being developed to improve image quality and accuracy. PET/MRI is also attracting a growing amount of interest and a prototype PET/MRI machine has already been built.

## Tumour imaging and therapy

A considerable part of nuclear medicine is the study of oncology and radionuclide therapy. Several radiopharmaceuticals are used for this purpose. The most recent developments have involved the use of receptor and antibody imaging.

### Radiolabelled receptors

A receptor is a molecule of integral protein in the cell membrane that can identify and attach to a specific molecule, such as a hormone or neurotransmitter, that has some function of that cell. A molecule that specifically binds to a receptor in this way is called a *ligand* for that receptor. When a receptor and ligand interact they can either inhibit or stimulate cell function. Hormone-dependent tumours have receptor sites typical of the tissue from which the tumour arose and sometimes to a greater degree than the normal tissue.

The ligand, or a biological analogue that does not cause cell activity, may be included in the molecule of the radiopharmaceutical. The radionuclide labelling the ligand has to have a half-life suitable for the accumulation and clearance rates of the individual ligand on the receptors. When injected into a patient the ligands will attach to the receptors and the distribution of radioactivity follows that of the receptor density. Increased density implies the presence of tumour tissue. The same technique can potentially be used with suitable radionuclides to target and destroy tumour cells.

One example of receptor imaging is the study of neuorendocrine tumours. Potentially three different radiopharmaceuticals may be used for this purpose: $^{111}$In-labelled octreotide, $^{123}$I-labelled mIBG (*meta*-iodobenzylguanidine) and $^{99m}$Tc-labelled depreotide. Neuroendocrine tumours vary in the type of receptors present in their cells and therefore the degree of uptake of each of these radiopharmaceuticals will vary. Two patients with the same type of neuroendocrine tumour may show different biodistribution for each of these radiopharmaceuticals. By replacing the radionuclide attached to each pharmaceutical with beta-emitting radionuclides, these radiopharmaceuticals can then also be used for therapeutic purposes; the avidity of the tumour for each radiopharmaceutical will help determine which radionuclide therapy treatment to administer. If different radiopharmaceuticals demonstrate different tumour biodistribution in the same patient, the patient may receive two different radionuclide treatment types. This is more common with octreotide- and mIBG-avid tumours.

Repeat treatments can also be administered if needed. This is especially important for tumour location or spread that cannot be dealt with surgically or by other means, particularly for those patients with widespread metastases.

### Radiolabelled antibodies

A similar methodology uses the body's own immune system. An antibody is a protein produced by the lymphocytes in response to the presence of a foreign substance or antigen. Many antibodies may be produced in response to one antigen but each lymphocyte produces a single type of antibody. Antigens may be expressed on the walls of tumour cells, and may be tumour specific or (more usually) typical of the tissue from which the tumour arose. When antibodies that attach to these antigens are radiolabelled and injected into a patient, their accumulation can be imaged. When labelled with a beta-emitting radionuclide, the use of radionuclide therapy also becomes possible.

Monoclonal antibodies are produced by the hybridoma technique and are usually murine (mouse) derived. A mouse is injected with the relevant antigen for the tumour being sought. Specific B lymphocytes are then taken from the animal's spleen or lymphoid tissue, and manipulated, isolated and radiolabelled. Hundreds of different antibodies have been produced in this way and are identified by letters and numbers, but not all are suitable for radiolabelling. Antibody fragments and subfragments, as well as full antibodies, are used for radiolabelling. These may be labelled with $^{99m}$Tc and $^{111}$In (which has a longer half-life of 2.8 days, and thus enables imaging over longer periods of time to allow the antibodies to accrue onto the tumour) and for therapeutic purposes, $^{131}$I (iodine: half-life 8.1 days) and yttrium-90 ($^{90}$Y). When used as a therapy agent, this approach is known as radio-immunotherapy. Current research is also looking at the possibility of radiolabelling antibodies with alpha particle-emitting radionuclides as therapy agents.[1]

Zevalin is one example of a monoclonal antibody that has been developed specifically to treat refractory B-cell non-Hodgkin's lymphoma. Zevalin is taken up at the CD20 receptor of normal and cancerous lymph cells. When labelled with $^{111}$In, a diagnostic image can be acquired showing biodistribution of the radiopharmaceutical. For therapeutic purposes, Zevalin may be labelled with $^{90}$Y. As $^{90}$Y is a pure beta emitter and excretion rates of this radiopharmaceutical are low, these patients are often treated on an outpatient basis. It is administered together with the drug rituximab to increase its efficacy. Unfortunately, the relatively high cost of this treatment has meant that it is currently underused, despite the fact that very good partial and complete response rates show it is an effective tool in fighting this disease.

Another, lesser-used approach is to administer a radiolabelled antibody before sending the patient for surgery to remove the tumour. A small probe detector system can be used to identify affected lymph nodes during the operation. By monitoring, but not imaging, radiation the surgeon can check directly if all tumour tissue has been removed from the area and adjacent nodes.

## Radiation protection considerations for radioactive substances

There are several pieces of legislation that govern the use of radioactive substances in the nuclear medicine environment. These acts are usually country specific. Most of what is covered in this section deals with acts published in the UK.

Administration of radioactive substances to patients requires legislation both for their protection and for the protection of the staff involved. Personnel have to be identified for the work. Under the Medicines (Administration of Radioactive Substances) Regulations 1978,[2] radiopharmaceuticals can only be administered by a doctor or dentist holding a Certificate from the Administration of Radioactive Substances Advisory Committee (ARSAC)[3] or people acting under their directions. These certificates are site specific and stipulate the range of work that can be carried out in a nuclear medicine department (including diagnostic, therapeutic and research applications). Storage and disposal of radioactive substances used in nuclear medicine departments are governed by the Radioactive Substances Act 1993. Other pieces of legislation include the Ionising Radiation (Medical Exposure) Regulations 2000[4] and the Ionising Radiation Regulations 1999.[5]

Potential radiation hazards can arise from the process of administering radioactive substances to patients, from the radiation emitted from these patients after administration and from their radioactive excreta. First, during administration there are risks of spillage of activity that can be minimised by the use of trays and absorbent materials wherever activity in syringes or drinks is handled. For intravenous administrations, lead or tungsten syringe shields are used to reduce the dose to the fingers of the person giving the injection, and protective clothing and gloves should always be worn. For oral administrations, capsules of $^{131}$I as NaI minimise the risk of spillage. There are various devices with which drinks or capsules can be administered to patients that maximise the shielding, and by remote handling of the active material also maximise distance.

**Radioactive patients**

Diagnostic levels of radionuclide do not require patients to be kept in isolation and the level of activity that they emit does not make them a 'mobile-controlled area', which would necessitate restricting contact with members of the public. Nevertheless, keeping the dose to the public *as low as reasonably practicable* (the ALARP principle) is in accordance with the regulations. Active patients should be advised to avoid close contact with small children (unless necessary for the child's wellbeing) and with pregnant women.

If a patient is an inpatient, ward staff must be informed of their radioactive condition and then they too will (hopefully) follow the prescribed protocols drawn up by the radiation protection adviser (RPA) to the nuclear medicine department. Generally, these patients' urine will be radioactive for a few hours. They can flush the toilet twice after use for a day but this is only really a problem with incontinent individuals (which includes small children). Care has to be taken by the person dealing with wet nappies – gloves and aprons should be worn. The waste should be stored away from busy areas before disposal. Saliva and vomit may also be slightly radioactive and need care in disposal. Patients should be advised not to breastfeed for a period dependent on the radiopharmaceutical used.

More research is needed as to the levels of radiation dose received by members of the public coming into contact with radioactive patients outside the hospital. Investigations have shown that presumed average times spent in contact with 'the public' are not always true and advice may be needed to minimise the time.

**High-activity patients**

The category *high activity* relates to patients containing quantities of radionuclide that have an activity × energy product >150 MBq MeV. For $^{131}$I, this is >400 MBq (a therapeutic dose).[6] These patients have a sufficiently high surface dose for their immediate surroundings to constitute a controlled area and are therefore treated as inpatients where they can be observed in a suitable environment. Systems are therefore necessary for their management. The guidance notes state that such a system should address the following points:

- Patient rooms: these should be specially designated and preferably single.
- Patient movements: these must be confined to the room/suite and rooms should be left only with permission from the RPA and with a suitably knowledgeable expert.
- Beds: these should be marked with radiation warning signs.
- Walls and floors: these must be easily cleaned.
- Bathroom and toilet: these should be exclusive or the patient should have exclusive use of bottles or bedpans. Disposable items are preferable.
- Crockery and cutlery: these should be separated from other utensils and the patient should wash these up if disposable items are not available.
- Waste and soiled linen storage: these should be segregated in little used areas.
- Contaminated bedding or personal clothing: these should be changed as soon as possible and the affected bedding/clothing segregated in little used areas.
- Protective clothing: staff should use gloves and aprons at all times.

**Table 15.1**  Restrictions on high-activity patients leaving hospital by category

| Category | Activity (MBq MeV) | Restrictions |
|---|---|---|
| 1 | <10 | Safe to leave hospital<br>No restrictions |
| 2 | 10–50 | Avoid prolonged contact with children and radiosensitive work |
| 3 | 50–150 | Do not return to work if close contact is involved<br>Avoid close contact generally, e.g. places of entertainment |
| 4 | 150–300 | Do not return to work<br>Do not use public transport |
| 5 | >300 | Cannot leave hospital |

- Contact time for nursing staff and visitors: this varies with radionuclide and activity and is determined individually by radiation protection staff. *It should, in any case, be the minimum consistent with proper nursing care.* Non-urgent nursing procedures should be postponed until the levels drop.
- Pregnant staff: should be allocated other duties wherever possible.

When patients travel home or move between hospitals, rules still apply. If they are transferred, information on levels of activity must go with them. There are four categories of activity levels that determine the allowable means of transport and restrictions on their activities (Table 15.1).[6]

An instruction card stating restrictions and the times for which they apply have to be issued where indicated. The times are calculated to reflect the time for the predicted level of activity in the body to decay to the next category down.

There are also procedures for patients dying with high levels of radioactivity in them in order to protect the public. (Further guidance in this area can be found in the *Medical and Dental Guidance Notes*.[7])

# Radiopharmaceutical dosimetry

Before giving radiopharmaceuticals to patients an idea of the radiation dose imposed is necessary. Radiation doses from internally administered radionuclides cannot be measured as such and have to be calculated. This is longwinded and involves many approximations. It is, however, based on relatively simple concepts. The factors involved are the half-life and characteristic energies of the nuclide used, the amount of activity administered, the rate of uptake and excretion from the body, the proportion of energy absorbed in each organ and the mass of the organ.

The equation for the absorbed dose to a target organ from an administered radionuclide looks complicated. Most commonly used is the American medical internal radiation dosimetry (MIRD) system, which still uses non-SI radiation units; there are different approaches to converting these for use in the formula. This can be done by expressing administered activity in microcuries ($1\,\mu Ci = 37\,kBq$) and converting the results from rads into grays, which is not arduous as 100 rads = 1 Gy.

The full equation is:

$$D_{(rt-rs)} = A \times t_{1/2} \times 1.44 \times \sum_i \Delta_i \varphi_{i(rt-rs)} / m_t$$

where $D_{(rt-rs)}$ is the dose from the *source* organ, i.e. the organ containing an amount of radionuclide, to the *target* organ (the organ for which the dose needs to be measured). Of course these may be the same organ but the same equation applies. $A$ is the amount of radioactivity resident in the organ and is determined from biodistribution measurements. It is the product of the *administered activity* (in microcuries) and the percentage uptake in that organ. When the amount of activity in an organ is decreasing by both radioactive decay and exponential clearance by the body, the combined rate of decrease is also exponential: $t_{1/2eff}$ is the *effective half-life*. This can be calculated from the formula:

$$\left[1/t_{1/2physical}\right] + \left[1/t_{1/2biological}\right] = \left[1/t_{1/2eff}\right]$$

$t_{1/2eff} \times 1.44$ is the *effective mean life*, which corresponds to the time that the activity would exist in the organ if it decayed at a constant rate over a period of time and then disappeared all at once, rather than reducing exponentially over the whole time period. This value can be proved mathematically and is expressed in hours.

$\tilde{A}$ is used for the product $A \times 1.44 \times t_{1/2eff}$ and is called the *cumulated activity*. This represents the total number of nuclear disintegrations occurring during the time that the radionuclide is in the organ under consideration and thus depositing their energy in it. The units can be seen to be $\mu Ci^{-1}$. This assumes instant uptake of the nuclide into the source organ, which is not always true but will give the highest dose value for that administration.

Therefore the equation simplifies to:

$$D_{(rt-rs)} = \tilde{A} \times \sum_i \Delta_i \varphi_{i(rt-rs)} / m_t$$

$\Delta$ is the *equilibrium absorbed dose constant* or the energy emitted per unit of activity. It must be calculated for each type of radioactive emission from the radionuclide because each will deposit different amounts of energy.

For each emission i, where $N_i$ is the relative frequency of each emission (number emitted per disintegration) and $E_i$ is the average energy:

$$\sum \Delta = \sum 2.13 N_i E_i \left(rads \, \mu Ci^{-1} h^{-1}\right)$$

Thus, $\Delta_i$ for all emissions has to be calculated and summed to produce a total $\Delta$. $\varphi$ is the *absorbed fraction* or the proportion of the energy from any emission which (1) is absorbed in the organ itself or (2) reaches and is absorbed in adjacent organs, e.g. bladder to gonads. The geometry and proximity of organs to each other has to be taken into account. If the energy of the photon is <10 keV, then all the energy is absorbed in the *source* organ, i.e. $\varphi = 1$ for the source organ and $\varphi = 0$ for all *target* organs, but for penetrating radiation, which is used in diagnosis, organ-to-organ doses need to be considered. A 'standard man' phantom has been constructed and successively modified to measure these absorbed fractions; $m_t$ is the mass of the organ concerned. Values are given per gram of source organ.

The value of $\Sigma_i \Delta_i \varphi_{i(rt-rs)}/m_t$ for all organ pairs has been computed for many nuclides and is published as mean dose per cumulated activity or '$S$'$_{(rt-rs)}$ values. These are published in tables and are in units of rads $\mu Ci^{-1} h^{-1}$.

Ultimately, therefore the equation simplifies dramatically to:

$$D_{(rt-rs)} = A \times S_{(rt-rs)}$$

## Self-test questions

### Multiple choice questions

1. Which of the following increase the rate of radioactive decay?
   (a) heat
   (b) magnetism
   (c) electricity
   (d) none of the above.

2. A becquerel (Bq) is a unit of measurement used in nuclear medicine. If 1 Bq equals one radioactive disintegration per second, how many disintegrations per second are in 1 megabequerel (MBq)?
   (a) 10
   (b) 1000
   (c) 1000 000
   (d) 1000 000 000.

3. The crystal contained within a nuclear medicine gamma camera is made of sodium iodide (NaI) and small amounts of which element?
   (a) thallium
   (b) lead
   (c) Perspex
   (d) neon.

4. What part of the gamma camera converts light signals into electrical signals?
   (a) sodium iodide (NaI) crystal
   (b) pulse height analyser
   (c) pre-amplifier
   (d) photomultiplier tube.

5. The crystal found in a gamma camera is said to be 'hygroscopic'. What does this mean?
   (a) It will easily absorb moisture from the surrounding air
   (b) It will easily absorb noise from surrounding sources
   (c) It will absorb light from surrounding sources
   (d) It is sensitive to temperature changes.

6. SPECT studies are used often in nuclear medicine. What does SPECT stand for?
   (a) single photon electric computed tomography
   (b) single photon emission computed tomography
   (c) separate photon emission computed tomography
   (d) single photon emission calculated tomography.

7. What benefit does SPECT imaging have over planar imaging for imaging?
   (a) SPECT provides better system spatial resolution
   (b) SPECT provides higher sensitivity of the gamma camera
   (c) SPECT allows for depth of organs to be taken into account
   (d) SPECT does not provide any benefits compared to planar imaging.

8. What advantage/s do multi-modality PET/CT systems have over single PET cameras?
   (a) PET/CT provides anatomical location
   (b) PET/CT incorporates attenuation correction
   (c) both of the above
   (d) None of the above.

9. A vial of $^{99m}$TcMDP is measured at 9am and contains 20 GBq of activity. If no doses are withdrawn from the vial, what will be the activity in the vial at 9pm?
   (a) 15 GBq
   (b) 10 GBq
   (c) 5 GBq
   (d) 2.5 GBq.

10. Patients undergoing radioactive Zevalin therapy are given what non-radioactive drug in conjunction with the therapy?
    (a) MIBG
    (b) aminophylline
    (c) Herceptin
    (d) rituximab.

### Definitions

Define the following terms:

11. Radioactive physical half-life

12. Metastable

13. Radiopharmacy

14. Gamma camera dead-time.

### Short answer questions

The next three questions relates to the following equation:

$$A = A_0 e^{-\lambda t}$$

15. What does 'A' represent?

16. What does '$A_0$' represent?

17. What does '$\lambda$' represent?

18. A radiopharmacist enters the radiopharmacy on a Thursday afternoon. The department has run out of $^{99m}$Tc, so the generator is to be re-eluted. What three (3) factors will determine how much $^{99m}$Tc will be present in the elution?

19. One type of hybrid imaging combines a PET camera with a CT machine for patient studies. What benefit does the CT component add to the PET study?

**Long answer**

20. The nuclear medicine gamma camera is made up of several components.

Table 15.2 lists each component. Complete the table by filling in the 'Role' section.

**Table 15.2**  Long answer

| Component | Role |
|---|---|
| Lead cover | |
| Collimator | |
| Scintillation crystal | |
| Optical coupling | |
| Photomultiplier tube (PMT) | |
| Preamplifiers | |
| Pulse height analyser (PHA) | |

# References

1. Goldberg DM. Targeted therapy of cancer with radiolabeled antibodies. *J Nucl Med* 2002; **43**: 693–713.
2. Her Majesty's Stationery Office. *The Medicines (Administration of Radioactive Substances) Regulations*. London: HMSO, 1978.
3. Her Majesty's Stationery Office. *Administration of Radioactive Substances Advisory Committee*. London: HMSO, 2006.
4. Her Majesty's Stationery Office. *Ionising Radiation (Medical Exposure) Regulations 2000*. London: HMSO, 2000.
5. Her Majesty's Stationery Office. *Ionising Radiation Regulations 1999*. London: HMSO, 2000.
6. Her Majesty's Stationery Office. *Guidance Notes for the Protection of Persons against Ionising Radiations Arising from Medical and Dental Use*. London: HMSO, 1988.
7. Institute of Physics and Engineering in Medicine. *Medical and Dental Guidance Notes*. York: Institute of Physics and Engineering in Medicine, 2002.

# Further reading

Christian PE, Bernier DR, Langan JK. *Nuclear Medicine and PET: Technology and techniques*, 5th edn. St Louis, MO: Mosby, 2003

Hamilton D. *Diagnostic Nuclear Medicine: A physics perspective*. Berlin: Springer, 2004.
Mettler FA, Guilberteau MJ. *Essentials of Nuclear Medicine Imaging*, 5th edn. Philadelphia, PA: Saunders/Elsevier, 2006.
Medical Internal Radiations Committee. Various pamphlets dealing with all aspects of radiation dosimetry. Society of Nuclear Medicine.
Powsner RA, Powsner ER. *Essential Nuclear Medicine Physics*. Oxford: Blackwell, 2006.
Saha GB. *Basics of PET Imaging: Physics, chemistry and regulations*. New York: Springer-Verlag, 2005.
Saha GB. *Physics and Radiobiology of Nuclear Medicine*, 3rd edn. New York: Springer-Verlag, 2006.
Sharp PF, Gemmell HG, Murray AD. *Practical Nuclear Medicine*, 3rd edn. London: Springer, 2005.
Wheldon TE. Radionuclide therapy of cancer: Particle range and therapeutic effectiveness. *Nuclear Med Commun* 1993; **14**: 409–10.
Workman RB, Coleman RE, eds. *PET/CT: Essentials for clinical practice*. New York: Springer-Verlag, 2006.

# Journals

*Nuclear Medicine Communications* (published by the British Nuclear Medicine Society)
*The Journal of Nuclear Medicine* (published by the Society of Nuclear Medicine)

*Journal of Nuclear Medicine Technology* (published by the Society of Nuclear Medicine)

*European Journal of Nuclear Medicine* (published by the European Association of Nuclear Medicine)

## Internet

A range of websites is available, including sites from various nuclear medicine communities.

www.bnms.org.uk (British Nuclear Medicine Society)

www.snm.org (Society of Nuclear Medicine)

www.eanm.org (European Association of Nuclear Medicine)

www.ipem.ac.uk (Institute of Physics and Engineering in Medicine)

www.sor.org (Society of Radiography, UK based)

# Chapter 16

# SEALED SOURCES IN RADIOTHERAPY

Tony Flynn and Bruce Thomadsen

## Aims and objectives

At the end of this chapter the reader should have:
- developed an understanding of the principles of the use of sealed radioactive sources used in medicine
- gained knowledge and understanding of the equipment used in afterloading techniques
- developed an understanding of the safety issues involved in brachytherapy procedures.

## Introduction

With the continual development of modern afterloading systems and the increasing importance of accurate localisation of sealed sources for dosimetry purposes, the radiographer is becoming increasingly involved in the delivery of brachytherapy. This chapter reviews aspects of the use of sealed sources in brachytherapy, particularly with regard to remote afterloading, and looks at some of the treatment delivery systems currently available, together with associated quality assurance procedures and safety issues. The use of manually inserted sources and manual afterloading techniques (e.g. traditional 'Manchester' gynaecological insertions, temporary low-dose rate iridium implants or permanent implants) are not covered, because radiographers are not usually involved with such techniques except, perhaps, in their localisation after insertion, and readers with an interest in these methods are referred to elsewhere.[1-4] Thomadsen et al.[5] provide a good overview of brachytherapy physics, and Thomadsen[6] and Kubo et al.[7] a comprehensive discussion of brachytherapy quality management.

It will be appreciated that this account of remote, or machine, afterloading is not exhaustive; rather it provides an indication of the types of technique and equipment that are available. It will be seen that some equipment and techniques have been designed to be site specific whereas others are more flexible in the way that they can be adapted for use in several body sites, and the technical and financial considerations of whether a particular afterloading machine or method is suitable in a particular institution depends, in part, on the anticipated number of applications and the case mix.

This chapter inevitably has to refer to trade names of sources and equipment, and also to the names of equipment suppliers. This should not be taken to imply any recommendation of the products of any individual company, but is done in the interest of clarity and brevity, because it is difficult to describe some of the techniques and equipment in purely generic terms. The reader will appreciate that machines that are similar (but not identical) in their mode of operation are available from various manufacturers and suppliers, e.g. the microSelectron-HDR (supplied by

Nucletron) and the Varisource (supplied by Varian). Reference to a particular brand name does not necessarily mean that there is no alternative to this equipment. It is the responsibility of the prospective purchaser to decide which particular machine is best suited to his or her purpose bearing in mind the cost, safety aspects, suitability of operating procedures, supplier's service record and all other appropriate considerations.

A good discussion of remote afterloading safety and quality assurance may be found in the American Association of Physicists in Medicine (AAPM) Report No 61.[7]

## Why use afterloading?

Most brachytherapy in the period before the 1960s entailed inserting a radioactive source directly into the patient, exposing all the operating room staff, radiographers and transport personnel to radiation from the sources, and particularly giving high doses of radiation to the hands of the radiation oncologist performing the insertion. In the early days of manual brachytherapy, from the 1930s to the early 1960s, large implants were performed using many radium needles which were inserted manually in the operating theatre, with the consequent radiation exposure of the clinicians and other staff, and there are both documented and anecdotal reports of radiation injury to the fingers of clinicians. In afterloading, the radiation oncologist inserts empty applicators into the patient, and only after the localisation procedures, inserting non-active 'dummy' markers into the applicator, and settling the patient into the room are the sources inserted into the applicators. This process is quick and exposures to people involved are low. The exposures to staff in the operating room, during localisation and in transport are eliminated. The afterloading of a radioactive source into carrier tubing is not a new technique: there is a report of it being performed in the USA in 1905, and later manual afterloading of radium into gynaecological applicators was performed by Suit et al.[8] Performing the localisation before insertion of the radioactive material allows repositioning of the applicator without exposure to the staff or a period of less than adequate dose delivery to the patient.

However, with manual afterloading the radiation protection advantage is gained only in the early part of the procedure and, eventually, the radioactive sources have to be inserted into the applicators by the operator and the patient has to be cared for by nursing and clinical staff, with radioactive sources in position, for the duration of the treatment. The use of remote afterloading further reduces the potential radiation hazard in that the sources are placed in the needles or applicators by the afterloading machine, thereby reducing the manipulation of radioactive sources by staff. In addition, the sources are transferred from the safe in the machine to the patient only when no staff are in the room, thereby extending the protection advantage to nursing and other clinical staff. Table 16.1 summarises the relative

**Table 16.1** Radiation protection advantages of afterloading

| Advantage to | Non-afterloaded (handling live sources) | Manual afterloading | Remote afterloading |
|---|---|---|---|
| Theatre staff | No | Yes | Yes |
| Medical staff | No | Yes | Yes |
| Radiographer | No | Yes | Yes |
| Technician | No | No | Yes |
| Nursing staff | No | No | Yes |

advantages of the different types of afterloading with regard to radiation protection.

Some modern treatment techniques would not be possible without the use of remote afterloading. For example, high-dose rate (HDR) and pulsed-dose rate (PDR) brachytherapy would be impossible (or at least highly inconvenient) without the use of afterloading machines. Also, 'optimised' brachytherapy using stepping or oscillating source positions are dependant on the availability of computer-controlled, accurate source positioning, which would not be possible without manual techniques.

## Brachytherapy dose rate

The effectiveness of radiation to produce an effect on tissue depends, among other things, on that type of tissue and the rate at which the dose is administered. A search of the literature reveals no general agreement about the boundaries of low, medium and high dose rates or even how the relevant dose rates are defined in relation to the treated volume. The International Commission for Radiological Units (ICRU)[9] and the American Association of Physicists in Medicine (AAPM)[10] both base their definitions on the dose rate at the prescription point or prescription isodose, but this varies depending on the dosimetry system being followed. The ICRU recognises three categories (Table 16.2), and the authors of ICRU 38[9] acknowledge that these definitions are debatable. On the other hand, the AAPM defines low-dose rate (LDR) saying 'conventional doses of about 10 Gy are delivered daily', which implies a prescription dose rate of about 0.5 Gy/h. The

**Table 16.2** ICRU 38 definitions of LDR, MDR and HDR

| Low dose rate (LDR) | 0.4–2 Gy/h |
|---|---|
| Medium dose rate (MDR) | 2–12 Gy/h |
| High dose rate (HDR) | >0.2 Gy/min (i.e. 12 Gy/h) |

AAPM HDR category is defined as having a prescription dose rate >0.2 Gy/min, which is the same as the ICRU definition of HDR. Medium-dose rate (MDR) is defined as being 'between LDR and HDR', but the boundary between LDR and MDR is not defined in the AAPM document.

Another set of definitions arises from radiation protection documentation, where the interest is the environmental levels of radiation around equipment rather than the clinical dose rates, e.g. the *Guidance Notes for the United Kingdom's Ionising Radiations Regulations 1985*[11] defines equipment giving a dose rate of <10 mGy/h at 1 m as LDR; radiation levels greater than this are HDR. This boundary corresponds approximately to a dose rate at point A of 0.4 Gy/min, which is not the same as the ICRU and AAPM boundary. An MDR category is not defined by this authority.

Biologically, HDR treatment is characterised by the absence of cellular repair of sublethal damage during the delivery of the radiation. External-beam treatments fall into HDR radiotherapy by this definition, and most treatments where the duration is less than about 30 min. On the other hand, for LDR treatments, the effect of repair remains constant until about 1 Gy/h when the rate of repair cannot keep pace with that at which the radiation damages cells. These distinctions may prove more useful than official definitions, even though they do not lend themselves as well to nice, clear tables. These differences in definition are somewhat academic in practice because HDR machines generally operate at dose rates well above these boundaries, typically at around 2 Gy/min, which is well within the HDR category as defined by all the aforementioned documents. Conventional LDR brachytherapy, at 0.5 Gy/h, falls clearly in the LDR region. The boundary between LDR and MDR is less well defined. In any event, the only safe practice when reporting radiotherapy is to state exactly the dose, dose rate and fractionation used, as recommended in the ICRU Report 38.[9]

It is interesting to note that the dose rate of about 1.5 Gy/h, which has been frequently used in cervical treatments with afterloaders since about 1980, biologically falls in the MDR range (although not by the definitions in Table 12.2) and it is generally accepted that radiobiological considerations require use of a dose-rate correction factor.

There is no formal definition of PDR brachytherapy. Although HDR brachytherapy has characteristics that make it desirable, the higher dose rates increase the sensitivity to radiation damage of normal tissues more than tumours. The principle of PDR is to replace continuous LDR (CLDR) brachytherapy by a series of 'pulses' of higher dose rate treatment. Brenner and Hall[12] and Fowler and Mount[13] have published in vitro studies of the radiobiology of these modalities, from which come recommendations that, in order to obtain an endpoint biologically equivalent to CLDR, the PDR treatment regimen should give the same overall dose in the same overall time as the CLDR, provided that the pulse interval is about 1 h, the length of each pulse should be not less than 10 min and each pulse should give a dose of about 0.5 Gy, i.e. a dose rate of not more than about 3 Gy/h within the pulse. Experience has shown PDR treatment to be equivalent to the LDR approach.[14-17] In addition to ameliorating the biological disadvantages of HDR brachytherapy, the main advantage of PDR is the improved ability to tailor the dose distribution to the needs of the patient compared with CLDR.

## Low-dose rate afterloaders

This section reviews some of the LDR afterloaders and their applications. Although not all the machines mentioned can still be purchased as new, the older equipment may still be in use in some hospitals.

### Curietron

The Curietron was designed and manufactured in France as one of the first remote afterloaders. The machine was designed for the treatment of the uterine cervix and in practice its use is limited to this site or others with relatively large access for an applicator. It uses pre-loaded flexible source trains, each train containing a series of caesium-137 sources and spacers in various configurations. The source arrangement in each train is determined by the requirements of the part of the applicator that it is intended to treat, i.e. the uterine canal or vaginal sources. The trains are mechanically coupled to drive motors, and up to four trains can be transferred to the applicators at the initiation of treatment in the current version of the device, three in the older models. The treatment exposure of each train is independently timed and the treatment can be readily interrupted to allow nursing care. The treatment unit contains a shielded safe to which the source trains are withdrawn during interruptions and at the end of treatment.

The capacity of the main treatment unit is limited to four source trains, so the Curietron also has a 'secondary' radiation sources safe, separate from the main treatment unit, which houses more source trains, thereby increasing the range of treatment dose distributions that may be obtained. When the applicators and treatment requirements for a particular application are known, the appropriate source trains are transferred to the main treatment unit, from where they are subsequently transferred to the applicators as described above.

The radioactive sources are caesium-137 pellets of physical length 5.2 mm and diameter 1.6 mm. Depending on the source strengths used, treatments with this device may be LDR or MDR brachytherapy. These sources are loaded into source holders, with spacers, to give a variety of active lengths. The use of this machine is described in the literature.[18]

### Selectron-LDR/MDR

This machine, manufactured by Nucletron BV (the Netherlands), became available in the late 1970s, and has been in extensive clinical use ever since, although recently it went out of production. There are reported to be over 100 installations around the world and there are many references in the literature relating to its clinical use. It was designed initially for the treatment of the uterine cervix[19] but it has also been used for intraluminal and surface applicator treatments.

The Selectron-LDR/MDR is available in either a three- or a six-channel version, so that one or two gynaecological treatments can be undertaken simultaneously, three channels being generally needed for each patient. The treatment dose rate generally falls into the MDR category; however, that depends on the actual activity of the sources.

Its principle of operation removes the restriction on number of active lengths in machines such as the Curietron. The Selectron allows the user the flexibility of constructing source trains as required for a particular insertion, at the time of programming the machine immediately before a treatment. To this end it contains up to 48 caesium-137 sources of external diameter 2.5 mm, together with a large number of inactive spacers, also of diameter 2.5 mm. The sources and spacers are initially stored in their respective compartments of the main safe. When a source train is programmed and composed by the user, the machine selects sources and spacers in the correct order, as required, and places them in a vertical column in the so-called 'intermediate safe'. This process is repeated for each channel until all the required channels have been composed. At this stage there are now up to six columns of sources and spacers in the intermediate safe. When all channels have been composed, and if the appropriate connections have been made between the machine and the applicator via flexible transfer tubes, the treatment may be initiated and the source trains are pneumatically driven through the transfer tubes into the applicators. The trains may be withdrawn into the intermediate safe when nurses enter the room to attend to the patient, under alarm conditions, and finally at the end of the treatment. Each channel may be independently timed.

Source activities between 20 mCi (740 MBq) and 40 mCi (1480 MBq) are available. Most users opt for the higher activity sources which typically give a dose rate to the Manchester Point A of about 1.5–1.7 Gy/h, putting it in the MDR category. The lower activity gives a Point A dose rate of about 0.8 Gy/h, which is in the LDR category, but is slightly higher than the traditional 'radium insertion' dose rate of about 0.5 Gy/h.

The gynaecological applicators for the Selectron are made of stainless steel tubing of external diameter 6 mm. They are available in various geometrical configurations following established 'systems' for the treatment of the uterine cervix, such as the Manchester set,[3] the Fletcher set (which incorporates shielding in the ovoids),[20,21] the Henschke set, and a Ring Applicator set in which the vaginal component is in the form of a ring of sources around the cervical os. There are also applicators for vaginal and endometrial treatments. The open ends of the applicators are mechanically coded to ensure that they connect to the correct transfer tubes.

The Selectron-LDR has also been used for the treatment of the oesophagus[22] and nasopharynx.[23]

## MicroSelectron-LDR

The microSelectron-LDR (Nucletron BV) is a LDR afterloading machine that can transfer simultaneously up to 18 radioactive line sources into treatment catheters. It is typically used for LDR implant or surface mould therapy. Either flexible catheters or rigid needles with an external diameter of 2 mm can be used for the implant in the patient. Flexible transfer tubes connect the catheters to the treatment unit. As with most other afterloaders, each catheter may be timed independently. The source drive mechanism is mechanical, each source train being attached to its own motor drive.

Originally, the microSelectron-LDR was used with iridium wires as the radioactive sources. These were made from the same type of iridium wire that is still is in common use in brachytherapy for non-remote afterloaded implants. This wire is supplied in coils containing 500 mm wire and is available in a variety of activities. For use in the microSelectron-HDR, the wires have to be cut to the required lengths and then attached to the drive cables, using a preparation station supplied with the machine. A range of lengths is made up to ensure that wires suitable for any proposed treatments are available.

The radiation safe of the microSelectron-LDR can store up to 18 wires, one in each channel. This is generally insufficient to cover all the combinations of lengths that may be required, so further sources are prepared and stored in a separate radiation safe, from where they can be transferred to the microSelectron-LDR itself when required, in a manner reminiscent of the Curietron. In this way an extra 45 wires can be made available. The main disadvantage of using iridium wires in the microSelectron-LDR is the relatively short half-life of iridium-192 (74 days), which means that a new set of sources has to be prepared every 6 weeks or so, in order to maintain clinically suitable treatment times. Also, individualised treatments, as is most common in modern brachytherapy, require separate sets of wires cut for each patient, and the wires have little likelihood of reuse. This disadvantage has been overcome by the introduction of miniature caesium-137 source trains. A disadvantage of both types of source, however, is that even with a full set of sources it is often difficult to ensure that the ideal lengths are available in sufficient numbers for each treatment. De Ru et al.[24] describes an example of the use of this system. This machine has now been largely superseded by HDR afterloaders and has been out of production for quite some time.

## Buchler system

This machine has been available in both LDR and HDR configurations, and in single- and three-channel versions, and is intended primarily for the treatment of the uterine cervix. It uses either caesium-137 or iridium-192 sources. Each channel is served by a single source, rather than a train of sources as used in the machines described above. All sources are attached to drive cables and are mechanically afterloaded. The central source of a three-channel unit (or the only source of a single-channel unit) is mechanically coupled to a drive system that moves the source in a controlled, predetermined, oscillating manner within its catheter, the range and pattern of the oscillation being used to generate the required dose distribution. The oscillating movement of this source is controlled by an eccentric cam within the drive system. The shape of the cam determines the position of the source at any instant. The main advantages of this system are its simplicity and reproducibility, it being necessary only to select and fit the appropriate cam corresponding to the dose distribution required. However, the cams have to be specially made (by the manufacturer) for each dose distribution required, so it is inflexible in use because changes in dose distribution cannot be implemented at short notice.

Typical source activities are 300 mCi (11.1 GBq) of caesium-137 for LDR use, but activities up to 4 Ci (148 GBq) of caesium-137 or 20 Ci (740 GBq) of iridium-192 have been used in HDR versions. This unit, also, has been out of production since the 1990s.

## High-dose rate afterloaders

HDR afterloading for both intracavitary and interstitial treatment is being used increasingly, leading to a relative reduction in the popularity of LDR techniques in recent years. HDR treatments have many advantages over LDR techniques. The first advantage is the delivery of treatments on an outpatient, or day-care, basis. The treatment proper usually takes less than 15 min, although if the procedure requires placement of an applicator and localisation, the whole procedure may require about 2 h. The short time of machine use increases the number of patients who can receive brachytherapy in a given week. In addition, in the case of uterine cervix treatments, the short treatment times allow rigid, fixed rectal retractors to be used, thereby reducing the rectal dose compared with LDR systems, and fixation of the applicator to the table minimises movement of the applicator in the patient between localisation and the completion of a treatment, neither of which would be acceptable with LDR. As the units use a single source (or possibly three sources) stepping through the applicator to deliver the dose, by adjusting the time the source stops along the path, very carefully tailored dose distributions can be created. However, these advantages are offset to some extent by the fact that, because of radiobiological considerations, the treatment has to be fractionated, so a patient will generally receive several of these albeit shorter treatments within a course of treatment. Also, there may be a clinical disadvantage in that a patient may need several anaesthetic episodes during the course of treatment, depending on the insertion or implantation procedure being performed. In addition, the treatment rooms required for HDR therapy equipment need to be shielded more substantially than for LDR equipment, due to the extra high source activities, making HDR installations generally more expensive.

Although this chapter does not intend to cover the clinical aspects of the provision of brachytherapy, it is important to be aware that the treatment regimens used in HDR brachytherapy are very different from those used for the equivalent LDR due to radiobiological considerations. In recent years much experience has been gained in the clinical applications of HDR brachytherapy and nowadays most new installations of afterloading equipment are of this type.

## Modern, stepping source units

Iridium-192 may be produced with a high specific activity. It is possible to manufacture iridium-192 sources that are physically small but that contain typically an activity of 10–20 Ci (370–740 GBq). This has led to the development of 'stepping source' treatment machines, in which a single iridium-192 source on the end of a computer-controlled cable sequentially moves through a series of dwell positions in each treatment applicator in turn. This technique avoids the need for several sources or source trains to be present in the machine because one source can simulate a series of sources effectively. Some units now use ytterbium-169 either instead of iridium-192 or as an option on a per-patient or per-catheter basis.

There are several machines of this type now available:

- The microSelectron-HDR (Nucletron BV)
- The Varisource (Varian, USA)
- The GammaMed (Varian)
- The Flexitron (Isodose Control BV, the Netherlands)
- Advanced Brachytherapy Services (USA).

Figure 16.1 shows a typical HDR unit.

After years of stability, the field recently has had new companies and many new products developed in a relatively short time. Although there are differences between the different systems, relating to source design, maximum catheter number and dimensions, number of dwell positions, detail of safety systems, etc., they are sufficiently similar to be dealt with generically here.

In parallel to the source, the machine also contains a 'check cable', which is essentially a dummy source on its own drive cable. The check cable is driven out through the transfer tubes and applicators before the source is transferred in order to check the correct connection of all the components and also for obstructions or tight curves. The check cable may also be used as a simulated source for radiography in some systems. The source and check cable are driven out and back, when appropriate, by stepper motors, with a positional accuracy of approximately ±1 mm. Such machines have the capacity to service a number of channels and applicators, e.g. up to 30 for the microSelectron-HDR, 24 for the Gammamed and 40 for the Flexitron. Within each channel the source is positioned sequentially in a number of dwell positions, e.g. up to 48 for the microSelectron-HDR and up to 40 for the Gammamed. The interval between the dwell

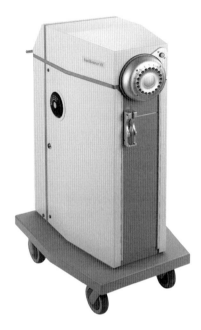

**Figure 16.1** The Nucletron microSelectron model V2: a typical HDR treatment unit. (Figure courtesy of Varian Brachy Therapy, Charlottesville, VA.)

positions may be fixed, e.g. 2.5 mm, 5 mm or 10 mm, or it may be variable and set by the planner for a given catheter, depending on the machine type.

The source diameter is small, typically about 1 mm or less, so the catheter lumen through which it travels can also be narrow; an external diameter of 1.3 mm (4 French gauge) or less is common. In addition, the length of travel of the source (and check cable) is long, from 1.5 m to 2 m depending on the machine. The combination of these two features makes this type of machine very adaptable, and it may be used for intraluminal, interstitial and intracavitary therapy. Each individual dwell time in each catheter may be different; this gives the user great flexibility to conform dose distributions to the target volume. However, it is emphasised that great care must be taken in the clinical situation if this flexibility is used to depart significantly from established dosimetry systems such as 'Manchester' and 'Paris', because the relationships between dose and volume irradiated will change. With older versions of these machines, data from the treatment planning computer has to be manually entered into the treatment unit; with multi-catheter treatments and many dwell positions per catheter this requires a large amount of data to be entered and is prone to human error. Current machines transfer the data via networks. Figure 16.2 shows a typical tandem and ovoid

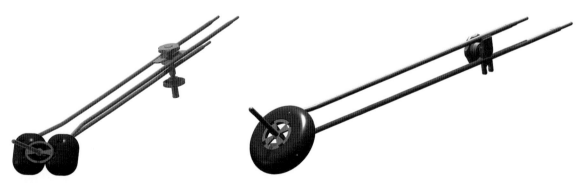

**Figure 16.2** A typical HDR tandem and ovoid (left) and the fixed geometry tandem and ring (right). (Courtesy of Nucletron International.)

set for an HDR unit (left) and a fixed geometry tandem and ring. The fixed geometry facilitates using a standard plan, reducing the planning time between applicator insertion and treatment.

Iridium-192 has a half-life of 74 days and source exchanges are required at (usually) 3-monthly intervals. The half-life of ytterbium-169 is only 32 days, so source exchanges may happen every month and a half.

### Pulsed-dose rate systems

At the time of writing the only PDR system generally available is the microSelectron-PDR (Nucletron BV), which is an adaptation of the microSelectron-HDR. It is similar in external appearance as are its mechanical and safety systems. However, there are two major differences. First, the radioactive source contains less radioactivity, typically having an activity of 0.5–1.0 Ci (37–18.5 GBq) of iridium-192. As a consequence, the source capsule is also physically smaller, having an active length of 0.5 mm and an overall length of 2.7 mm. Second, the operating software is different, allowing the source movement to be programmed for the pulsed nature of the treatment as described above.

### Safety issues in brachytherapy

As with any form of radiotherapy, safety is an important issue. It is particularly so in brachytherapy because the treatments and machine programming are complex and often done under the pressure of having to work quickly in an operating theatre environment. It is vitally important, therefore, that all staff groups are adequately trained and practised in the techniques, there are sufficient staff to allow appropriate checking of machine programming, etc., and procedures are standardised wherever possible. In addition, robust quality assurance procedures for the equipment need to be in place.

## Treatment protocols in brachytherapy

Brachytherapy facilities should have written procedures to cover the methods of treatment for the various conditions. The risk of an error occurring is much reduced when treatments are given according to a documented protocol whenever possible. Each treatment site and method of application should have its own protocol, which should include a description of localisation procedures on imaging equipment (including any radiographic markers, operating theatre procedure, treatment planning method, treatment delivery, and verification and recording procedures). The documentation should be clear and unambiguous. Care should be taken to ensure that the interface between the various personnel is clarified to avoid errors in the transmission of information from one person to another.

### Treatment prescription

The radiographer requires a signed instruction about the treatment to be given. This is the treatment prescription, which should be clear, complete and unambiguous, and specify exactly the treatment machine and technique to be used. Diagrams should be used routinely and particularly where this aids clarity. The type and size of applicators, radiation sources, prescribed radiation dose and dose location should be clearly indicated. The prescription should be clearly signed and dated by the prescribing clinician. Any additional information on the prescription sheet, e.g. treatment planning information (perhaps provided by a physicist) or calculations of the dwell or treatment times (perhaps performed by a radiographer), should be signed, and then checked and countersigned by a second suitably qualified person.

The treatment prescription sheet should provide unambiguous information relevant to the treatment, such as the treated region, left or right side, and any patient and applicator position information, e.g. the length of insertion and the treated active length should be described for intraluminal applicators, and gynaecological applicators should be described to permit reproducibility for fractionated treatments and to allow correct reconstruction for dosimetric purposes. The prescription sheet should also record the radiation dose given to critical organs, where appropriate.

One of the difficulties with HDR treatments is that there is often only a short period of time available between the insertion of the applicators and the start of the treatment fraction. This is, of course, desirable from a clinical point of view because the patient may be intubated and anaesthetised while awaiting the start of the treatment. However, it does mean that the treatment parameters have to be determined and entered into the treatment machine in a short space of time, with the staff working under considerable pressure. These are conditions in which errors are likely to occur. This task is made easier and safer if information on the current source strength, radioactive decay tables and treatment times are readily available in the treatment machine control area.

## Treatment planning

It is beyond the scope of this chapter to discuss treatment planning safety issues in any detail (see Chapter 10). However, it is worthwhile to note briefly three of the safety issues to be addressed in this component of the treatment process.

### Transfer of information
When not using a standard plan, the requirements of the plan (treatment volume, prescribed dose, critical organ constraints, dose fractionation, etc.) must be transmitted unambiguously to the planning staff. A convenient and safe way to do this is to make use of the prescription sheet. It is worthwhile spending time carefully designing prescription sheets for the various applications so that the appropriate information can be written easily and clearly. It is not enough to rely on information transmitted verbally; all relevant information should be in written form and its authorship should be clear.

### Physical data
The accuracy of the treatment plan depends on the quality and provenance of the physical data used for its production. It is important to ensure that the origins of the data for particular types of radiation source, individual sources and other physical parameters are properly researched, well documented and of proven accuracy. The origin of 'in-house' produced tables and graphs should be referenced and documented. Although in a busy department it is tempting to assume that the commercial software writers have got it right, it is, of course, ultimately the responsibility of the user to be certain that the algorithms operate correctly and that the values of the various physical constants and other parameters used by the software are correct and used appropriately.

### Checking computed treatment plans
Each computed treatment plan must be checked before being used for treatment. Preferably, a written checklist should be followed and a record of the checks filed. Where practicable, a quantitative check of some consistency index should be made, preferably by a second qualified person, independent of the original calculation.[6]

Quality assurance checks on the treatment planning system are beyond the scope of this chapter and readers are referred to the literature.[6,25]

## Transfer of information to the treatment unit

The completed treatment plan provides the information necessary for the correct treatment of the patient. With modern HDR systems, this may be either by a direct connection between the two components through a network or by the use of a diskette or program card. With older units, this information may be transcribed onto the prescription sheet from the treatment plan and from there into the treatment unit, increasing the risk of transcription errors, particularly for multi-catheter treatments. Alternatively, the planning computer printout may be attached to the prescription sheet, but in this case it must be clear that the computer printout refers to the correct patient, whose name and identification must be prominently displayed. When automated, the correct operation of the data transfer should be checked as part of the treatment planning and treatment unit quality assurance programs, and at each clinical use the data printout should be checked by an appropriate person. It is unwise to rely on the verbal transmission of data and all printouts and written information should be signed by the person from whom it originated.

## Treatment machine quality assurance in brachytherapy

Each treatment machine must have a fully documented quality assurance programme, which should consist of a series of specific tests, at defined repetition intervals with appropriate record keeping. Typically, checks of the machine operation and selected safety features are performed on a daily and 3-monthly basis. In most institutions this is set up by the physics department and physicists perform most of the checks. It is not appropriate here to define the details of these because they depend on the type of machine, local circumstances, frequency of use of the equipment, etc. However, it is useful (and reassuring) for the radiographer to be involved in performing the daily or pre-treatment checks, which should include, for example, a source position check, and a check on the normal operation of the machine.

### Self-test questions

1. Define the term 'afterloading'.
2. Define the terms 'HDR' and 'LDR'.
3. Name three types of radioactive sources used in afterloading procedures.
4. What is meant by the term 'source train'?
5. What is the ICRU?

## References

1. Pierquin B, Wilson JF, Chassagne D. *Modern Brachytherapy*. Paris: Masson, 1987.
2. Godden TJ. *Physical Aspects of Brachytherapy*. Bristol: Adam Hilger, 1988.
3. Tod M, Meredith WJ. Treatment of cancer of the cervix uteri – a revised 'Manchester method'. *Br J Radiol* 1953; **26**: 252.
4. Blasko JC, Ragde H, Schumacher D. Transperineal percutaneous iodine-125 implantation for prostatic carcinoma using trans-rectal ultrasound and template guidance. *Endocurietherapy/Hyperthermia Oncol* 1987; 3: 131–9.
5. Thomadsen B, Rivard M, Butler W. *Brachytherapy Physics*. Madison, WI: Medical Physics Publishing, 2005.
6. Thomadsen B. *Achieving Quality in Brachytherapy*. London: Taylor & Francis, 1999.
7. Kubo H, Glasgow G, Pethel T, Thomadsen B, Williamson J. *American Association of Physicists in Medicine Report 61*: High dose-rate brachytherapy treatment delivery. *Med Physics* 1998;**25**: 375–403.
8. Suit HD, Moore EB, Fletcher GH, Worsnop B. Modification of Fletcher ovoid system for afterloading using standard radium tubes. *Radiology* 1963; **81**: 126.
9. International Commission on Radiation Units and Measurements. *Dose and Volume Specification for Reporting Intracavitary Therapy in Gynaecology*. ICRU Report 38. Bethesda, MA: ICRU, 1985.
10. Glasgow GP, Bourland JD, Grigsby PW, Meli JA, Weaver KA. American Association of Physicists in Medicine. *Remote Afterloading Technology Report 41*. New York: American Institute of Physics, 1993.
11. National Radiological Protection Board. *Guidance Notes for the Protection of Persons against Ionising Radiations Arising from Medical and*

*Dental Use*. Didcot: National Radiological Protection Board, 1988.

12. Brenner DJ, Hall EJ. Conditions for the equivalence of continuous to pulsed low dose rate brachytherapy. *Int J Radiat Oncol Biol Phys* 1991; **20**: 181–90.

13. Fowler JF, Mount M. Pulsed brachytherapy: the conditions for no significant loss of therapeutic ratio compared with traditional low dose rate brachytherapy. *Int J Radiat Oncol Biol Phys* 1992; **23**: 661–9.

14. Mazeron JS, Boisserie G, Gokarn N, Bailiet F. Pulsed LDR brachytherapy: current clinical status. In: Mould RF, Batterman JJ, Martinez AA, Speiser BL (eds), *Brachytherapy from Radium to Optimisation*. Veenendaal, The Netherlands: Nucletron BV, 1994: 246–53.

15. Swift PS, Fu KK, Phillips TL, Roberts LW, Weaver KA. Pulsed low dose rate interstitial and intracavitary therapy. In: Mould RF, Batterman JJ, Martinez AA, Speiser BL (eds), *Brachytherapy from Radium to Optimisation*. Veenendaal, The Netherlands: Nucletron BV, 1994: 254–9.

16. Bachtiary B, Dewitt A, Pintilie M et al. Comparison of late toxicity between continuous low-dose-rate and pulsed-dose-rate brachytherapy in cervical cancer patients. *Int J Radiat Oncol Biol Phys*. 2005; **63**, 1077–82.

17. Harms W, Krempien R, Hensley FW, Berns C, Fritz P, Wannenmacher M. 5-year results of pulsed dose rate brachytherapy applied as a boost after breast-conserving therapy in patients at high risk for local recurrence from breast cancer. *Strahlenther Onkol* 2002; **178**: 607–14.

18. Jackson AW, Davies ML. Brachytherapy. In: Bleehan N, Glatseine E, Haybittle J (eds), *Radiation Treatment Planning*. New York: Marcel Dekker, 1983.

19. Wilkinson JM, Moore CJ, Notley HM, Hunter RD. The use of Selectron afterloading equipment to simulate and extend the Manchester system for intracavitary therapy of the cervix uteri. *Br J Radiol* 1983; **56**: 404–14.

20. Fletcher GH, Shalek RJ, Cole A, Cervical radium applicators with screening in the direction of bladder and rectum. *Radiology* 1953; **60**, 77.

21. Marbach JR, Stafford PM, Delclos L, Almond PR. A dosimetric comparison of the manually loaded and Selectron remotely loaded Fletcher–Suit–Delclos utero-vaginal applicators. In: Mould RF (ed.), *Brachytherapy 1984*. Veenendaal, The Netherlands: Nucletron BV, 1985: 255–65.

22. Rowland CG. Treatment of carcinoma of the oesophagus with a new Selectron applicator. In: Mould RF (ed.), *Brachytherapy 1984*. Veenendaal, The Netherlands: Nucletron BV, 1985: 235–54.

23. Flores A D. Remote afterloading intracavitary irradiation for cancer of the nasopharynx. In: Mould RF (ed.), *Brachytherapy 1984*. Veenendaal, The Netherlands: Nucletron BV, 1989: 404–11.

24. de Ru VJ, Hofman P, Struikmans H et al. Skin dose due to breast implantation for early breast cancer. In: Mould RF, Batterman, JJ, Martinez AA, Speiser BL (eds), *Brachytherapy from Radium to Optimisation*. Veenendaal, The Netherlands: Nucletron BV, 1994: 239–45

25. Institution of Physics and Engineering in Medicine and Biology. *A Guide to Commissioning and Quality Control of Treatment Planning Systems*. IPEMB Report No. 68. York: Institution of Physics and Engineering in Medicine and Biology, 1996.

# Appendix
# SELF-TEST ANSWERS

## Chapter 1

1. 1.80 Gy.
2. Three from:
   - they are composed of transverse electric and magnetic waves
   - they travel at the speed of light in a vacuum
   - in free space they travel in straight lines
   - in free space they obey the inverse square law.
3. When a magnet is moved through a coil of wire a current is induced in the coil. The opposite is also true: a current passing through a coil generates a magnetic field through the centre of the coil. This is known as electro-magnetic induction.
4. The wave- and particle-like properties of electromagnetic radiation can be related. From the wave-like properties, it is known that the wave can be described by the following relationship:

   If particle-like properties are considered, it can be shown that the energy carried by the particles or photons is given by:

   $$E = h\upsilon$$

5. Electron orbits also have an energy associated with them. This is known as the binding energy and is dependent on the force of attraction between the nucleus and the orbiting electrons. The binding energy associated with the K-shell is greater than for shells further away from the nucleus because the force of attraction on the K-shell electrons will be greater.

   It is the binding energy that must be overcome if an electron is to be removed from its shell. The potential energy associated with shells further from the nucleus will be greater than for those shells close to the nucleus, which is analogous to the greater potential energy associated with an object the further it is away from the earth.

## Chapter 2

1. (a) The cathode produces a focused beam of electrons. It is made up of two parts: the filament and the focusing cup. Electrons are released from the filament and this electron beam is shaped into a small area on the target by the focusing cup. The cathode is negatively charged.
   (b) The anode consists of two metal parts: a copper disc with the target embedded in it. The target is the area where the electron beam hits the anode and interacts. The target is usually made of tungsten

but can be other metals such as molybdenum or rubidium. The copper disc provides a support for the target and also dissipates heat away from the target during X-ray production.

The housing around the X-ray tube is surrounded in lead, to provide shielding from X-rays everywhere except the exit window. The housing protects the user from the high voltage within the tube, and is also used to support filters and beam modification devices.

2. Tungsten has:
   • a high melting point; both the anode and cathode are excessively heated and they need to be able to withstand very high temperatures
   • high thermal conductivity: this means that for the target any heat produced is quickly dissipated away to the copper anode; for the filament this means that it can heat and cool quickly, allowing it to be heated for thermionic emission without becoming damaged
   • a high atomic number: this is important during X-ray production because it increases the probability of an electron interacting. This in turn increases the probability of an X-ray being produced. The high atomic number means that the filament will have a long lifetime because it has a high number of electrons available for thermionic emission.

3. The actual focal spot size is the area of the target that interacts with the electron beam. This area is much larger than the area that the X-ray beam covers when it exits the tube window. This area is the effective focal spot size, and is smaller than the actual focal spot size due to the target being positioned at an angle.

4. A filament of tungsten is heated to a very high temperature. The energy supplied as heat to the tungsten atoms liberates electrons from the surface of the filament. This process is similar to boiling a liquid.

5. It is necessary to maintain the glass or metal envelope at vacuum pressure so that there are minimal molecules present between the cathode and the anode. This means that the electrons travelling from the cathode will not unnecessarily lose kinetic energy through collisions with air molecules.

6. Characteristic X-rays are produced when a projectile electron interacts with an orbital electron of a target atom. If the projectile electron imparts enough energy to eject the target electron and ionise the atom, a vacancy is left in this shell. An outer shell electron jumps to fill this vacancy, releasing the energy required as a characteristic X-ray. The energy of the X-ray produced is equal to the difference in binding energy between the two shells.

7. Bremsstrahlung X-rays are produced when a projectile electron interacts with the nucleus of the target atom. The electron slows down and changes direction, due to the influence of the electrostatic force of the target atom. The energy lost by the electron during this process is emitted as an X-ray. Bremsstrahlung X-rays can have a range of possible energies from $0\,kV$ to the kV setting of the X-ray tube.

8. X-ray tubes are thought of as inefficient because 95–99% of the energy of the electron beam is converted into heat, which is a non-useful by-product of the X-ray tube, and only 1–5% of interactions result in X-ray production. In order to dissipate this heat added energy is used by the X-ray tube system in powering a rotating anode.

9. The X-ray intensity is dependent on:
   • the mA of the X-ray tube, which is linearly proportional to the mA
   • the kV, which varies with $kV^2$
   • the distance from the tube; the intensity reduces with distance according to the inverse square law
   • filtration: adding any attenuating material into the path of the beam reduces the beam output intensity.

10. The quality of an X-ray spectrum is used to describe how well a polyenergetic beam penetrates a material. It describes the spectrum because high-energy X-rays are more penetrating than low-energy X-rays.

11. Beam quality is determined by measuring the half-value layer (HVL) of aluminium of the beam. The HVL is measured by placing a radiation detector into the useful beam, which has been collimated down to a small area. A reading is taken over a short time with nothing in the beam. A 1 mm sheet of Al foil is placed in the beam and another reading is taken. This is repeated adding a 1 mm Al foil for each reading. By plotting these readings on a graph the thickness of Al needed to reduce the intensity of the beam by half can be found. This thickness is the HVL of the tube.

12. The kV setting on a console control determines the amount of voltage across the X-ray tube. This in turn determines the amount of kinetic energy gained by the electrons emitted by the cathode. This energy determines the maximum amount of energy that a bremsstrahlung photon can have and the $kV_p$ of the output spectrum.

13. If the kV setting is increased the amount of kinetic energy of the electrons in the tube is increased. This causes an increase in the maximum amount of energy that a bremsstrahlung X-ray can have.

14. The mA setting on the console is related to the current passing through the cathode filament and this controls the number of electrons that are released by the cathode. The number of electrons released by the cathode determines the number of electrons that interact with the target and therefore the number of X-rays emitted by the tube.

15. If the mA is increased the number of electrons hitting the target is increased. This means that the number of X-rays produced (and the amount of heat produced) increases. The intensity of the beam increases.

16. (a) $I \propto kV_p^2$ therefore $I = c\,kV_p^2$ where $c$ is a constant
$$I_1 = c\,kV_{p1}^2 \text{ and } I_2 = c\,kV_{p2}^2$$
$$\frac{I_2}{kV_{p2}^2} = \frac{I_1}{kV_{p1}^2}$$
$$I_2 = \frac{I_1}{kV_{p1}^2}kV_{p2}^2$$
$$= I_1\left(\frac{kV_{p2}}{kV_{p1}}\right)^2$$
$$= 75 \times \left(\frac{100}{80}\right)^2$$
$$= 75 \times \left(\frac{5}{4}\right)^2$$
$$= 117.2\,\mu Gy$$

(b) $I \propto mA$ therefore $I = c\,mA$ where $c$ is a constant
$$I_1 = c\,mA_1 \text{ and } I_2 = c\,mA_2$$
$$\frac{I_2}{mA_2} = \frac{I_1}{mA_1}$$
$$I_2 = I_1\left(\frac{mA_2}{mA_1}\right)$$
$$= 75 \times \left(\frac{300}{500}\right)$$
$$= 75 \times \left(\frac{3}{5}\right)$$
$$= 45\,\mu Gy$$

17.

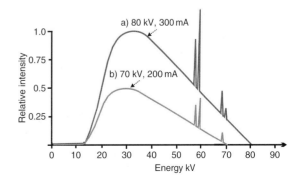

Reducing the kV of the tube reduces the maximum intensity to about three-quarters. If the mA is reduced by one-third, from 300 mA to 200 mA, this will not change the shape of the spectrum, but will reduce the intensity by one-third, from three-quarters to half of the original intensity.

18. Reducing the $kV_p$ from 80 kV to 70 kV reduces the intensity by a factor of $(70/80)^2$. Reducing the mA from 300 mA to 200 mA reduces the intensity by a factor of (200/300). Therefore an original intensity of 100 μGy will be reduced to:

$$100\,\mu Gy \times \left(\frac{70}{80}\right)^2 \times \left(\frac{200}{300}\right) = 57.4\,\mu Gy$$

19.

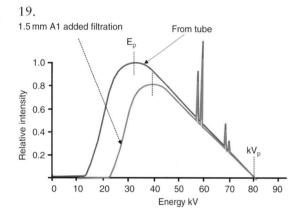

20. If there is no added shielding placed over the exit beam of an X-ray tube all of the low-energy X-rays are absorbed by the patient. These X-rays do not contribute to the image and result in an unnecessary dose being received by the patient.

**Chapter 3**

1. Gray.
2. Minute temperature changes in the irradiated medium.
3. Mass of the material concerned.
4. The secondary standard is the dosimeter used in clinical practice and is calibrated against the primary absolute standard dosimeter at NPL.
5. The term 'kerma' stands for kinetic energy released per unit mass.
6. Doping is a process whereby impurities are deliberately introduced into a semiconductor material to create excess positive holes or excess electrons in its structure.
7. Semiconductor, TLD.
8. Thimble chamber, semiconductors.
9. Compton effect, photoelectric effect, pair production.
10. Bremsstrahlung process.
11. Size, voltage and limited range of energies that it can measure in practice.
12. Thimble chamber or parallel plate.
13. Bragg cavity theory.
14. 5–50 MeV.
15. To directly compare the effects of the radiation dose in tissue.
16. Sensitive, accurate, robust, linear equivalent to dose, suitable physical size.
17. When the material is heated up the release of light photons from the electrons returning to the ground state is proportional to the amount of radiation absorbed.
18. Lithium fluoride.
19. Tissue equivalent properties, low fading, energy independent.

20.

| Advantages | Limitations and disadvantages |
|---|---|
| Re-usable | Precision can be affected by poor handling and storage |
| Automated read-out | Immediate read out is not possible |
| Energy independent over a wide range of the energies | 'Fading'– unintentional release of trapped electrons, may be caused by exposure to heat or light (particularly UV) |
| Similar atomic number to soft tissue (except those containing calcium) | Some types may liquefy if left in humid conditions |
| Capable of measuring over a wide range of doses | Scratches on the surface of the TLD or reduction in mass will affect the light emission characteristics |
| Small physical size | May become contaminated by grease or adhesives |

## Chapter 4

1. Intensity: rate of flow of photon energy through a unit area lying at right angles to the path of the beam.
2. Attenuation: reduction in intensity of the radiation beam that occurs when that beam of radiation travels through a medium.
3. Absorption: transference of energy from the photons to the atoms of the material as a beam of radiation passes through a medium and interacts with the atoms of that medium.
4. Scattering: deflection of photons from their original path as they pass through a medium and interact with the atoms of that medium.
5. Transmission X-rays contribute to the radiographic image and the exit dose of radiotherapy beams.
6. The intensity has been reduced to 12.5% of the original value.

7. (a) $m^{-1}$; (b) $m^2/kg$
8. HVL is related to the linear attenuation coefficient ($\mu$) by the equation $\mu = 0.693 \div HVL$.
9. Photoelectric absorption, Compton scatter and pair production.
10. Lower kV energies, i.e. between 120 and 500 keV.
11. Interaction between incoming photon and inner shell electron resulting in absorption of incoming photon and production of photoelectron and characteristic radiation.
12. Iodine: $Z = 53$; barium: $Z = 56$.
13. Proportional to $Z^3$.
14. At the surface of the attenuating material due to the backscatter produced.
15. Collision interaction between an incident photon and a free electron.
16. Not dependent on $Z$.
17. $E = mc^2$ where $m$ = mass, $E$ = energy and $c$ = velocity of light.
18. 1.022 MeV.
19. Interaction between incoming photon and electric field of nucleus resulting in production of negatron and position, followed by recombination of particles and release of annihilation radiation.
20. For example, lead, concrete.

## Chapter 5

1. The seven effects of X-rays: fluorescence, photographic, penetration, ionisation, excitation, chemical, biological.
2. No photons would reach the imaging device and all the energy would be absorbed by the patient, thus resulting in no image being created; therefore there would be no density differences to create a contrast between adjacent structures.
3. Three methods: cathode ray tube, liquid crystal and flat screen systems.
4. CT numbers/hounsfield units are a set of nominal values that represent different materials. They represent the attenuation of the beam that has occurred in a voxel. Water is

given an HU or CT number of 0 and the value for gas = −1000. The value for bone = +1000 and these values represent the transition from black through the various shades of grey to white (i.e. from air, to water and then to bone).

5. ROI stands for region of interest. It allows us to obtain a finite measurement for a specific area so that definitive CT numbers can be established. In doing so, a clearer representation of the image is formulated so that we can be certain of the tissue type at a certain point.

6. Third-generation CT scanners have an arc of detectors opposite the X-ray tube which rotate at the same time. This means that both the X-ray tube and the detectors rotate around the patient during an exposure. This allows the scan data to be collected according to the speed at which the gantry system rotates.

7. Slip rings allow for continual rotation of the X-ray tube and detectors while the patient is moved through the beam. Their use means that the problem of unwinding the cables is overcome and so the tube and detectors can rotate as the table moves, thus continuously corkscrewing through the area of interest.

8. Hydrogen atoms are the most readily available in the body (contained in water and fat) and they also have one single proton that gives them a strong magnetic signal.

9. MRI has to be fused with CT data because it does not provide the electron density information required by planning computer algorithms to calculate dose distributions within a target volume.

10. The brain–blood flow which represents cortical activity/brain function.

11. Patients and personnel should ensure that they do not have any magnetic materials/objects within them or about their person (pacemakers, other metallic objects in their body, hairpins, watches, scissors, etc.).

12. Longitudinal direction.

13. Piezoelectric effect: contraction and expansion of the crystals as a result of application of an alternating current.

14. The acoustic impedance ($Z$) of tissues is a function of the density of the tissues and the speed of sound within them.

15. Doppler ultrasonography can be used for imaging red blood cells.

16. Positron and electron.

17. Fluorodeoxyglucose (FDG).

18. Neoplastic tissue can be discerned from healthy tissues in PET imaging due to the unregulated growth of malignant cells and higher glucose consumption.

19. Image registration is the process of superimposing two or more images from different imaging modalities, into one single image with just one coordinate ($x$, $y$, $z$) system.

20. Distortion occurs as a result of co-registering images automatically and thus before acceptance of registered images a manual check should occur to ensure the superimposed images are aligned accurately.

## Chapter 6

1. Cathode, filament, target, anode, borosilicate glass envelope, tube casing.
2. A clear plastic sheet with intersecting black lines indicating beam central axis.
3. The autotransformer.
4. Measures the maximum load of $kV_p$, mA and exposure time, which may be safely applied to a tube.
5. Picture archiving and communication system.

## Chapter 7

1. To achieve accuracy and reproducibility of treatment on a daily basis.
2. Can the immobilisation device be accommodated through the CT bore? Is the device compatible with both the CT couch and the treatment couch?

3. Availability of mould room facilities, cost, treatment intent (radical versus palliative), patient compliance.
4. The patient should have a reduced number of visits to the department. For the patient it is a less claustrophobic experience.
5. Supraorbital ridge, nose/nasion, chin, clavicles.
6. Ability to add surface landmarks such as isocentre, beam entry points, field borders and match lines. Provides base for addition of build-up.
7. To move the tongue out of the treatment field or to keep the mouth open during treatment.
8. Lack of skin sparing can potentially increase skin reactions (erythema, moist desquamation, etc.).
9. Ensure immobilisation material is not excessively thick. Limit reactions by cutting out shell in the region of the treatment fields.
10. The incline results in the sternum lying horizontally to the couch top. This prevents the need for collimator angulation.
11. Mobility of breast tissue in the supine and lateral direction, resulting in the potential need to move lateral field border posteriorly. This could result in increased lung volume being treated.
12. Possibly consider the use of a prone position or consider immobilising the breast itself via the use of an immobilisation brassière.
13. Patient should be positioned in the arms-up position in order to accommodate oblique fields while avoiding the arms. A dedicated chest-board or body mould system may be used.
14. Pelvic vacuum bag or body mould; ankle stocks, leg stocks or knee supports. An external fixation shell may also be used.
15. Limits movement of the prostate, pushes the rectum posteriorly, resulting in decreased rectal volume in high-dose regions.
16. Use of dedicated breathing control system, e.g. ABC. This can restrain the patient in the breath-held position.
17. Achievement of a treatment 'corridor' to reduce potential lymphoedema. Abduction of arm to keep away from thorax. Suitable position used to permit CT planning can be carried out.
18. Patient's head should be supported using sand bags, vacuum bag or equivalent. A lead cut-out should be constructed. A nasal septum shield may be required to protect the nasal mucosa.
19. The patient may be seated for treatment using a dedicated treatment chair. The head may be immobilised using a head strap.
20. Patient can be positioned on a vacuum-bag support or custom-made mould. Head position is retained via the use of a bite block system.

## Chapter 8

1. The ionisation chambers and mirror: if the wedge was placed above the ionisation chambers it would be smaller, which would be an advantage; however, the chamber would record a reduced dose rate and the beam would not be flat and the interlock would probably stop the unit. Both (d) and (e) could be correct; placing a physical wedge in position (e) would block the light beam and so would have to be the last operation of the set-up.
2. Prevent cobalt from escaping, filter out β particles. Cobalt decays to nickel, another solid so no gas is present and the decay scheme only includes γ rays and β particles so no α particles are produced. The γ rays are required for treatment and, although there will be minor attenuation in the steel walls this is not desired. β particles, being electrons, would contribute only to the skin dose and so need to be removed and we don't want the radioactive cobalt to escape.
3. Longer treatment times, larger focal spot, lower beam energy, larger penumbra. The treatment times are longer and need adjusting on a monthly basis; the source size is

larger than the focal spot a linear accelerator (17 mm compared with 5 mm) which will give rise to a larger penumbra. The penumbra will also be larger due to the lower energy where there is more sideways scatter of the beam. The beam is roughly equivalent to a 2 MeV linear accelerator, much lower than most linear accelerators, and although the source change is costly it usually takes place every 3 years, not annually.

4. Magnetron, ion pump, focusing coils. All the above use magnets, the magnetron to force the electrons into a circular orbit, the ion pump to cause the ions to spiral, increasing their path length, and the focusing coils to move the electron bunches in the accelerating structure to the optimum position for acceleration. The electron gun uses an electrostatic charge to focus the electrons not a magnet and the ionisation chambers collect the electrons by use of a potential difference.

5. Motorised, manual and virtual.

6. Beam-flattening filter, ion pump. The other devices are found on other equipment, the reflection target for kilovoltage units and the simulator, the quality filter on the kilovoltage unit and the stator on a rotating anode X-ray tube. The ion pump is used to maintain the vacuum of the accelerating structure whereas the beam-flattening filter produces a flat beam profile.

7. Gold. The efficiency of X-ray production at all energies is proportional to the atomic number of the target material. Gold has a much high atomic number compared with the other materials listed. Its atomic number is greater than tungsten, 79 compared with 74, and so is a better target material than tungsten. It is not used at lower energies because of the larger amount of heat produced in the target, the melting point of gold being 1064 °C, approximately a third of that of tungsten (3422 °C).

8. 5.26 years. Fact, this is a constant and cannot be changed.

9. Electron gun: scattering foils scatter the existing thin stream of electrons, whereas the magnetron and klystron produce the RF wave, both use electrons but do not emit electrons into the waveguide structure. The oscillator is attached to the klystron and produces the RF wave.

10. Maintain a vacuum: ion pumps work well only at high vacuums and cannot produce a vacuum from normal atmospheric pressure because they would overheat. A standard vacuum pump lowers the pressure sufficiently for the ion pump to work. It could be argued that they accelerate electrons, because they can cause ionisation of atoms and then removal of the ions by attracting them towards an electrode across a potential difference, but this is not their function.

11. Stop the electrons diverging in the waveguide: focusing coils produce a magnetic field along the length of the accelerating waveguide that prevents the electrons from diverging due to the radial component of the RF wave.

12. It uses the energy of the electrons to add power to the RF wave: klystrons tend to be used in higher energy units, the reverse of (a). The klystron is an amplifier; it amplifies RF wave produced by the oscillator. The head of the linear accelerator is compact and does not contain the klystron; rather it tends to be situated in the stand of the unit and connected to the accelerating structure by a series of hinged waveguides. These waveguides contain $SF_6$ to quench arcing, but if the gas were present in the klystron the electrons would lose energy through collisions, which would be undesirable. The electrons lose kinetic energy that is given to the RF wave increasing its power.

13. Decrease. The production of X-rays is approximately 30%. With the removal of the target there would be a lot more electrons exiting the linear accelerator compared with photons when in X-ray mode. This repre-

sents a large increase in the dose rate, which is undesirable. Fewer electrons need to be produced and so the gun current is reduced.

14. It does not generate an RF wave. It uses the energy of the electrons to add power to the RF wave. Klystrons are used in high-energy linear accelerators and are usually situated in the stand not the head of the unit. If gas were present in the klystron, the electrons would collide with the gas molecules and lose energy, a situation that is not desirable. The klystron is an amplifier; it amplifies RF waves produced by the oscillator, and this amplification is achieved by using the kinetic energy of the electrons.

15. Standing; travelling.

16. Primary collimator, tungsten alloy pre-collimator, source bushing assembly, secondary collimator. The beam channel is made up of a source bushing assembly, pre-collimator, primary and secondary collimator. The helmet just functions as a locator for the secondary collimator.

17. Two. Other than the MLCs there are two pairs of collimators, one in each plane. One set of collimators will collimate the beam and the other move in just behind the MLCs to reduce the amount of radiation leaking between the leaves.

18. X-ray contamination contributes to dose at a depth greater than the range of the electrons. X-ray contamination tends to be along the central axis of the beam and although small (<5%) it can lead to a significant dose when treating large areas of the body such as with TBI. As a scattering foil is placed in the beam to scatter electrons it will produce a small amount of X-rays and so this method produces greater X-ray contamination. The true statement relates to the greater range of the photons that will give a dose at a depth, beyond the range of the electrons.

19. Flattening filter. The variation in beam energy across the field is much lower than in conventional radiotherapy units, <5%,

which is the consequence of the absent flattening filter.

20. Beam bending magnet, magnetron, ion pumps.

## Chapter 9

1. Applicator size, thickness of underlying tissue, beam quality, use of a lead cut-out. Backscatter is dependent on two factors. The volume of tissue irradiated, as any change in the volume means a change in the amount of scatter produced. The volume is dependent on the area irradiated (applicator and cut-out affect this) and the thickness of tissue. The other factor affecting the amount of backscatter is beam energy; the higher the energy the more forward the scatter, so high-energy beams have less backscatter than low-energy beams.

2. Applicator factor, backscatter factor, stand-off factor, cut-out factor. At kilovoltage energy we do not use the term 'field size factor' because applicators are always used that define field size so an applicator factor is used. The use of cut-outs will effectively further affect the field size irradiated, so must be included if used. The dose at any point will be affected by the amount of backscatter because dose is deposited by scatter as well as the primary beam. The dose received is also affected by any change in treatment distance, which is accounted for in the stand-off factor.

3. Absorb X-rays produced outside the focal spot. When electrons interact with the target some will be scattered backwards, and then because of the potential difference will again be attracted back towards the anode. These electrons can strike any part of the anode giving rise to unwanted X-rays, which the hood will absorb.

4. Atomic number. The k absorption edge depends on the atomic number of the material; the higher the atomic number, the

greater the k absorption edge value. In the photoelectric effect the chance of an interaction is greatest at and just above the binding energy of the electrons. This value therefore represents a point where the K-shell electrons can take place and absorption of X-rays increases; below this point there will be considerably less absorption because the K-shell electrons cannot play a part and there is effectively a window letting the X-rays through. Using the filters in the order of atomic number allows the subsequent filter to remove the absorption edge of the previous filter.

5. 20 cm. This is a simple application of the inverse square law (see Figure 9.9).

6. Tin, copper, aluminium. The order depends on atomic number; see the answer to question 4.

7. Trim the penumbra. As a result of the large focal spot the penumbra could be quite large; however, the penumbra is also dependent on the distance of the collimators from the patient, so adding lead here to trim the beam reduces the penumbra size.

8. Conduction. Heat is primarily removed through conduction. This is aided by the anode being made of copper, as a good thermal conductor, having a wide cross-sectional area and maintaining a high thermal gradient by use of cooling systems.

9. Choosing a material with a high thermal conductivity – see above.

10. 30°. The target angle is kept high to reduce the anode heel effect.

11. Superficial, low energy. Low-energy beams are defined as beams with a HVL of between 1 and 8 mm of aluminium which covers beams generated between 50 and 160 kV; this corresponds to superficial beams that covered the energy range 50–150 kV. Supervoltage beams were not mentioned in the text, but is a term used to cover beams generated at a voltage between 500 and 1000 kV.

12. High atomic number. X-ray production is directly proportional to the atomic number of the target material. The other factors are not important in the choice of a target material.

13. Remove low-energy X-rays. Filters harden the beam by increasing the average energy of the beam through preferential removal of low-energy X-rays.

14. Isocentric. Kilovoltage units do not have isocentric mountings, but are free to move in three dimensions.

15. Stator, electron gun. Stators are found in the rotating anode tube. They produce a magnetic field that causes the anode to rotate. Kilovoltage tubes are of a stationary tube design and are not required to rotate. The electron gun is part of the linear accelerator; it differs from the cathode in that it has its own anode, through which pulses of electrons can be produced.

16. Target angle, generating voltage. The lower the target angle the greater the degree of self-attenuation (see Figure 9.5). If the electrons have greater energy they can travel further into the target before producing X-rays, again enhancing the effect.

17. Generating voltage and the HVL. Both HVL and generating voltage describe the beam quality, but not until both are put together do we get the proper picture. Different units may have different inherent filtrations and so beams are not directly comparable; the same is true of inherent filtration in that it tells you nothing of the added filtration.

18. Door interlock, treatment unit movements, emergency off button.

19. Skin apposition is when the end of the applicator is parallel to the skins surface giving a uniform treatment distance and dose rate. When you don't have skin apposition you will have stand-off on at least one side of the treatment field. This change in distance affects the dose received at this point (inverse square law).

20. Beryllium is a metal with an atomic number of 4. X-ray interaction at this energy is predominantly photoelectric which is dependent on atomic number $(Z^3)$. A low atomic number material means that most X-rays will pass through the window without interacting, which is what we want. There are three elements with a lower atomic number but all are unsuitable, two are gases (hydrogen and helium) and one is a soft metal (lithium) that is very reactive.

## Chapter 10

1. A uniform dose to the PTV, of +7% and −5% of the prescribed dose, keeps organs at risk within tolerance levels.

2. PDD requires the phantom position to remain at a constant distance from the source while the radiation detector moves to the point of measurement, whereas for TMR the detector remains at a constant distance from the source and the phantom (or surface) moves to provide measurement at depth.

3. The build-up region and penumbra regions of the photon field have high dose gradients.

4. Beam wedges, bolus material, intensity modulators using step and shoot MLC or dynamic MLC.

5. Oblique incidence correction, tissue heterogeneity correction, SSD correction.

6. The pattern of energy, or dose deposition around a very narrow electron or photon beam.

7. Divide field into 36 sectors by drawing radii at 10° intervals from calculation point. Divide each sector into lengths of $d$ cm. The contribution from each of the resultant sections to the calculation point depends upon its size and distance from the point, and can be determined from tabulated data. The equivalent square field size is the square field that results in the same scatter contribution as the sum of the sections' contributions.

8. Scattered dose is poorly accounted for; approximate corrections for inhomogeneities, etc., applied after the dose to water calculated; corrections mainly consider the changes in primary photon attenuation, particularly poor performance in the absence of electronic equilibrium.

9. Beam angle selection, field shaping, overlay of structures, fields and DRRs.

10. Discrepancies between the algorithms used in the inverse planning and the forward dose calculation. The optimisation is guided by the inverse planning algorithm and adjusts field fluences based on its calculations, which tend to use large approximations. When a more accurate algorithm is used to calculate the final dose distribution, the actual doses can be significantly different from those predicted by the less accurate one.

## Chapter 11

1. Radiographs can provide only 2D data.

   CT scans provide electron density data that can be directly loaded into the treatment planning system. Can be digitally reconstructed to produce volumetric images leading to 3D planning. The patient must be positioned in the treatment position before the CT scan, and needs to have an identical table top to the treatment machine. Aperture has to be wide enough to allow immobilisation devices to pass through easily. The images have to be able to be transferred electronically to the treatment planning system.

   MR scans can be taken in multiple planes. Better for imaging brain tumours. Table tops have to be identical to treatment table top. Greater tissue contrast. There are circumstances when patients would not be suitable for MRI.

   Image fusion – fusing PET images with CT images can enhance treatment planning options as tissue function can be considered.

CT and MRI data is stored electronically so it is possible to manipulate the images and fuse the two together, allowing better visualisation of tumour.

2. MLCs have several functions in terms of beam direction and delivery. They conform the shape of the beam to closely match the 3D contour of the tumour and treatment volume, allowing the irradiated volume to closely resemble the planning target volume, thereby sparing normal tissue and increasing the therapeutic ratio. MLCs are also the tools to allow IMRT to be delivered because they act as the shaping and shielding for the 'fieldlets' that gradually build up the high dose/low dose regions of the IMRT treatment plan.

3. Definition of isocentre: a fixed point in air, usually 100 cm from the source of radiation, around which the gantry, collimators and couch can be rotated without affecting its position. This is usually visualised within the treatment room as the point at which the lateral and sagittal lasers intersect, where the optical distance scale reads 100 cm and meets the central axis of the radiation beam.

4. Information on the treatment plan to aid in accurate beam direction includes: beam direction information – gantry angles, collimators angles, field size, isocentre depth, patient contour details. The plan also has details of dose distribution and treatment volume/organs at risk; these also influence beam direction accuracy.

5. Electrons are negatively charged and will naturally repel each other as they travel towards the patient. If they were collimated close to the head of the machine then, because of the repelling properties, the beam shape would be distorted by the time it reached the patient. By collimating the electrons close to the patient it is more representative of the beam that will reach the patient, therefore making beam shaping and delivery more accurate. The electron applicator acts as an aid to achieving a perpendicular beam delivery and also as a carrier for the electron end frame that will shape the beam to that required by the recipient.

## Chapter 12

1. The difference between the two modalities is hadrons deposit their energy at an increased depth in tissue. The hadrons' increased energy means that they penetrate tissue at considerable depth before delivering their maximum dose.

2. The build-up region is much larger than that associated with photon beams and furthermore there is no dose delivered after the Bragg peak. This is because, unlike photon treatments, there is no X-ray dose penetrating the tissue. Once the particles deposit their energy, they stop.

3. Stereotactic, meaning spatial movement.

4. A tomotherapy unit is a linear accelerator and an associated megavoltage imaging system is mounted in a sealed ring gantry; it can be moved safely around the patient at high speeds.

5. This allows for an increased number of beam angles to be used for treatment and for rapid megavoltage CT image acquisition. Thus the equipment combines the conformality of IMRT treatment with the confidence provided by inherent IGRT capability.

## Chapter 13

1. A systematic error is one that arises due to discrepancies between the planning and treatment processes and thus, if undetected, remains fixed throughout the course of treatment. A random error is unpredictable and may vary between fractions (interfraction) and/or during a treatment fraction (intrafraction).

2. Poor immobilisation, poor set-up, patient movement, movable skin marks and organ motion.

3. True because random error varies between fractions; it must be corrected for on the same day, before the treatment is delivered, because it may change again the next day.

4. Offline correction is where an image is acquired and then reviewed after treatment delivery. Any error is corrected for in subsequent fractions.

5. False; it will provide only a snapshot of that fraction and does not allow a clear picture of the average error occurring to be determined.

6. The photodiodes (each representing a pixel of the resulting image) absorb the light and convert this into an electric charge. When a voltage is applied, the accompanying TFTs act as a switch, allowing the current to flow between the diodes and an electronic readout to be taken.

7. Conventional portal imaging based on bony anatomy alone will not allow the visualisation of the target itself. Although the external set-up may be deemed as accurate based on bony landmarks, the target position relative to this may have moved due to organ motion. Therefore IGRT, where the target itself is visualised, is preferred.

8. Ultrasonography: no ionising radiation dose.

   EPID and markers: relatively cheap, can be used together with existing MV EPIDS; minimal training, relative to other techniques; marker registration is not subject to interobserver variability.

   CBCT: matches like for like, can visualise the target and its contour.

9. Ultrasonography: probe pressure may move the target, relatively poor image quality can limit the accuracy of contouring and alignment.

   EPID and markers: radiation dose, markers may migrate.

   CBCT: radiation dose, as with ultrasound contour and anatomy-based registrations are subject to interobserver variability.

10. Thermoluminescent dosimeters, semiconductor diodes, MOSFETS and EPIDs.

11. They measure only point doses and are therefore limited for verifying the accuracy of dose fluence across IMRT fields.

12. Verification data gathered for a specific patient may indicate a change from what was originally planned, e.g. using verification the error may be reduced to the point where the original PTV margin could be decreased. Another example may be where changes in the size, position and shape of the CTV are detected. In both these scenarios the treatment is re-planned based on this new data. The ultimate rationale behind adaptive radiotherapy is the maximisation of the therapeutic ratio.

13. They initially removed the random transcription errors associated with the manual entry of treatment parameters each day for treatment, but were still reliant on the accurate entry of treatment data at the planning stage. Modern systems utilise the DICOM network to allow direct transfer of the planned treatment parameters and thus remove this potential for a systematic transcription error.

14. They cannot verify everything; not all aspects of the treatment set-up are computer controlled. The computer-based systems themselves must still be subject to QA checks to monitor their inherent accuracy. Radiographer diligence is essential to avoid becoming over reliant on such systems.

## Chapter 14

1. They are random in nature with no 'threshold' dose.

2. The Ionising Radiation Regulations (1999) and the Ionising Radiation (Medical Exposures) Regulations 2000.

3. Anything contributing to an exposure.

4. When working unsupervised.

5. The employer.

6. The practitioner.
7. The radiation protection adviser.
8. The radiation protection supervisor.
9. The sievert.
10. 1 mSv.
11. Controlled.
12. Reducing normal tissue exposure.
13. Using the least dose possible to obtain clear images, using the referrer's data, avoiding re-imaging.
14. To ensure that local rules and procedures are effective.
15. Primary beam, scatter and leakage.
16. Primary beams are more penetrating than scattered radiation.
17. Beam energy, workload, room size, barrier material, use of room beyond barrier.
18. Room size, maximum field size, collimator rotation.
19. Visible barrier, space saving, absorption of neutrons at high energies.
20. Sharing of primary barriers is possible.

## Chapter 15

1. a
2. c
3. a
4. d
5. a
6. b
7. c
8. c
9. c
10. d
11. The time required for the radioactivity level of a source to decay to exactly 50% of its original value.
12. An excited state of an atom with a measurable half-life *or* a nucleus that takes time to decay.
13. The preparation and supply of safe and effective radiopharmaceuticals for diagnosis or treatment of disease.
14. Time it takes the camera to generate and process a reading from a single photon interaction. During dead-time, no other photons can be detected.
15. Amount of radioactivity present at a given/desired time.
16. Initial amount of radioactivity present.
17. The transformation (or decay) constant.
18. Time since last elution:
    • size of generator (related to activity of parent)
    • age of generator (related to activity of parent).
19. Allows the application of non-uniform attenuation correction to the PET image and for co-registration of both modalities so that areas of radionuclide uptake can be more accurately localised.
20.

| Component | Role |
|---|---|
| Lead cover | Prevents background radiation from interacting with the crystal and providing false information |
| Collimator | Allows only those gamma rays travelling in an appropriate direction from the patient/background to reach and interact with the crystal |
| Scintillation crystal | Interacts with gamma rays to emit a small amount of light that is detected by PMTs |
| Optical coupling | Couples crystal to front face of PMTs |
| Photomultiplier tube (PMT) | Converts light signals received from the scintillation crystal into electrical signals |
| Preamplifiers | Sits between PMT and PHA (or between detector and amplifier). Increases the size of signal from the PMT |
| Pulse height analyser (PHA) | Accepts input from pre-amplifier and categorises the pulses on basis of signal strength |

## Chapter 16

1. Where inactive guides/applicators are positioned accurately in the area to be treated, the position verified and radioactive sources are then loaded into the guide wires or applicator.

2. High dose rate and low dose rate.
3. Caesium-137, iridium-192, ytterbium-169.
4. A mechanically operated flexible tube containing a series of caesium-137 sources and spacers in various configurations.
5. The International Commission for Radiological Units.

# INDEX